Introduction to Deep Learning for Healthcare

Cao Xiao • Jimeng Sun

Introduction to Deep Learning for Healthcare

Springer

Cao Xiao
Seattle, WA, USA

Jimeng Sun
San Francisco, CA, USA

ISBN 978-3-030-82186-9 ISBN 978-3-030-82184-5 (eBook)
https://doi.org/10.1007/978-3-030-82184-5

This Springer imprint is published by the registered company Springer Nature Switzerland AG
The registered company address is: Gewerbestrasse 11, 6330 Cham, Switzerland

Preface

> Life can only be understood backwards, but it must be lived forwards.
>
> *Søren Kierkegaard*

Deep learning models are multi-layer neural networks that have shown great success in diverse applications. This is a book describing deep learning models in the context of healthcare applications.

Story 1 When we took an artificial intelligence class many year ago, many topics were covered, including neural networks. The neural network model was presented as a supervised learning method. However, it was considered a practical failure compared to other more effective supervised learning methods such as decision trees and support vector machine. The common explanation about neural networks at the time involves two aspects: (1) Multi-layer neural networks can approximate any arbitrary functions and hence is a theoretically powerful model. (2) In practice, they don't work well due to the ineffective learning algorithm (i.e., backpropagation method). When we asked why backpropagation doesn't work well, a typical answer was about the accumulated errors across layers, which will eventually become too big to lead to an accurate model. Of course, the understanding of neural networks has evolved greatly in the past few years. When big labeled datasets and parallel computing infrastructure such as graphic processing units (GPU) finally become available, the power of deep neural networks will be unleashed. These days, deep learning models have become the most popular and standard machine learning models.

Story 2 When we first got into machine learning for healthcare many years ago, we spoke with a senior medical doctor about the potential impact of machine learning and artificial intelligence (AI) in medicine in the future. Specifically, we asked him about the possibility of creating AI algorithms to mimic the practice of real-world doctors. He was very pessimistic about the possibility because he believes doctors largely depend on medical "intuition" to do their job, which is impossible to be learned by algorithms. Of course, now we know it is not only possible, but often AI algorithms can outperform human experts in various clinical pattern recognition tasks such as diagnosis. Even commercial medical devices have now become available (e.g., atrial fibrillation detection algorithm in Apple Watch). Many rely on deep learning models. Before we finished the book, we saw that doctor's profile on LinkedIn listed as an innovator in AI for healthcare.

Seattle, WA, USA
Cao Xiao

Champaign, IL, USA
Jimeng Sun

Contents

Chapter 1
Introduction

Humans are the only species on earth that can actively and systematically improve their health via technologies in the form of medicine. Throughout history, human knowledge is the driving force for the progress of medicine and healthcare. Humans created new technologies such as diagnostic tests, drugs, medical procedures, and devices. As the life expectancy increases, healthcare cost is growing dramatically over the years to be deemed unsustainable. For example, the US healthcare cost in 2019 alone is over 3.6 trillion dollars and accounts for 17.8% of gross domestic product (GDP). Within the gigantic spending in healthcare, there is enormous waste that should be avoided. The estimated total annual costs of waste were $760 billion to $935 billion [135].

Meanwhile, mountains of new medical knowledge are being created, making human doctors' knowledge quickly outdated. Moreover, human doctors are struggling to catch up with the increasing volume of patient visits. Physician burnout is a serious issue that affects all doctors in the age of electronic health records due to the overwhelming patient data for doctors to review and complex workflows, including tedious documentation tasks. Patients are also dissatisfied with limited interactions and attention from doctors during their short clinical visits. Quality of care is often sub-optimal, with over 400K preventable medical errors in hospitals each year [78].

With the rise of artificial intelligence (AI), can new healthcare technology be created by machine directly? For example, can machines provide more accurate diagnoses than human doctors? In the center of the AI revolution, deep learning technology is a set of machine learning techniques that learn multiple layers of neural networks for supporting prediction, classification, clustering, and data generation tasks. The success of deep learning comes from

- *Data:* Large amounts of rich data, especially in images and natural language texts, become available for training deep learning models.
- *Algorithms:* Efficient neural network methods have been proposed and enhanced by many researchers in recent years.

C. Xiao, J. Sun, *Introduction to Deep Learning for Healthcare*,
https://doi.org/10.1007/978-3-030-82184-5_1

- *Hardware:* Advances in parallel computing, especially graphic process units (GPUs), have enabled a fast and affordable computing engine for deep learning workload.
- *Software:* Scalable and easy-to-use programming frameworks have been developed and released via open source projects to the public. Most of them, including TensorFlow and Pytorch, have strong support from the technology industry.

This book explains the first two ingredients: rich health data and neural network algorithms that can effectively model those health data. The advance in relevant hardware and deep learning software will not be covered in this book as those topics are largely independent of healthcare applications.

Healthcare Data Among all healthcare technologies, electronic health records (EHRs) had vast adoption and a huge impact on healthcare delivery in recent years. One important benefit of EHRs is to capture all the patient encounters with rich multi-modality data. Healthcare data include both structured and unstructured information. Structured data include various medical codes for diagnoses and procedures, lab results, and medication information. Unstructured data contain (1) clinical notes as text, (2) medical imaging data such as X-rays, echocardiogram, and magnetic resonance imaging (MRI), and (3) time-series data such as the electrocardiogram (ECG) and electroencephalogram (EEG). Beyond the data collected during clinical visits, patient self-generated/reported data start to grow thanks to wearable sensors' increasing use. It was estimated over 100 Zettabytes of health-related data are being created [38].

Deep Learning Models Neural network models are a class of machine learning methods that have a long history. Deep learning models are neural networks of many layers, which can extract multiple levels of features from raw data. As large labeled data sets and modern hardware (especially GPU) become available, deep neural networks with many layers start to show significant performance advantages over other machine learning methods. For example, AlexNet using convolutional neural networks (a popular deep learning model) won the ImageNet competition by reducing the error rate to 15.3%, more than 10% points lower than that of the runner up [90]. Deep learning applications are in many domains, such as computer vision [46, 90], speech recognition [70, 128], and natural language processing [33, 79, 166]. Deep learning applied to healthcare is a natural and promising direction with many initial successes [44, 61].

1.1 Motivating Applications

Deep learning has great successes in the technology industry. Very hard technical problems had amazing performance improvements such as image classification, machine translation, and speech recognition. There are various promising deep learning applications in healthcare, including medical imaging analysis, waveform sleep analysis, inpatient outcome prediction, outpatient disease risk prediction, treatment recommendation, clinical trial matching, and molecule generation for drug discovery. Next, we briefly present some concrete healthcare applications using deep learning. More detailed applications will be presented in each chapter later.

1.1.1 Diabetic Retinopathy Detection

Diabetic retinopathy (DR) is a deadly complication of diabetes that can cause blindness. DR affects 4.2 million adults. Suppose detected early DR can be treated. However, in its early stage, patients often do not realize any symptoms. But without timely treatment, DR can cause permanent vision damage. The gold standard diagnosis is to have ophthalmologists (eye doctors) perform manual grading of retinal photographs. The cost and accessibility for such diagnoses are challenging, especially in the low resource environment. Deep learning models, in this case, convolutional neural networks, have demonstrated initial successes in the automatic diagnosis of DR based on the same retinal photographs also scored by ophthalmologists [61]. According to this study, the deep learning models trained on over 100K images can achieve expert-level accuracy over 99% area under the ROC curve (AUC)[1] Accurate automated diagnosis tools like this can potentially assist ophthalmologists in speeding up the diagnosis process and quickly identifying the patients who need the most help (Fig. 1.1).

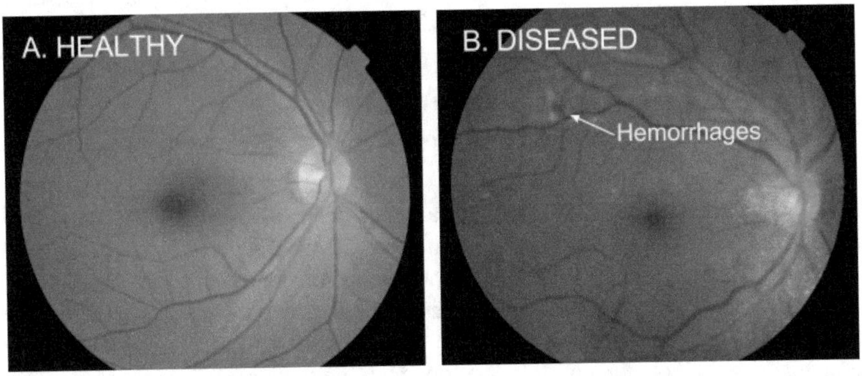

Fig. 1.1 Example retinal photos from a healthy individual and a disease patient. Credit to https://ai.googleblog.com/2016/11/deep-learning-for-detection-of-diabetic.html

[1] AUC is a common classification metric that will be described in details in Section "Real-Value Prediction for Classification".

1.1.2 Early Detection of Heart Failure

Heart failure (HF) is another deadly disease that affects approximately 5.7 million people in the United States and has over 825,000 new cases per year with around 33 billion dollars total annual cost. The lifetime risk of developing HF is 20% at 40 years of age [2]. HF has a high mortality rate of about 50% within 5 years of diagnosis [5]. There has been relatively little progress in slowing HF progression because there is no effective means of early detection of HF to test interventions. Choi et al. [30] used a deep learning model called recurrent neural networks to model longitudinal electronic health records to accurately predict the onset of HF 6 to 18 months before the actual diagnosis.

1.1.3 Sleep Analysis

Scoring laboratory polysomnography (PSG) data remains a manual task by sleep technologists. They need visually process the entire night of sleep data and annotate different diagnostic categories, including sleep stages, sleep disordered breathing, and limb movements. Attempts to automate this process have been hampered by PSG signals' complexity and physiological heterogeneity between patients. Biswal et al. [7] used a combination of deep recurrent and convolutional neural networks for assigning sleep stages, detecting sleep apnea and limb movement events. Their models achieved PSG diagnostic scoring for sleep staging, sleep apnea, and limb movements with accuracies of 87.6%, 88.2%, and 84.7%, respectively.

1.1.4 Treatment Recommendation

Medication error is the third leading cause of death in the US. The Food and Drug Administration (FDA) receives more than 100,000 reports each year related to suspected medication errors. To ensure medication safety, different medication recommendation methods have been proposed using deep learning methods. For example, researchers have attempted to build predictive models for suggesting treatments based on patient information, including diagnoses, procedures, and medication history, with the abundant longitudinal electronic health record data. LEAP [174] and GAMENet [134] are examples of such models using deep learning, particularly sequence-to-sequence models and memory networks.

1.1.5 *Clinical Trial Matching*

Clinical trials play important roles in drug development but often suffer from expensive, inaccurate, and insufficient patient recruitment. The availability of electronic health records (EHR) and trial eligibility criteria (EC) bring a new opportunity to develop computational models for patient recruitment. One key task named patient-trial matching is to find qualified patients for clinical trials given structured EHR and unstructured EC text (both inclusion and exclusion criteria). How to match complex EC text with longitudinal patient EHRs? How to embed many-to-many relationships between patients and trials? How to explicitly handle the difference between inclusion and exclusion criteria? COMPOSE [50] and DeepEnroll [176] are two deep learning models for patient-trial matching. They search through EHR data to identifying the matching patients based on the trial eligibility criteria described in the natural language.

1.1.6 *Molecule Property Prediction and Generation*

Drug discovery is about finding the molecules with desirable properties for treating a target disease. Traditional drug discovery heavily depends on high throughput screening (HTS), which involves many costly wet-lab experiments. Given large molecule databases and their associated drug properties (e.g., from drugbank), machine learning models, especially deep learning models, have shown great potentials in identifying promising drug candidates. For example, some deep learning models were proposed to predict drug property given the input molecule structures [105, 139]. Some were introduced to produce brand new molecules with desirable properties [48, 80].

1.2 Who Should Read This Book?

Most deep learning books focus on computational methods where algorithms and the underlying mathematics are described—however, few books focus on the applications in specific domains. We take a method-oriented approach with a target application domain in healthcare. The main targets are graduate students and researchers who want to learn about deep learning methods and their healthcare applications. Ideally, the audience should have a basic machine learning background, but we provide a short overview of machine learning in Chap. 3. The audience does not need to have a healthcare or medical background to read this book. The other target audience is healthcare researchers and data scientists who want to learn about the use cases of deep learning in healthcare. Finally, experienced machine learning researchers and engineers can benefit from this book if they want to learn more healthcare data and analytic problems.

This book does not require any computer programming knowledge and can be used as a textbook for the concepts of deep learning and its applications. We deliberately do not cover the programming details so that our readers can be broadened. Also, we realize the fast pace of deep learning software evolution, which will likely outdate what we wrote on that programming topic very quickly. Nevertheless, the hands-on exercises of deep learning are essential to gain practical knowledge of the topic. We encourage readers to supplement this book with other hands-on programming exercises, online tutorials, and other books on deep learning software packages.

1.3 Who Are the Authors?

When we completed the book in Apr 2021, here is our background.

Dr. Cao "Danica" Xiao is the senior director, data science and machine learning at Amplitude. Before that, she was the director of Machine Learning in the Analytics Center of Excellence (ACOE) of IQVIA, located in Cambridge, Massachusetts. Before joining IQVIA, she got her Ph.D. degree from University of Washington, Seattle and was a research staff member in IBM Research. Her work focuses on developing machine learning and deep learning models to solve real-world healthcare challenges.

Dr. Jimeng Sun is a Professor at the Computer Science Department and Carle's Illinois College of Medicine at the University of Illinois Urbana-Champaign. Before Illinois, he was an associate professor in the College of Computing at the Georgia Institute of Technology. His research focuses on artificial intelligence (AI) for healthcare, including deep learning for drug discovery, clinical trial optimization, computational phenotyping, clinical predictive modeling, treatment recommendation, and health monitoring. He was recognized as one of the Top 100 AI Leaders in Drug Discovery and Advanced Healthcare by Deep Knowledge Analytics.

1.4 Book Organization

We organize chapters based on the neural network techniques. In each chapter, we first introduce the specific neural network techniques then present concrete healthcare case studies of those techniques. We organize the book into core and advanced parts. The core part includes health data (Chap. 2), machine learning basics (Chap. 3), and fundamental neural network architectures, namely deep neural networks (DNN) (Chap. 4), embedding (Chap. 5), convolutional neural networks (CNN) (Chap. 6), recurrent neural networks (RNN) (Chap. 7), and autoencoder (AE) (Chap. 8).

- Chapter 2 covers the various healthcare data ranging from structured data such as diagnosis codes to unstructured data such as clinical notes and medical imaging data. This chapter also introduces important health data standards such as international classification of diseases (ICD) codes.
- Chapter 3 provides a primer of machine learning basics. We present the fundamental machine learning tasks, including supervised and unsupervised learning and some classical examples (e.g., logistic regression and principal component analysis). We also describe evaluation metrics for different tasks such as the area under the receiver operating characteristic curve (AUC) for classification and mean squared error for regression.
- Chapter 4 presents the deep neural networks (DNN) called a feed-forward neural network or multi-layered perceptron (MLP). In particular, we cover the basic components of DNNs, including neurons, activation functions, loss functions, and forward/backward passes. Of course, we also introduce the famous backpropagation algorithm for training DNN models. We also present two case studies: hospital re-admission prediction and drug property prediction.
- Chapter 5 illustrates the idea of embedding using neural networks, including popular algorithms such as Word2Vec and other domain-specific embeddings for EHR data such as Mec2Vec and MiME.
- Chapter 6 introduces convolutional neural networks (CNN) designed for grid-like data such as images and time series. We will present the important operation of CNNs, such as convolution and pooling, and some popular CNN architectures. We will also describe the application of CNNs on medical imaging data and clinical waveforms such as the electrocardiogram (ECG).
- Chapter 7 covers recurrent neural networks (RNN) designed to handle sequential data such as clinical text. We present important variants of RNN, including Long short-term memory (LSTM) and gated recurrent unit (GRU). The RNN case studies include heart failure prediction and de-identification of clinical notes.
- Chapter 8 describe the autoencoder model, an unsupervised neural network model. We also present case studies of autoencoder including phenotyping EHR data.

The advanced part covers the attention model (Chap. 9), graph neural networks (Chap. 10), memory networks (Chap. 11), and generative models (Chap. 12).

- Chapter 9 introduces attention models, which creates the foundation for many advanced deep learning models. We illustrate the attention model in several healthcare applications, including disease risk prediction, diagnosis code assignment, and ECG classification.
- Chapter 10 presents another foundation of advanced deep learning models, namely graph neural networks (GNN). Graph data are common in many healthcare tasks such as medical ontology and molecule graphs. GNN models are a set of powerful neural network models for graph data. The case studies focus on drug discovery.
- Chapter 11 presents memory network-based models, a set of powerful models for embedding complex data (such as text and time series). We will introduce

the idea behind original memory networks and their powerful extensions, such as Transformer and BERT models. We demonstrate memory networks on medication recommendation tasks.
- Chapter 12 presents deep generative models, including generative adversarial networks (GAN) and variational autoencoder (VAE). We show their applications in synthetic EHR data generation and molecule generation for drug discovery.

1.5 Exercises

1. Present an example data science application for lower healthcare cost, specify the datasets needed for building such machine learning models, and describe the evaluation metrics.
2. Which type of healthcare data are considered large in terms of data volume?
   (a) Genomic data
   (b) Medical imaging data
   (c) Clinical notes
   (d) Medical claims
3. Which type of healthcare data are considered fastest in velocity?
   (a) Real-time monitoring data from intensive care units
   (b) Medical imaging data
   (c) Structured electronic health records
   (d) Clinical notes
4. Which one is NOT a drug discovery and development application?
   (a) Sepsis detection
   (b) Molecule property prediction
   (c) Clinical trial recruitment
   (d) Molecule generation
5. Which one is NOT a drug discovery and development application?
   (a) Sepsis detection
   (b) Molecule property prediction
   (c) Clinical trial recruitment
   (d) Molecule generation
6. Which one is a public health application?
   (a) Mortality prediction in ICU
   (b) Patient triaging application
   (c) Treatment recommendation for heart failure
   (d) Predicting COVID19 cases at different locations in the US

Chapter 2
Health Data

Health data are diverse with multiple modalities. This chapter will introduce different types of health data, including structured health data (e.g., diagnosis codes, procedure codes) and unstructured data (e.g., clinical notes, medical images). We will also present the popular health data standards for representing those data.

2.1 The Growth of Electronic Health Records

Over the past decade, more and more health service providers worldwide have adopted electronic health record (EHR) systems to manage data about patients and records of health care services. For example, Fig. 2.1 shows the increase of national basic and certified EHR adoption rate over time according to the American Hospital Association Annual Survey. Here the basic EHR adoption curve corresponds to the EHR systems having basic EHR functions such as patient demographics, physician notes, lab results, medications, diagnosis, clinical and drug safety guidelines. A certified EHR just has to cover essential EHR technology that meets the technological capability, functionality, and security requirements adopted by the Department of Health and Human Services. From Fig. 2.1, we can see nearly all reported hospitals (96%) possessed a certified EHR technology by 2015. In 2015, 84.8% of hospitals adopted at least a Basic EHR system; this represents a ninefold increase since 2008. Thanks to the wide deployment of EHR systems, many healthcare institutions have collected diverse health data. This chapter provides an overview of health data: what different data types are available and how the data are collected, and by whom. All these data are potential inputs for training deep learning models for supporting diverse healthcare tasks.

C. Xiao, J. Sun, *Introduction to Deep Learning for Healthcare*,
https://doi.org/10.1007/978-3-030-82184-5_2

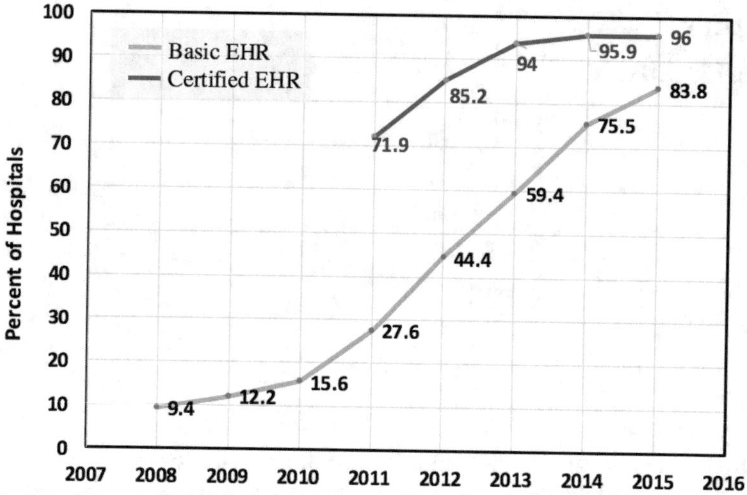

Fig. 2.1 Percentage of EHR system adoption over time. Basic EHR means EHR systems with a set of required functionalities such as patient demographics, physician notes, lab results, medications, diagnosis, clinical and drug safety guidelines. A certified EHR system means the hospital has the essential EHR technology certified by Department of Health and Human Services. Source: American Hospital Association Annual Survey

2.2 Health Data

Shifting from the traditional paper-based records to electronic records has generated a massive collection of health data, which created opportunities for enhanced patient care, data-driven care delivery, and accelerated healthcare research. According to the definition from Centers for Medicare & Medicaid Services (CMS)—a federal institution that administers government-owned health insurance services, EHR is "an electronic version of a patient's medical history, that is maintained by the provider over time, and may include all of the key administrative, clinical data relevant to that person's care under a particular provider, including demographics, progress notes, problems, medications, vital signs, past medical history, immunizations, laboratory data, and radiology reports".[1] From the modeling perspective, EHR can be viewed as a longitudinal record of comprehensive medical services provided to patients and documentation of patient medical history. There are several important observations of EHR data:

1. EHR data are mostly managed by providers (although there is an ongoing movement to enable patients to augment additional data into their EHRs);
2. Each provider manages their own EHR systems; as a result, partial information about the same patient may scatter across EHR systems from multiple providers;

[1] https://www.cms.gov/Medicare/E-Health/EHealthRecords/index.html.

3. The main purpose of EHR data is to support accurate and efficient billing services, which creates challenges for other secondary use of EHR data such as research.

2.2.1 The Life Cycle of Health Data

Let us first introduce the key players in the healthcare industry and the life cycle of health data from the perspectives of those key healthcare players.

Key Healthcare Players There are diverse healthcare institutions that generate and manage health data.

- **Providers** are hospitals, clinics, and health systems, which provide healthcare services to patients. Providers use electronic health records (EHR) systems to capture everything that happened during patient encounters, such as diagnosis codes, medication prescription, lab and imaging results, and clinical notes. Providers interact with other players such as payers, pharmacies, and labs.
- **Payers** are entities that provide health insurance. They can be private insurance companies such as United Healthcare and Anthem. Or they can be public insurance programs owned by government entities such as MEDICARE and MEDICAID. Payers reimburse the full or partial cost associated with healthcare services to providers. Payers interact with providers and pharmacies via claims. More specifically, providers and pharmacies submit claims to corresponding payers from which they have medical insurance. Claims are usually structured data with diagnosis, procedure, and medication codes, and associated cost information.
- **Pharmacies** prepare and dispense medications often based on medication prescriptions. Pharmacies know what and when patients actually fill medications. Pharmacies produce pharmacy claims, which are also sent to payers of the patients for reimbursement.
- **Pharmaceutical companies** discover, develop, produce, and market drugs. They conduct clinical trials to validate new drugs. Pharmaceuticals generate experimental data for drug discovery and clinical trials data.
- **Contracted Research Organizations (CROs)** provide outsourced contract services to pharmaceutical companies such as pre-clinical and clinical research and clinical trial management. Depending on the services line, CROs produce various datasets that support pharmaceutical companies to get their drugs to market.
- **Government agencies** play multiple roles in the healthcare ecosystem. Food and Drug Administration (FDA) is the most important regulator to approve new drugs and monitor existing drugs. Centers for Disease Control and Prevention (CDC) is a public health institution focusing on monitoring, controlling, and preventing diseases. For example, government agencies worldwide have been collecting the reports from Spontaneous Reporting Systems (SRS) submitted by pharmaceutical companies, healthcare professionals, and consumers to facilitate

post-market drug surveillance. These SRSs have served as a cornerstone for post-marketing drug surveillance, and the FDA Adverse Event Reporting System (FAERS) is one of the most prominent SRSs.

- **Patients** are at the center of healthcare, who interact with all the other players. For example, the healthcare benefits of patients are usually covered by their payers. Patients are also increasingly empowered to produce and manage their own health-related data. Most EHR systems provide patient portals (e.g., Web-based or Apps) for patients to assess their own EHR data and interact with their healthcare providers. For example, with wearable sensors such as wristbands and smartphones, more people can have activity monitoring data such as movement and heart rates, which are essential to monitoring individual health.
- **Researchers** are an important group of individuals that try to push the frontier of medical and healthcare research. Healthcare researchers can have a diverse background, including medicine, biology, chemistry, engineering, and data science. On one end, they can be conducting basic research in biology and chemistry that can help discover new drugs in the future or understand the basics of disease mechanisms. On the other end, they can be analyzing EHR data to produce translational insights that immediately change clinical practice. Researchers produce medical literature and clinical guidelines, which are important data in itself.

Life Cycle of Health Data When a patient comes to a clinic or a hospital, an electronic health record will be created about this clinical encounter or visit. This record will be documented by doctors or nurses (or generally healthcare providers) to describe what happened during this visit. A **clinical note** will be created to describe the visit in narrative text. Then various **medical codes** will be assigned to this visit, including diagnosis codes, procedure codes, and medication prescriptions. **Lab and imaging tests** may be ordered, which are done either at the clinic or sent to an external lab. The **lab report** contains both structured data and unstructured text. After the clinical visit, a **medical claim** containing most structured medical codes will be filed to the payer, usually by the provider on behalf of the patient. Then the payer will verify and reimburse the associated cost to the providers or patients. Meanwhile, the patient may take the medication prescription to a pharmacy to fill their medication. The corresponding medication will be dispensed to the patient. Then pharmacy may file a **pharmacy claim** to the payer to obtain reimbursement of the medication. In parallel, to invent new drugs, pharmaceutical companies (pharma) often work with providers to recruit patients to participate in clinical trials. Many **clinical trials** are managed by external CRO for pharma. Once patients are enrolled in the trials, various measurements related to the drug's efficacy and safety will be collected as part of the trial results. The complete results and their analysis will be submitted to the FDA for approval. The new drugs can only be widely distributed once three phases of trials are conducted with positive results and the corresponding FDA's approval is acquired. Different kinds of health data and the associated players are illustrated in Fig. 2.2.

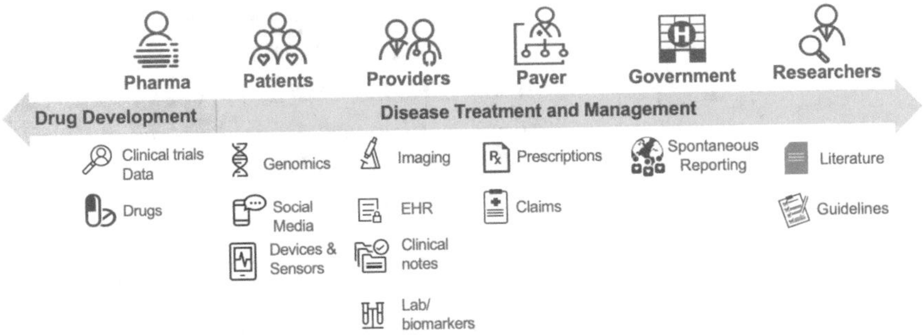

Fig. 2.2 Important players and the life cycle of health data

2.2.2 *Structured Health Data*

Structured data are common in healthcare, which are often represented as medical codes.

Various **medical codes** are used in both EHR and claim data, which usually follow common data standards. For example, diagnosis codes follow international disease classification (ICD); procedures use current procedure terminology (CPT) codes. The number of unique codes from each data standard is large and growing. For example, ICD version 9 (ICD-9) has over 13,000 diagnosis codes, while ICD-10 has over 68,000 diagnosis codes. Each encounter is only associated with a few codes. The resulting data are high-dimensional but sparse. A simple and direct way to represent such data is to create a *one-hot vector* for a medical code and a *multi-hot vector* for the patient with multiple codes as shown in Fig. 2.3. For example, to represent diagnosis information in an encounter, one can create a 68,000-dimensional binary vector where each element is a binary indicator of a corresponding diagnosis code. If only one dimension is one and zeros otherwise, we call it *one-hot vector*. If multiple ones are present, it is a *multi-hot vector*. As we will show in later chapters, such multi-hot vectors can be improved with various deep learning approaches to construct appropriate lower-dimensional representation.

Most medical codes follow certain standards such as ICD for diagnosis, CPT for procedures, and NDC for drugs, which will be explained later in Health data standards. Most of these medical codes are organized in hierarchies defined by medical ontologies such as CCS codes. These hierarchies are instrumental in constructing more meaningful and low-dimensional input features for the deep learning models. For example, instead of directly treating each ICD-10 code as a feature, we can group them into a few hundred CCS codes,[2] higher disease categories and treat each CCS code as a feature.

[2]https://www.hcup-us.ahrq.gov/toolssoftware/ccs/ccs.jsp.

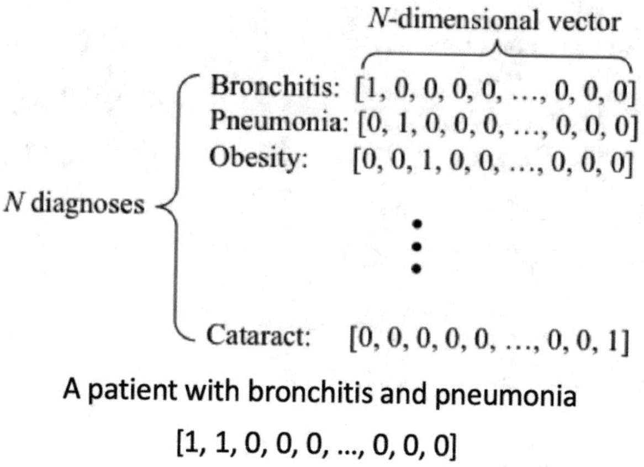

Fig. 2.3 Examples of one-hot vectors of medical codes, a multi-hot vector for a patient. Here 1 or 0 indicates the presence or absence of a particular diagnosis

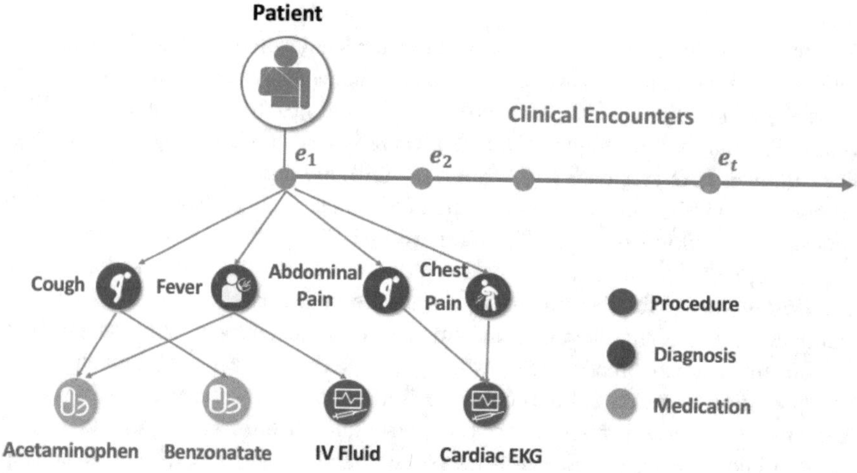

Fig. 2.4 In EHR data, medical codes are structured hierarchically with heterogeneous relations, e.g., medication *Acetaminophen* and procedure *IV fluid* are correlated, while both occur due to the same diagnosis *Fever*

All medical codes are interconnected in a hierarchical way within an encounter, as depicted by Fig. 2.4. In particular, EHR data can be seen as a collection of individual patient records, where each patient has a sequence of encounters over time. Within an encounter, multiple interrelated medical codes are assigned. Once a diagnosis code is assigned, the corresponding medication orders and procedure orders are then created. Each medication order contains information such as the medication code, start date, end date, and instructions. Procedure orders contain the procedure code and possible lab results. As shown by Fig. 2.4, procedures such

Table 2.1 Structured data in EHR

Codes	Standard	Example
Diagnoses	International Classification of Disease (ICD)	S06.0x1A
Procedures	Current Procedural Terminology (CPT)	70010
Labs	Logical Observation Identifiers Names & Codes (LOINC)	5792-7
Medication	RxNorm, ATC	
Demographics	NA	Gender, age
Vital signs	NA	Numeric
Behavioral status	NA	Smoking status

Table 2.2 Unstructured components of EHRs

Component	Description	Format
Discharge summary	Summary of an encounter	Text
Progress notes	Timestamped detailed description	Text
Radiology report	Summary of imaging test	Image+text
Electroencephalogram (EEG)	Brain activity monitoring	Time series
Electrocardiogram (ECG)	Heart monitoring	Time series

as *Cardiac EKG* come with several results (QRS duration, Q-T interval, notes), but *IV Fluid* does not. Note that some diagnoses might not be associated with any medication or procedure orders.

Other Structured Data In addition to medical codes, there are other structured data such as patient demographics (e.g., age and gender), vital signs (e.g., blood pressure), and social history (e.g., smoking status). These are also stored as structured fields in the EHR database. Various data standards are used for documenting different medical codes, as summarized in Tables 2.1 and 2.2.

Challenges Several challenges exist in analyzing structured data:

1. *Sparsity:* Raw data such as medical codes are often high dimensional and extremely sparse. For example, with 68,000 possible ICD-10 codes, each patient encounter may have only a few codes present;
2. *Temporality:* Health data often have an important time aspect that needs to be modeled. For example, EHR data of a patient may contain multiple visits over time. Discovering temporal relations is crucial for making an accurate assessment or prediction of any health outcome.

2.2.3 Unstructured Clinical Notes

Clinical notes are recorded for various purposes, either for the documentation of an encounter in discharge summaries, describing the reason and use of prescriptions in medication notes, interpreting the results of medical images with radiology reports, or analyzing the results from lab tests pathology reports. The reports include different sets of functional components, thus yield various difficulties in understanding. There are growing interests in using machine learning for these unstructured clinical notes, especially deep learning methods for automated indexing, abstracting, and understanding. Also, some works focus on automated classification of clinical free text to standardized medical codes, which are important for generating appropriate claims for that visit [114]. For example, a progress note is one type of clinical note commonly used in describing clinical encounters. A progress note is usually structured in four sections with the acronym SOAP:

- *Subjective* part describes what the patient tells you;
- *Objective* part presents the objective findings such as lab test results and imaging rests;
- *Assessment* part provides the diagnosis of the encounter;
- *Plan* part describes the treatment plan for the patient.

There are many different types of notes, including Admission notes, Emergency department (ED) notes, Progress notes, Nursing notes, Radiology reports, ECG reports, Echocardiogram reports, Physician notes, Discharge summary, and Social work notes. Each type can be written in a very different format with different lengths and quality.

Challenges Several key technical challenges exist in mining clinical text data:

1. *High dimension*—the number of unique words in clinical text corpus is large. Many words are acronyms, which are important to understand using their context.
2. *External knowledge*—in addition to clinical text in EHR data, there is a large amount of medical knowledge encoded in the text, such as medical literature and clinical guidelines. It is important to be able to incorporate that knowledge in modeling EHR data.
3. *Privacy*—Besides technical challenges, it is challenging to access clinical text due to privacy concerns as the data are very sensitive and affect individual privacy. As a result, very limited clinical notes are openly accessible for method development. And the volume of the shared data is also limited due to largely privacy concerns.

2.2.4 Continuous Signals

With an increasing number of new medical and wellness sensors being created, there will be more continuous signals as part of health data. Most commonly collected continuous signals in clinics include electrocardiogram (ECG) and electroencephalogram (EEG). ECG measures the electrical activities by placing electrodes on the chest, arms, and legs. In contrast, EEG measures the electrical activities of a brain via electrodes that are placed on the scalp. Both ECG and EEG are routine clinical measurements captured by multiple sensors (multi-channel) in high frequency (e.g., 200 Hz). Human doctors currently conduct most interpretations of ECG and EEG recordings (sometimes with machines' help). Beyond clinical signals like ECG and EEG, there are also consumer-grade wearables that monitor movement and heart rate. Several such sensors, including an accelerometer, gyroscope, and heart rate sensor, are already built into a typical smartphone.

Challenges Two significant challenges involved in analyzing continuous signals:

1. *Noise*—Sensor data often contain a significant amount of noises, making many simple models fail. For example, ECG and EEG signals can easily interfere with physical movement and power lines.
2. *Lack of labels*—To create direct clinical values, the continuous signals have to be mapped to meaningful phenotypes such as disease diagnoses. However, learning such a mapping requires sufficient labeled data that map continuous signals to phenotypes, which can be difficult to obtain. Because it may require significant time from human experts to produce the labels. Sometimes the data generated by new types of sensors are not well studied before, making it difficult for anyone to produce accurate labels.

2.2.5 Medical Imaging Data

Medical imaging is about creating a visual representation of the human body for diagnostic purposes. Various imaging technologies have been introduced, such as X-ray radiography, computed tomography (CT), magnetic resonance imaging (MRI), ultrasound (e.g., echocardiography). The resulting data are 2D images or 3D representations from multiple 2D images and videos. Medical imaging data are stored and managed by a separate system called *Picture archiving and communication system* (PACS). The images themselves are stored and transmitted in DICOM format (Digital Imaging and Communications in Medicine). Given the raw imaging data, radiologists read and mark the images and write a text report (radiology reports) to summarize the findings. The radiology reports are often copied into the EHR systems so that clinicians and patients can access the findings of the imaging tests. Thanks to the digitization of the radiology field, a large number of high-resolution images and their corresponding phenotypes (labels) are available for modeling. Thus there is tremendous excitement in using deep learning for radiology tasks [65, 101].

Challenges Data quality and lack of reliable and detailed labels are still challenges in analyzing such data. As the raw input images are very large (high-dimensional), it demands a sufficient sample size to train accurate and generalizable models.

2.2.6 *Biomedical Data for In Silico Drug Discovery*

In silico drug discovery is about using computational methods to create and select molecule compounds for new drugs. The data used *in silico* modeling include molecule compound graphs or sequences, protein target sequences, genome sequences, and disease-related knowledge graphs. For a molecule compound, a molecular graph represents the structural formula of the compound in terms of nodes (atoms) and edges (chemical bonds). Many computational models are not directly conducted on their original graph form but using specialized encodings:

- **SMILES**: A special string encoding called simplified molecular-input line-entry system (SMILES) is used to represent the chemical compounds.
- **ECPF/FCFP**: One can describe the compound using the functional connectivity fingerprints, including the Extended Connectivity Fingerprint (ECPF), which is a list of integer identifiers or a fixed-size bit string, where each identifier and bit corresponds to a neighbor substructure; and similarly the Functional-Class Fingerprint (FCFP), which is a variant of ECFP, integrates the functional features to the ECFP fingerprint.
- **Functional genes** are characterized by a unique gene identifier in a gene database such as GeneBank. There are also text descriptions of gene functions.

More generally, various knowledge graphs are constructed to represent the relations among entities within and/or across different data types. For example, the human disease network is a taxonomy of diseases themselves, the disease-drug network, disease-gene network. These networks describe the association between disease and drugs, as well as diseases and genes.

Challenges Several significant challenges in analyzing data associated with *in silico* studies.

1. *Incorporating domain knowledge*—Data for in-silico studies are mainly chemical data and various knowledge graphs. All the representations have a precise meaning in their domains. It is crucial to understand and incorporate their domain knowledge.
2. *Interpretable models*—Since the purpose of such data is to support drug discovery, it is important to provide more convincing evidence and interpretable explanation of each prediction.

2.3 Health Data Standards

Next, we overview a set of commonly used standards in healthcare data.

- **ICD** stands for International Classification of Diseases, which is a set of codes that represents diseases, symptoms, and clinical procedures [12]. ICD codes follow a hierarchical structure where related codes can be grouped into a higher level category. ICD codes are a widely used international standard maintained by World Health Organization (WHO). The latest version is ICD-11 as of 2020. Most of the world is currently using ICD-10. For example, "I50" corresponds to the ICD-10 category for heart failure, I50.2 is Systolic (congestive) heart failure, and I50.21 is Acute systolic (congestive) heart failure. ICD codes are used to represent disease diagnosis in EHR and claims data. Most EHR data will have ICD codes either in ICD-9 or ICD-10 format. An ICD9 code has up to 5 digits. The first digit is either alphabetic or numeric, and the remaining digits are numeric. For example, the ICD-9 code for *Diabetes mellitus without mention of complications* is 250.0x. The first three digits of an ICD-9 code corresponding to the disease category. And the last 1 or 2 digits reflect the subcategories of the disease. Besides numeric codes, ICD-9 codes can have an initial letter of V or E. For example, V85.x is an ICD-9 code for body mass index (BMI). In particular, V85.0 corresponds to BMI$<$19, V85.1 BMI between 19 and 25, and V85.2x indicates BMI$>$25. ICD-10 codes are more granular than ICD-9 codes. Each ICD-10 code has up to 7 digits. The first digit is always a letter; the second digit is always numeric; the third to seventh digits are alphanumeric. For example, E10.9 is the ICD-10 code for *Type 1 diabetes mellitus without complications*.

- **CPT** corresponds to Current Procedural Terminology, which is a standard created and copyrighted by American Medical Association. CPT codes represent medical services and procedures that doctors can document and bill for payment. CPT codes also follow a hierarchical structure. For example, CPT codes between 99201 and 99215 correspond to Office/other outpatient services, while a high-level category 99201–99499 corresponds to codes for evaluation and management. Like ICD codes, CPT codes are commonly present in structured EHR data.
- **NDC** codes are 10- or 11-digit national drug codes, which are managed by Food and Drug Administration (FDA). It consists of three segments: labeler, product, and package. For example, 0777-3105-02 is an NDC code where 0777 corresponds to labeler Dista Products Company, 3105 maps to the product Prozac, and 02 indicates the package of 100 capsules in 1 bottle. The same drugs with different packages will have different codes. From an analytic modeling perspective, NDC codes are probably too specific to be used directly as features.
- **LOINC** is a terminology standard for lab tests. LOINC stands for Logical Observation Identifiers Names and Codes (LOINC). Like other standards, LOINC has LOINC codes and associated descriptions of the code. To support lab tests, LOINC description follows a specific format with six parts: (1) COMPONENT (ANALYTE): The substance being measured or observed; (2) PROPERTY: The characteristic of the analyte; (3) TIME: The interval of time of the observation; (4) SYSTEM (SPECIMEN): The specimen upon which the observation was made; (5) SCALE: How the observation is quantified: quantitative, ordinal, nominal; (6) METHOD: how the observation was made (which is an optional part). For example, LOINC code 806-0 is the lab test of the manual count of white blood cells in the cerebral spinal fluid specimen. The different parts of the description are Component:Leukocytes, Property:NCnc (Number concentration),

Time:Pt(Point in time), System:CSF (Cerebral spinal fluid), Scale:Qn (Quantitative), Method:Manual count. LOINC codes demonstrate even structured data can encode multiple aspects of information.

- **SNOMED CT** is a comprehensive ontology of all medical terminologies. SNOMED CT stands for Systematized Nomenclature Of Medicine Clinical Terms. The core components of SNOMED include concept codes (or SNOMED ID), concept description, and the relationships between concepts. For example, 22298006 is the SNOMED code for a heart attack; there are various heart attack descriptions, including Myocardial infarction, Infarction of heart, Cardiac infarction, and Heart attack, Myocardial infarction (disorder), and Myocardial infarct. There are many associated relationships to heart attacks, such as a parent relationship to Ischemic heart disease (disorder), a child relationship to Acute myocardial infarction (disorder), an associated-morphology relation to infarct, and a finding-site relation to myocardium structure. Computationally SNOMED CT provides a large knowledge graph that connects many clinical terminologies, which can be extremely useful to combine with EHR data for predictive model building.

In addition to the data standards, various mapping software packages can process different types of healthcare data.

- **CCS** codes are a hierarchical categorization of ICD and CPT codes maintained by the Healthcare Cost and Utilization Project (HCUP). The purpose of CCS codes is to aggregate detailed ICD and CPT codes into clinically meaningful groups to support better statistical analysis. CCS codes have much fewer categories than the original ICD and CPT codes. For example, there are about a few hundred CCS codes, while ICD and CPT have tens of thousands of codes. From a machine learning modeling perspective, CCS codes can often be more informative than raw ICD and CPT codes.
- **RxNorm** is a terminology system for drugs and the associated software for mapping various mentions of drugs to normalized drug names. RxNorm group synonyms of drug expressions into drug concept. Each concept is assigned with a normalized name. In addition to drug name normalization, RxNorm also creates relations for each drug. For example, The drug "Naproxen 250 MG Oral Tablet" has a dose relation to "Oral Tablet", an ingredient relation of "Naproxen" and an *is-a* relation to "Naproxen Oral Tablet."
- **UMLS** standards for Unified Medical Language System, which integrates many biomedical terminologies. UMLS has three knowledge sources: (1) **Metathesaurus** integrates many terminologies including ICD, CPT, LOINC, SNOMED, and RxNorm, normalizes concepts and provides concept unique identifiers (CUIs) for each concept; (2) **Semantic Network** specifies all the relations among concepts; (3) **Lexical Tools** normalizes strings, handles lexical variants and provides basic natural language capability for biomedical text.

2.4 Exercises

1. What are the most useful health data for predicting patient outcome (e.g., mortality)?
2. What are the most accessible health data? And why?
3. What are the most difficult health data (to access and to model)?
4. What are the important health data that are not described in this chapter?
5. Which of the following is NOT true about electronic health records (EHR)?
   (a) EHR data from a single hospital consists of complete clinical history from each patient.
   (b) Outpatient EHR data are viewed as point events
   (c) EHR data contain longitudinal patient records.
   (d) Inpatient EHR data are viewed as interval events.
6. Which of the following is not true about clinical notes?
   (a) They can provide a detailed description of patient status.
   (b) Most EHR systems provide clinical notes functionality.
   (c) Clinical notes can contain sensitive protected health information.
   (d) Because of its unstructured format, it is easy for computer algorithms to process the notes
7. Which of the following are the limitations of claims data?
   (a) Coding errors can commonly occur in the claims data.
   (b) Since claims data are for billing purposes, they do not accurately reflect patient status.
   (c) Claims data are rare and difficult to find.
   (d) Claims data of a patient are often incomplete because they can go to different hospitals.
8. Which of the following is not true?
   (a) EHR are richer than claims.
   (b) EHR captures the medication prescription information but does not capture whether the prescription are filled.
   (c) Continual signals are rarely collected in hospitals.
   (d) Continuous signals provide objective assessments of patients.
9. Which of the following are not imaging data?
   (a) X-rays
   (b) Computed tomography
   (c) Electrocardiogram
   (d) Magnetic resonance imaging
10. What is true about medical literature data?
   (a) They are difficult to parse because of the natural language format.

(b) They are noisy and often low in quality.
(c) They often contain sensitive patient identifiers.
(d) They are in a machine-friendly format.

11. Which of the following is a medical ontology for medications?

    (a) CPT codes
    (b) RxNorm
    (c) SNOMED codes
    (d) MESH terms

12. Which of the following is not clinical trial data?

    (a) Trial protocols
    (b) Trial eligibility criteria
    (c) Data in clinical trial management systems
    (d) Electronic health records

13. Which of the following is not true about drug data?

    (a) Drugs are often represented in molecule structures.
    (b) Drug data are standard.
    (c) Drug data are often encoded in 3D molecule structures.
    (d) ChEMBL is a large bioactivity database.

Chapter 3
Machine Learning Basics

Machine learning has changed many industries, including healthcare. The most fundamental concepts in machine learning include (1) *supervised learning* that has been used to develop risk prediction models for target diseases and (2) *unsupervised learning* that has been applied to discover unknown disease subtypes. Both supervised and unsupervised learning expect to model various patient features as demographic features, including age, gender and ethnicity, and past diagnosis features (e.g., ICD codes). The key difference is the presence of labels in supervised learning and the absence of labels in unsupervised learning. A label is a gold standard for a target of interest, such as a patient's readmission status for training a readmission predictive model.

As we will describe in later chapters, most of the deep learning successes are in supervised learning. In contrast, the potential for unsupervised learning is immense due to the availability of a large amount of unlabeled data. This chapter will present the predictive model pipeline, basic models for supervised and unsupervised learning, and various model evaluation metrics. Table 3.1 defines notations used in this chapter.

3.1 Predictive Modeling Pipeline

A predictive modeling pipeline is a process of building prediction models from observational data. And predictive modeling pipelines are common use cases for supervised learning. As shown in Fig. 3.1, such a pipeline is not a single algorithm but a sequence of computational steps involving the following steps:

1. We first define the **prediction target**. For example, we may want to predict a future diagnosis of heart failure. An appropriate prediction target should be important for the application and feasible to achieve, given the available data.

C. Xiao, J. Sun, *Introduction to Deep Learning for Healthcare*,
https://doi.org/10.1007/978-3-030-82184-5_3

Table 3.1 Notation table

Notation	Definition
$\boldsymbol{x} \in \mathbb{R}^M$	M-dimensional feature vector
$\boldsymbol{x}_+$	Index set of data points of positive class
$\boldsymbol{x}_-$	Index set of data points of negative class
$y_i \in \{1, 2, \ldots, K\}$	Label for data point i
$(\boldsymbol{x}_i, y_i)$	A data point for supervised learning
$\boldsymbol{x}_i$	A data point for unsupervised learning
N	Number of data points
$\boldsymbol{X} \in \mathbb{R}^{M \times N}$ $\boldsymbol{y} \in \mathbb{R}^N$	Feature matrix and label vector
$\boldsymbol{w}$	weight vectors

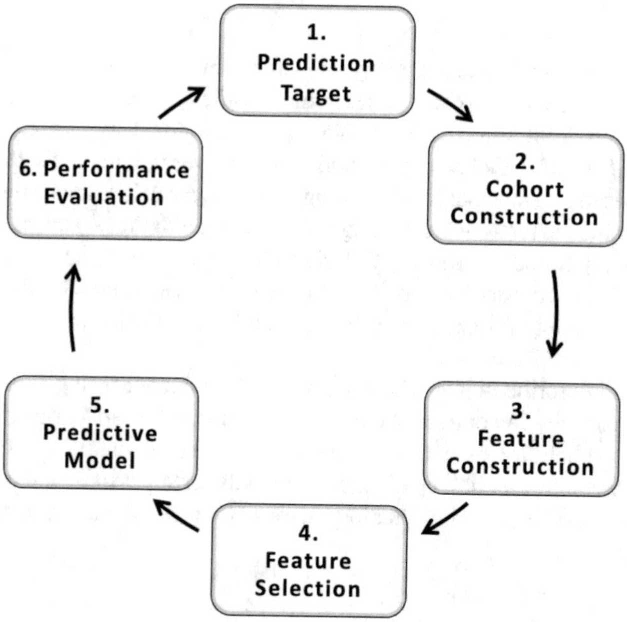

Fig. 3.1 Predictive modeling pipeline

2. We then need to **construct the patient cohort** for this study. For example, we may include all patients with an age greater than 45 for a heart failure study. There are many reasons why cohort construction is needed when building healthcare predictive models: (1) there might be the financial cost associated with acquiring the dataset based on the cohort; (2) we may want to build the model for a specific group of patients instead of a general population; (3) the full set of all patients may have various data quality issues.
3. Next, we will **construct all the features** from the data and **select those relevant features** for predicting the target. In a traditional machine learning pipeline, we

often have to consider both feature construction and selection steps. With the rise of deep learning, the features are often created and implicitly selected by the multiple layers of neural networks.
4. After that we can build the **predictive model** which can be either classification (i.e., discrete labels such as heart failure or not) and regression (i.e., continuous output such as length of stay).
5. Finally we need to **evaluate the model performance** and iterate.

3.2 Supervised Learning

We will start with the problem of disease classification as one major supervised learning task in healthcare applications: given a set of patients and their associated patient data, assign each patient with a discrete label $y \in \mathcal{Y}$, where $\mathcal{Y}$ is the set of possible diseases. This problem has many applications, from studying electroencephalography (EEG) time series for seizure detection to analyzing electronic health records (EHR) for predicting heart failure diagnosis. Supervised learning tasks such as disease classification are also a building block throughout many complex deep learning architectures, which we will discuss later.

Supervised learning expects an input of a set of N data points; each data point consists of m input features $\boldsymbol{x}$ (also known as variables or predictors) and a label $y \in \mathcal{Y}$ (also known as a response, a target or an outcome). Supervised learning aims to learn a mapping from features $\boldsymbol{x}$ to a label y based on the observed data points. If the labels are continuous (e.g., hospital cost), the supervised learning problem is called a *regression* problem. And if the labels are discrete variables (e.g., mortality status), the problem is called a *classification* problem. In this chapter, the label y are categorical values of K classes (i.e., $y \in \{1, 2, \ldots, K\}$).

3.2.1 Logistic Regression

Logistic regression is one popular binary classification model.[1] Logistic regression is actually the simplest neural network model, which is also known as the perceptron. Next, let us explain logistic regression with a healthcare example.

Suppose we want to predict the heart failure onset of patients based on their health-related features. In this example, the label $y = 1$ if the patient has heart failure and $y = 0$ if the patient does not have heart failure. Each patient has a M-dimensional feature vector $\boldsymbol{x}$ representing demographic features, various lab tests,

[1] Maybe a confusing name as logistic regression is for classification not for regression. But the naming choice will become meaningful after we explain the mathematical construction.

and other disease diagnoses. The classification task is to determine whether a patient will have heart failure based on this M-dimensional feature vector $\boldsymbol{x}$.

Mathematically logistic regression models the probability of heart failure onset $y = 1$ given input features $\boldsymbol{x}$, denoted by $P(y = 1|\boldsymbol{x})$. Then the classification is performed by comparing $P(y = 1|\boldsymbol{x})$ with a threshold (e.g., 0.5). If $P(y = 1|\boldsymbol{x})$ is greater than the threshold, we predict the patient will have heart failure; otherwise, the patient will not.

One building block of logistic regression is the log-odds or logit function. The odds are the quantity that measures the relative probability of label presence and label absence as

$$\frac{P(y = 1|\boldsymbol{x})}{1 - P(y = 1|\boldsymbol{x})}.$$

The lower the odds, the lower probability of the given label. Sometimes we prefer to use log-odds (natural logarithm transformation of odds), also known as the logit function.

$$logit(\boldsymbol{x}) = \log\left(\frac{P(y = 1|\boldsymbol{x})}{1 - P(y = 1|\boldsymbol{x})}\right).$$

Now instead of modeling probability of heart failure label given input feature $P(y = 1|\boldsymbol{x})$ directly, it is easier to model its logit function as a linear regression over $\boldsymbol{x}$:

$$\log\left(\frac{P(y = 1|\boldsymbol{x})}{1 - P(y = 1|\boldsymbol{x})}\right) = \boldsymbol{w}^T\boldsymbol{x} + b \tag{3.1}$$

where $\boldsymbol{w}$ is the weight vector, b is the offset variable. Equation (3.1) is why logistic regression is named logistic regression.

After taking exponential to both sides and some simple transformation, we will have the following formula.

$$P(y = 1|\boldsymbol{x}) = \frac{e^{\boldsymbol{w}^T\boldsymbol{x}+b}}{1 + e^{\boldsymbol{w}^T\boldsymbol{x}+b}} \tag{3.2}$$

With the formulation in Eq. (3.2), the logistic regression will always output values between 0 and 1, which is desirable as a probability estimate.

Let us denote $P(y = 1|\boldsymbol{x})$ as $P(\boldsymbol{x})$ for brevity. Now learning the logistic regression model means to estimate the parameters $\boldsymbol{w}$ and b on the training data. We often use maximum likelihood estimation (MLE) to find the parameters. The idea is to estimate $\boldsymbol{w}$ and b so that the prediction $\hat{P}(\boldsymbol{x}_i)$ to data point i in the training data is as close as possible to actual observed values (in this case either 0 or 1). Let $\boldsymbol{x}_+$ be the set of indices for data points that belong to the positive class (i.e., with heart failure), and $\boldsymbol{x}_-$ one for data points that belong to the negative class (i.e., without heart failure), the likelihood function used in the MLE is given by Eq. (3.3).

$$\mathcal{L}(\mathbf{w}, b) = \prod_{a_+ \in \mathbf{X}_+} P(\mathbf{x}_{a_+}) \prod_{a_- \in \mathbf{X}_-} (1 - P(\mathbf{x}_{a_-})) \tag{3.3}$$

If we take the logarithm to the MLE, we will get the following formula for log-likelihood in Eq. (3.4).

$$\log(\mathcal{L}(\mathbf{w}, b)) = \sum_{i=1}^{N} [y_i \log P(\boldsymbol{x}_i) + (1 - y_i) \log(1 - P(\boldsymbol{x}_i))] \tag{3.4}$$

Note that since either y_i or $1 - y_i$ is zero, only one of two probability terms (either $\log P(\boldsymbol{x}_i)$ or $\log(1 - P(\boldsymbol{x}_i))$) will be added.

Multiplying a negative sign to have a minimization problem, what we have now is the negative log-likelihood, also known as (binary) cross-entropy loss.

$$J(\mathbf{w}, b) = -\sum_{i=1}^{N} [y_i \log P(\boldsymbol{x}_i) + (1 - y_i) \log(1 - P(\boldsymbol{x}_i))] \tag{3.5}$$

To maximize the log-likelihood is the same as to minimize the cross-entropy loss. We can use the gradient descent method to find the optimal $\boldsymbol{w}$ and b.

3.2.2 *Softmax Regression*

We sometimes want to classify data points into more than two classes. For example, given brain image data from patients that are suspected of having Alzheimer's disease (AD), the diagnoses outcomes include (1) normal, (2) mild cognitive impairment (MCI), and (3) AD. In that case, we will use multinomial logistic regression, also called softmax regression to model this problem.

Assuming we have K classes, the goal is to estimate the probability of the class label taking on each of the K possible categories $P(y = k|\boldsymbol{x})$ for $k = 1, \cdots, K$. Thus, we will output a K-dimensional vector representing the estimated probabilities for all K classes. The probability that data point i is in class a can be modeled by Eq. (3.6).

$$P(y_i = a|\boldsymbol{x}_i) = \frac{e^{\boldsymbol{w}_a^T \boldsymbol{x}_i + b_a}}{\sum_{k=1}^{K} e^{\boldsymbol{w}_k^T \boldsymbol{x}_i + b_k}} \tag{3.6}$$

where $\boldsymbol{w}_a$ is the weight for a-th class, $\boldsymbol{x}_i$ is the feature vector for data point i, $\boldsymbol{w}_a$ and b_a are the weight vector and the offset for class a, respectively. To learn parameters for softmax regression, we often optimize the following average cross-entropy loss over all N training data points:

$$J(w) = -\frac{1}{N}\sum_{i=1}^{N}\sum_{k=1}^{K} I(y_i = k)\log(P(y_i = k|\boldsymbol{x}_i))$$

where K is the number of label classes (e.g., 3 classes in AD classification), $I(y_i = k)$ is binary indicator (0 or 1) if k is the class for data point i. And $P(y_i = k|\boldsymbol{x}_i)$ is the predicted probability that data point i is of class k.

3.2.3 Gradient Descent

Gradient descent (GD) is an iterative learning approach to find the optimal parameters based on data. For example, for softmax regression parameter estimation, we can use GD by computing the derivatives

$$\nabla_{\boldsymbol{w}} J(\boldsymbol{w})$$

and update the weights in the opposite direction of the gradient like the following rule

$$\boldsymbol{w} := \boldsymbol{w} - \eta\nabla_{w_k} J(\boldsymbol{w})$$

for each class $k \in \{1, \cdots, K\}$ and η is the learning rate, which is an important hyperparameter that needs to be adjusted. The gradient computation and weight update are iteratively performed until some stopping criterion is met (e.g., maximum number of iterations reached). Here ∇ is a differentiation operator which transforms a function $J(\boldsymbol{w})$ into its gradient vector along each feature dimension x_i. For example, $\boldsymbol{x} = [x_1, x_2, x_3]$, then the gradient vector is

$$\nabla J(\boldsymbol{w}) = \left\langle \frac{\partial J(\boldsymbol{w})}{\partial x_1}, \frac{\partial J(\boldsymbol{w})}{\partial x_2}, \frac{\partial J(\boldsymbol{w})}{\partial x_3} \right\rangle$$

3.2.4 Stochastic and Minibatch Gradient Descent

The gradient descent is a method to optimize an objective function $g(\boldsymbol{\theta})$ parameterized by model parameters $\boldsymbol{\theta} \in R^d$ by updating the parameters in the opposite direction of the gradient of the objective function $\nabla_{\boldsymbol{\theta}} g(\boldsymbol{\theta})$ with respect to the parameters. The full gradient can be very expensive to compute on a large data set because it has to process all data points. Several gradient descent variants reduce the computational cost, e.g., stochastic gradient descent (SGD) and mini-batch gradient descent.

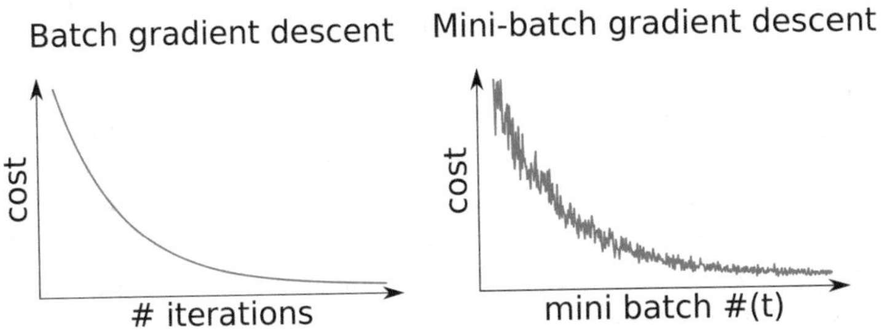

Fig. 3.2 Objective function changes for batch gradient descent and mini-batch gradient descent

The SGD performs parameter updating for every single data point in the training set. Given data point $\boldsymbol{x}_i$ with label y_i, the SGD does the following update:

$$\theta = \theta - \eta \nabla_{\boldsymbol{\theta}} g(\boldsymbol{\theta}; < \boldsymbol{x}_i, y_i >) \tag{3.7}$$

where η is the learning rate and $g(\boldsymbol{\theta}; < \boldsymbol{x}_i, y_i >)$ is the objective function evaluated on one data point $< \boldsymbol{x}_i, y_i >$. By updating one data point at a time, SGD is computationally more efficient. However, since SGD updates based on one data point at a time, it can have a much higher variance that causes the objective function to fluctuate. Such behaviors can cause SGD to deviate from the true optimum. There are several ways to alleviate this issue. For example, we can slowly decrease the learning rate as it empirically shows SGD would have similar convergence behavior as batch gradient descent (Fig. 3.2).

The mini-batch approach inherits benefits from both GD and SGD. It computes the gradient over small batches of training data points. The mini-batch n is a hyperparameter, and the mini-batch gradient descent does the following update.

$$\theta = \theta - \eta \nabla_{\boldsymbol{\theta}} g(\theta; < \boldsymbol{x}_i, y_i >, \ldots, < \boldsymbol{x}_{i+n-1}, y_{i+n-1} >) \tag{3.8}$$

where $< \boldsymbol{x}_i, y_i >, \ldots, < \boldsymbol{x}_{i+n-1}, y_{i+n-1} >$ are the n data points in a batch. Here the gradient is iteratively computed using batches of data points. Via such a mini-batch update, we reduce the variance of the parameter updates and solve the unstable convergence issue seen by SGD.

3.3 Unsupervised Learning

In many healthcare applications, labels are not available. In such cases, we resort to unsupervised learning models. Unsupervised learning models are not used for classifying (or predicting) towards a known label y. Rather we discover patterns or clusters about the input data points $\boldsymbol{x}$. Next, we briefly introduce some popular unsupervised learning methods.

3.3.1 Principal Component Analysis

Suppose we want to study N data points of M features represented by a matrix $\boldsymbol{X} \in \mathbb{R}^{N\times M}$. The number of features M can be large in many healthcare datasets. For example, there are 68,000 ICD-9 codes where each code can be a separate binary feature. Principal component analysis (PCA) can be applied to reduce the data dimensionality from M to a much lower dimension R. More specifically, PCA is a linear transformation:

$$\boldsymbol{Y} = \boldsymbol{X}\boldsymbol{W} \tag{3.9}$$

where $\boldsymbol{X}$ is the original data matrix, $\boldsymbol{Y} \in \mathbb{R}^{N\times R}$ is the low-dimensional representation after PCA, $\boldsymbol{W} \in \mathbb{R}^{M\times R}$ is the orthogonal projection matrix. The objective of PCA is to minimize the reconstruction error:

$$\min_{\boldsymbol{W}} \|\boldsymbol{X} - \boldsymbol{X}\boldsymbol{W}\boldsymbol{W}^\top\|^2$$

where $\boldsymbol{X}\boldsymbol{W}\boldsymbol{W}^\top = \boldsymbol{Y}\boldsymbol{W}^\top$ is the reconstruction matrix. The solution of PCA relates to another matrix factorization named singular value decomposition (SVD).

$$\boldsymbol{X} \approx \boldsymbol{U}\boldsymbol{\Sigma}\boldsymbol{W}^\top$$

where $\boldsymbol{U} \in \mathbb{R}^{M\times R}$ and $\boldsymbol{W} \in \mathbb{R}^{N\times R}$ are orthogonal matrices[2] that contain left and right singular vectors and $\boldsymbol{\Sigma} \in \mathbb{R}^{R\times R}$. Connecting to PCA, if $\boldsymbol{X}$ is the high-dimensional data matrix, the low-dimensional representation $\boldsymbol{Y} = \boldsymbol{U}\boldsymbol{\Sigma} = \boldsymbol{X}\boldsymbol{W}$.

In practice, PCA can be used as a feature extraction method for generating features from high-dimensional data such as neuroimaging data. For example, neuroimaging data such as Magnetic Resonance Imaging (MRI) or functional MRI includes many voxels, whose high dimensionality brings many challenges for diagnostic classification tasks. If we consider brain voxels as a raw feature, we can apply PCA to generate low-dimensional features to support downstream classification tasks. For instance, [86] showed that PCA features combining with a support vector machine (SVM) classifier provided good discriminative power in early diagnosis of Alzheimer's disease.

To summarize, as an unsupervised learning method, PCA provides low-dimensional linear representation to approximate the original high-dimensional features. In fact, PCA can be achieved by a neural network via autoencoders with linear activation. In later chapters, we can see more details about how neural networks expand the idea of PCA to low-dimensional nonlinear embedding using methods such as autoencoder.

[2]This means $\boldsymbol{U}\top\boldsymbol{U} = \boldsymbol{I}$ where $\boldsymbol{I}$ is the identity matrix.

3.3.2 Clustering

Besides dimensionality reduction, clustering is another major topic in unsupervised learning. Clustering methods aim to find homogeneous groups (or clusters) from a dataset, such that similar points are within the same cluster but dissimilar points in different clusters. For example, researchers have applied a clustering algorithm on EHR data to find disease subtypes of type II diabetes patient group into three clusters [97].

One popular clustering method is K-means, which tries to group data into K clusters where users specify the number K. The clustering assignments are achieved by minimizing the sum of distances (e.g., Euclidean distances) between data points and the corresponding cluster centroid (or the mean vectors). The K-means method is described in the following procedure:

Algorithm 1 The K-means algorithm

Input: (1) data points $\boldsymbol{x}_1, \cdots, \boldsymbol{x}_N$; (2) number of clusters K
Until convergence
DO
  Initialize K centers.
  WHILE not converged, **DO**
    Assign each $\boldsymbol{x}_i$ to the closest center $\arg\min_{k\in 1,2,\ldots,K} \|\boldsymbol{x}_i - \boldsymbol{\mu}_k\|$;
    Compute $\mathcal{L}$ for this observation $(\boldsymbol{x}, t)$;
    Update K centers $\boldsymbol{\mu}_k := \frac{1}{|S_i|}\sum_{i\in S_i} \boldsymbol{x}_i$.
RETURN
    Disjoint clusters $S_1, S_2, \ldots, S_K$.

Following the aforementioned procedure, we finish clustering all samples. Figure 3.3 provides a visualization of the iterative clustering procedure, where we apply k-means clustering over a set of points with cluster number $K = 2$.

3.4 Evaluation Metrics

In this section, we will introduce some common performance measures and evaluation strategies in machine learning.

3.4.1 Evaluation Metrics for Regression Tasks

The mean squared error (MSE) is the most basic performance metric for regression models. The formulation of MSE is given in Eq. (3.10).

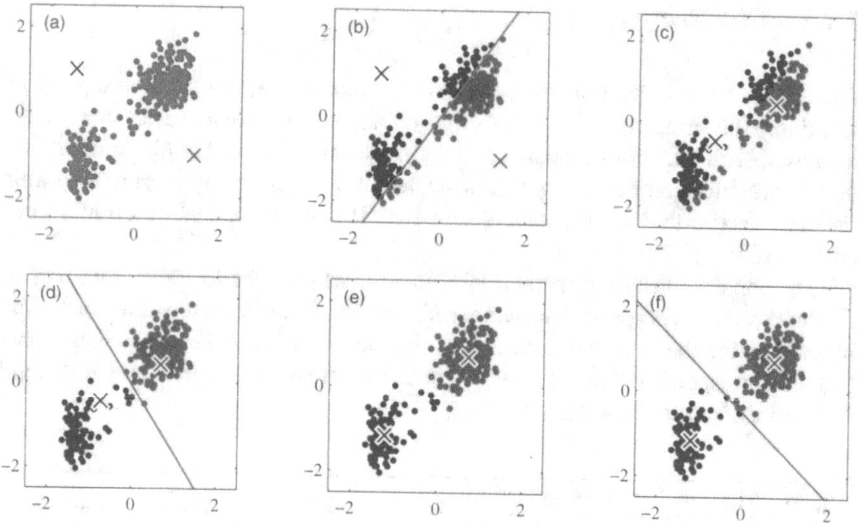

Fig. 3.3 k-Means clustering over a set of points with $K = 2$. From left to right, top to bottom, we firstly initialize two cluster centers with a blue cross and a red cross. After a few iterations, all blue (red) points are assigned to the blue (red) cluster, completing the K-means clustering procedure

$$MSE = \frac{1}{N}\sum_{i=1}^{N}(f(\boldsymbol{x}_i) - y_i)^2 \tag{3.10}$$

where $f(\boldsymbol{x}_i)$ is the predicted value for the i-th data point. Small MSE means the prediction is close to the true observation on average. Thus the model has a good fit. We can take the squared root of MSE to obtain another popular metric called root mean squared error (RMSE):

$$RMSE = \sqrt{\frac{1}{N}\sum_{i=1}^{N}(f(\boldsymbol{x}_i) - y_i)^2} \tag{3.11}$$

RMSE and MSE are commonly used in neural network parameter tuning. For example, the authors in [150] built a feedforward neural network model to find prognostic ischemic heart disease patterns from magnetocardiography (MCG) data. In training the model, RMSE was calculated as the evaluation metric to help to choose the model parameters, such as the number of nodes in the hidden layer and the number of learning epochs (see Fig. 3.4). Hyperparameters leading to the lowest RMSE was then chosen in the final model.

Another measure for regression problem is the coefficient of determination (also called as R^2) that measures the correlation between the predicted values $\{f(\boldsymbol{x}_i)\}$ and actual observations $\{y_i\}$. The R^2 is computed using Eq. (3.11).

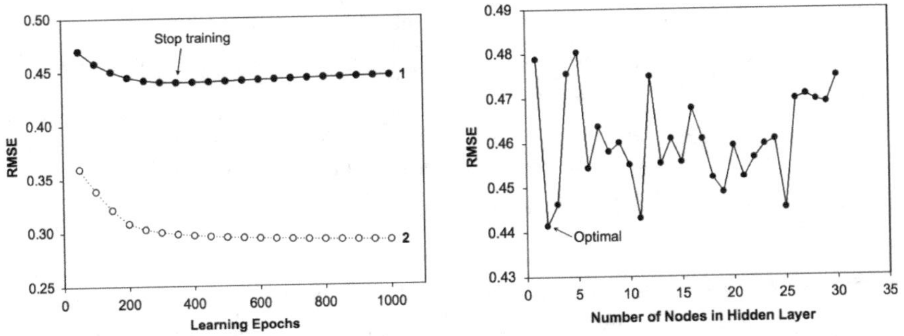

Fig. 3.4 In [150], to train the neural network model, RMSE was used as the evaluation metric in parameter tuning, including the number of learning epochs and the number of nodes in the hidden layer. Parameters exhibiting the lowest RMSE were chosen for the final model

$$R^2 = 1 - \frac{\sum_{i=1}^{N} (f(\boldsymbol{x}_i) - y_i)^2}{\sum_{i=1}^{N} (\bar{y} - y_i)^2} \tag{3.12}$$

where $\bar{y} = \frac{1}{N} \sum_i^N y_i$ is the sample mean of the target observation y_i.

The R^2 measures the "squared correlation" between the observation y_i and the estimation $f(\boldsymbol{x}_i)$. If R^2 is close to 1, then the model's estimations closely mirror true observed outcomes. If R^2 is close to 0 (or even negative), it means the estimation is far from the outcomes. Note that R^2 can become negative, in which case the model fit is worse than predicting the simple average of y_i regardless of the value of $\boldsymbol{x}_i$.

3.4.2 *Evaluation Metrics for Classification Tasks*

For binary classification, the label y_i can be either 1 or 0. For example, $y_i = 1$ indicates patient i is a heart failure patient (*case*) and $y_i = 0$ indicates a patient without heart failure (*control*). There are many performance metrics for classification models. For binary classification, prediction scores can be real values (e.g., probability risk scores between 0 and 1) or binary values.

Binary Prediction for Classification

If the predictions are binary values, we can construct a 2-by-2 confusion matrix to quantify all the possibilities between predictions and labels. In particular, we count the following four numbers: the number of case patients that are correctly

Table 3.2 Confusion matrix and performance metrics for classification

Total	Actual cases	Actual controls	Accuracy = (TP+TN)/Total
Predicted cases	True positive (TP)	False positive (FP)	Precision
Predicted controls	False negative (FN)	True negative (TN)	= TP/(TP+FP)
	Recall=Sensitivity =TP/(TP+FN)	Specificity=1-FPR =TN/(FP+TN)	False Positive Rate FPR=FP/(FP+TN)

predicted as cases is the true positive (TP); the number of case patients that are wrongly predicted as controls is the false negative (FN); the number of control patients that are correctly predicted as controls is the true negative (TN); and the number of control patients that are wrongly predicted as cases is the false positive (FP) (Table 3.2).

A few important performance metrics can be derived from the confusion matrix, including accuracy, precision—also known as positive predictive value (PPV), recall—also known as sensitivity, false positive rate, specificity, and F1 score:

Accuracy is the fraction of correct predictions over the total population, or formally:

$$Accuracy = \frac{TP + TN}{TP + TN + FP + FN}.$$

However, accuracy does not differentiate true positives (TP) or true negatives (TN). If there are many more controls (e.g., patients without the disease) than cases (patients with the disease), the high accuracy can be trivially achieved by classifying everyone as controls (or negatives). Other metrics address this class imbalance challenge indirectly, such as precision and recall, by focusing on the positive class.

Precision or positive predictive value (PPV) is the fraction of correct case predictions over all case predictions:

$$precision = \frac{TP}{TP + FP}. \tag{3.13}$$

While recall, also known as sensitivity and true positive rate (TPR), is the fraction of cases that are correctly predicted as cases

$$recall = \frac{TP}{TP + FN}. \tag{3.14}$$

Since precision and recall are often a trade-off, the F1 score is a popular measure that combines them by treating false positives and false negatives as equally important. More specifically, the F1 score is defined as the harmonic mean of precision and recall, given by the following formula:

$$F1 = 2 \times \frac{precision \times recall}{precision + recall}. \tag{3.15}$$

A more detailed explanation about the F1 score can be found at [130].

Specificity is also called the true negative rate, which measures the proportion of controls (negative samples) that are correctly predicted as controls:

$$specificity = \frac{TN}{FP + TN}$$

A related measure is the false positive rate (FPR), which is 1-specificity.

Real-Value Prediction for Classification

Most classifiers output a soft prediction score x between 0 and 1 instead of binary values. In those cases, one often has to define a classification threshold θ. That is, the classifiers output 1 if $x \geq \theta$, otherwise output 0. However, the right classification threshold value is often unknown. To avoid choosing values of θ, one can evaluate the average performance across different θ.

We will introduce the **area under the Receiver Operating Characteristic curve**, called ROC-AUC or AUROC. Before describing ROC-AUC, we need to understand the Receiver Operating Characteristic curve (ROC), which has the true positive rate (TPR) or recall or sensitivity as the y-axis and the false positive rate (FPR) or 1-specificity as the x-axis. The ROC-AUC is commonly used in model comparison and can be interpreted as the probability that the classifier will assign a higher score to a randomly chosen positive example than a randomly chosen negative example. A model with higher ROC-AUC is considered a better model. The advantage of ROC-AUC over accuracy is that it does not require choosing a classification threshold. In this manner, ROC-AUC is more robust against class imbalance.

A similar metric is an **area under the precision-recall curve**, called PR-AUC or AUPR. The precision-recall (PR) curve uses recall as x-axis and precision as y-axis. The area under the precision-recall curve has a very similar interpretation as the ROC-AUC but has a different visual representation of the curves. Looking at PR curves can expose differences between algorithms that are not apparent in ROC curves. For example, Fig. 3.5 shows performance comparison using ROC and PR curves. The figure is from [167] where the authors built machine learning models to predict adverse drug reactions using drugs' molecular structure data. In the performance comparison, results indicated the proposed model (denoted as "lda-dummy" in both figures) that incorporates medical ontology achieved the best performance in both ROC-AUC and PR-AUC.

The goal in ROC space is to be in the upper-left-hand corner, and when we look at the ROC curves in Fig. 3.5 the baseline model "lasso" appears to be fairly close to the best model "lda-dummy". In PR space, the goal is to be in the upper-right-hand

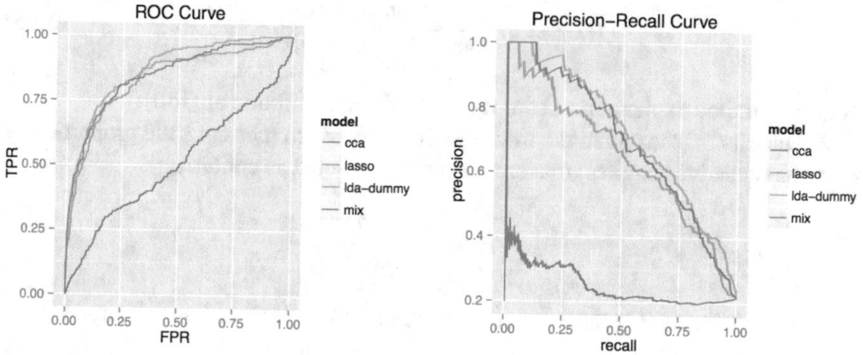

Fig. 3.5 In [167] where the authors built machine learning models to predict adverse drug reactions using drugs' molecular structure data. In the performance comparison, results indicated the model that incorporate medical ontology achieved the best performance in both ROC-AUC and PR-AUC

corner, and the PR curves in Fig. 3.5 show that there is still a significant gap between the performance of "lasso" and "lda-dummy".

Similar effects have been observed and discussed in [35], where the authors provided the following insights: "this difference exists because in this domain the number of negative examples greatly exceeds the number of positives examples". Consequently, a large change in the number of false positives can lead to a small change in the false positive rate used in ROC analysis. Precision, on the other hand, by comparing false positives to true positives rather than true negatives, captures the effect of a large number of negative examples on the algorithm's performance". In healthcare applications, since we often have many negative samples (e.g., controls), PR curve, and PR-AUC can be more meaningful to ROC-AUC.

Multi-Class Classification

Beyond binary classification, such as heart failure prediction, there are many scenarios we have multiple classes such as disease prediction, where each disease is a separate class. Thus each class becomes a separate binary classification task, which leads to a separate set of performance metrics such as precision and recall. When evaluating the multi-class classification's overall performance, people often have to average those performance metrics from different classes. There are two general approaches for computing average performance: **macro-average** or **micro-average**.

Suppose we have K classes, let TP_k, FP_k, TN_k, FN_k denote the number of data points that belong to true positive prediction, false positive prediction, true negative prediction, and false negative prediction in class k respectively ($k \in \{1, \cdots, K\}$). For each class k, we can compute aforementioned metrics such as F1 score using (3.15), denoted as $F1_k(TP_k, FP_k, TN_k, FN_k)$ since F1 score is a function of the four values in the confusion matrix. Then the macro-F1 is a simple averaging across all K classes given by Eq. (3.16).

$$\text{macro-F1} = \frac{1}{K}\sum_{k=1}^{K} F1_k(TP_k, FP_k, TN_k, FN_k). \tag{3.16}$$

Micro-averaged metrics are computed differently. We will first sum up the counts of true positives, false positives, true negative, and false negatives of the model for different classes to construct a new confusion matrix where we have

$$\begin{aligned} TP &= \frac{1}{K}\sum_{k=1}^{K} TP_k, \quad FP = \frac{1}{K}\sum_{k=1}^{K} FP_k \\ TN &= \frac{1}{K}\sum_{k=1}^{K} TN_k, \quad FN = \frac{1}{K}\sum_{k=1}^{K} FN_k \end{aligned} \tag{3.17}$$

Then we can use Eqs. (3.13) and (3.14) to calculate micro-precision and micro-recall. Then by plugging in both measures into Eq. (3.15) we can find micro-F1, which is also a function of the new measures produced in Eq. (3.17):

$$\text{micro-F1} = F1(TP, FP, TN, FN).$$

We can follow the same procedure to compute other micro-averaged and macro-averaged measures. In general, macro-averaging gives each class equal weight, whereas micro-averaging gives each data point equal weight. As a result, the micro-averaged metric is a measure of effectiveness in the large classes. To observe performances on small classes, macro-averaged metrics will be needed.

3.4.3 Evaluation Metrics for Clustering Tasks

A clustering algorithm usually aims at achieving high intra-cluster similarity (i.e., similarity within a group) and low inter-cluster similarity (i.e., similarity across groups). Here the similarity is usually represented by distance measures such as Euclidean distance and cosine distance.

One popular metric for clustering tasks is **silhouette coefficient**, which measures how similar each data point is to its own cluster compared to other clusters. The silhouette coefficient is computed as follows. Let $d_0(i)$ be the average distance between a data point i and all other data within the same cluster, let $d_1(i)$ be the lowest average distance of data point i to all data points in any other cluster where i does not belong to, silhouette coefficient is given by Eq. (3.18).

$$s(i) = \frac{d_1(i) - d_0(i)}{\max\{d_1(i), d_0(i)\}} \tag{3.18}$$

The range of $s(i)$ is $[-1, 1]$. A silhouette coefficient close to 1 indicates that the data point is appropriately clustered. And a silhouette coefficient close to -1 means the data point is wrongly clustered. Then the overall clustering performance can be the average silhouette coefficient of all points.

If ground truth clustering assignments are known, we can also use other metrics such as **rand index**, **mutual information** and **normalized mutual information** to evaluate the cluster results. Given C the clustering assignments, and C^* the ground-truth clustering assignments, we can define the following metrics to evaluate the clustering assignment C:

- **Rand index (RI)** defines as $\frac{a+b}{n(n-1)/2}$ where a is the number of data point pairs that belong to the same cluster in C and C^*, b is the number of data point pairs that belong to different clusters in C and C^*, and n is the number of data points. The rand index is a score between 0 and 1, where 0 indicates C and C^* do not agree on any clustering assignments, and 1 indicates C and C^* agree completely.
- **Mutual information (MI)** is another way to measure clustering quality. Mutual information is a concept from information theory, which measures the mutual dependence of two random variables.

$$MI(C, C^*) = \sum_{x \in C} \sum_{y \in C^*} p(x, y) \log \frac{p(x, y)}{p(x)p(y)}$$

  where x is a particular cluster with clustering assignment C and y is a particular ground-truth cluster in C^*, and $p(x, y)$ computes the probability of a data point in both cluster x and y.
- **Normalized mutual information (NMI)** is a normalized version of MI between 0 (no mutual information) and 1 (perfect correlation).

$$NMI(C, C^*) = \frac{MI(C, C^*)}{\sqrt{H(C)H(C^*)}}$$

  where $MI(C, C^*)$ is the mutual information, $H(C)$ and $H(C^*)$ are the entropy measure. For example, $H(C) = \sum_{x \in C} p(x) \log p(x)$ where x is a cluster in C and $p(x)$ is the proportion of the cluster x.

3.4.4 Evaluation Strategy

A cross-validation strategy is commonly used to evaluate the performance of regression and classification models. The general idea is to split the entire dataset into training and testing sets iteratively. We then use the testing set to evaluate the model's performance constructed from the training set. A common practice is to have most data used as the training set while a small portion is used as the test set (e.g., 90-10 split).

A popular variant is called K-fold cross-validation. We randomly split the entire data set into K non-overlapping partitions or folds of equal size in that strategy. When performing the split, one should ensure a non-overlapping partition to avoid information leaking. For example, to predict heart failure risk on patients where multiple visits of the same patient can occur, it is important to partition the patients' data so that no patients are shared across partitions. Each time we use onefold as the test set and the remaining folds as the training set. We learn a model using the training data and compute the model's performance measures on the testing data. We iterate K times until all folds have been used as a test set once. We then calculate the average performance measures across the K folds, which becomes the overall model performance. Another well-known strategy is called leave-one-out cross-validation (LOOCV) is, in fact, a special form of k-fold cross-validation, where each partition contains only one data point. LOOCV is typically only used for small datasets due to its expensive computation cost.

In deep learning, the data sets become huge, and the model training and parameter tuning become expensive. It becomes computationally too expensive to perform cross-validation, mainly due to model hyperparameters tuning. Instead, the evaluation strategy is shifted toward a single random split of the large data set into three partitions: training, validation, and test. A typical setup can be 80% training, 10% validation, and 10% test. First, we iteratively train the models with different hyperparameters (e.g., number of layers and number of neurons) on the training set and check the model performance on the validation set to decide the best hyperparameters setting. Then we use the best hyperparameters setting to train another model on the combination of training and validation set and check the model performance on the test set. The final performance on the test set will be used as the estimate of the true model performance.

3.5 Exercises

1. If you have a classification problem on 500 10-dimensional patient records, what algorithms would you try first? What algorithms would you try last?
2. If you have to cluster a large patient dataset (e.g., one billion data points), what algorithms would you use? what steps would you try to speed up the process?
3. What are the steps in a clinical predictive modeling pipeline?
4. How do you know if a prediction target is possible?
5. Which of the following are standard/good practice for building clinical predictive models?

   (a) Cross-validation are most commonly used for evaluating deep learning models.

		Ground Truth	
	TOTAL POPULATION	Condition Positive	Condition Negative 935
Prediction	Prediction Outcome Positive 155	True Positive	False Positive 100
	Prediction Outcome Negative	False Negative 10	True Negative

Fig. 3.6 Classification evaluation exercise

(b) For training deep learning models, it is important to keep validation and test sets large.
(c) Validation and Test sets can be small but should contain realistic samples with high-quality labels.
(d) Training data can be large and flexible, even with potentially noisy data.

6. What is the time complexity of K-means algorithm given n is the number of points, k is the number of clusters, d is the dimensionality of each point, and i is the number of clustering iterations?
7. Calculate the following statistics: Total Population, Condition Positive, True Positive, Prediction Outcome Negative, True Negative (Fig. 3.6).
8. Continue with the previous question, calculate True Positive Rate, False Positive Rate, False Negative Rate, True Negative Rate.

Chapter 4
Deep Neural Networks (DNN)

Neural networks are a family of machine learning models that consist of connected function units called neurons. They are built as powerful function approximators that accurately map input data $\boldsymbol{x}$ to output y (i.e., to learn a function $f(\boldsymbol{x}) \approx y$) through multiple layers of nonlinear transformations. Such a design enables neural networks to perform tasks like classification and regression.

The neurons in a neural network are organized into three interconnected layers: input, hidden, and output layers. When a neural network has one or more layers of hidden units, it can be regarded as a deep neural network (DNN). Based on different types of input data, multiple variants of DNN are invented. For example, the convolutional neural networks (CNN or ConvNet) are suitable for modeling grid data such as images or continuous time series. The recurrent neural networks (RNN) are appropriate for modeling sequential data such as text and clinical event sequences. Moreover, these variants have demonstrated great performance in solving real-world healthcare problems, for instance, CNN for automatic classification of skin lesions from image data [45], and RNN for clinical event prediction from patients longitudinal electronic health data [25, 30]. We will describe different DNN variants in later chapters. In this chapter, our focus is the basic deep neural networks (DNN). We summarize notations used throughout this chapter in Table 4.1. We first describe the structure and the training method of a single neuron and then move on to a general DNN, where neurons are organized in multiple interconnected layers.

4.1 A Single Neuron

To describe a deep neural network, we start with a simplest one that comprises of a single neuron. The neuron is a computational unit that takes n input values $\boldsymbol{x} = [x_1, \cdots, x_n]$ and their associated weights $\boldsymbol{w} = [w_1, \cdots, w_n]$. Then, a neuron takes

C. Xiao, J. Sun, *Introduction to Deep Learning for Healthcare*,
https://doi.org/10.1007/978-3-030-82184-5_4

Table 4.1 Notations for deep neural networks

Notation	Definition
$\boldsymbol{x}$	Input feature vector
x_i	ith input feature
$\boldsymbol{y}$	Output layer
y_i	ith output feature
L	Number of layers
l	Index of hidden layers
$\boldsymbol{W}^{(l)}$	Weight matrix of the lth layer
$w_{ji}^{(l)}$	Weight associated with unit i of the lth layer and unit j of the $(l+1)$th layer
$\boldsymbol{b}^{(l)}$	Bias vector for the lth layer
$b_j^{(l)}$	Weight of lth layer bias associated with jth unit of the $(l+1)$th layer
$g^{(l)}(\cdot)$	Activation function for the lth layer
$\boldsymbol{z}^{(l)}$	Output vectors of the lth layer
$z_j^{(l)}$	Output value of the jth unit of the lth layer
$\boldsymbol{a}^{(l)}$	Output vectors of the activation of the lth layer
$a_j^{(l)}$	Activated output value of the jth unit of the lth layer

a linear transformation of the inputs as $z = \boldsymbol{w}^T\boldsymbol{x} = \sum_{i=1}^{n} w_i x_i$, and follows with a nonlinear activation function $g(z)$. The output $g(z)$ can be used in machine learning tasks such as classification, with additional evaluation using loss functions. Thus two key components in this computation are activation functions and loss functions.

4.1.1 *Activation Function*

The activation functions, denoted as $g(\cdot)$, are the main components that perform a nonlinear transformation. Although we can use simple linear activation functions such as $g(x) = x$, the neural network's power often comes from the nonlinear activation functions such as Sigmoid, Tanh, and Rectified Linear Unit (ReLU). They are plotted on Fig. 4.1 for comparison.

Sigmoid as given by Eq. (4.1) outputs real values bounded in the range of (0, 1), making it a popular choice for binary classification due to the results can naturally be interpreted as the probability of an event, for example, the probability of having heart diseases.

$$g(x) = \frac{1}{1+e^{-x}} \tag{4.1}$$

However, since the gradient around either end of the function $g(x)$ (i.e., when x is very large or very small) is very close to zero, the output values toward either end

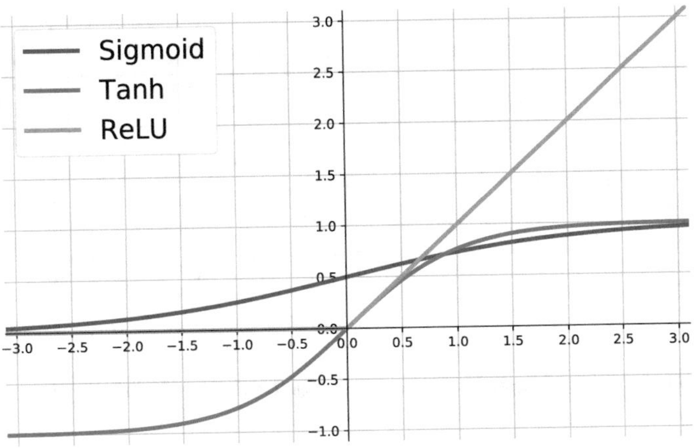

Fig. 4.1 The activation functions: Sigmoid, Tanh, and ReLU

tend to have less response to changes in input x, which is referred to as the *vanishing gradient* problem. The vanishing gradient causes gradient descent optimization to slow down dramatically, which is one of the most challenging problems in deep learning. In particular, the vanishing gradient becomes a major concern when using sigmoid activation. The gradient for the logistic activation function can be derived as below.

$$\begin{aligned}\frac{\partial}{\partial x}\left(\frac{1}{1+e^{-x}}\right) &= \frac{e^{-x}}{\left(1+e^{-x}\right)^2} \\ &= \frac{1+e^{-x}-1}{\left(1+e^{-x}\right)^2} \\ &= \frac{1+e^{-x}}{\left(1+e^{-x}\right)^2} - \left(\frac{1}{1+e^{-x}}\right)^2 \\ &= g(x)(1-g(x))\end{aligned}$$

Tanh as given by Eq. (4.2) is an alternative to the Sigmoid function.

$$g(x) = \frac{e^x - e^{-x}}{e^x + e^{-x}} = \frac{2}{1+e^{(-2x)}} - 1 = 2\text{sigmoid}(2x) - 1. \tag{4.2}$$

It is easy to see Tanh is a scaled and shifted Sigmoid function: with the scaling, the derivatives are much steeper, while the shift makes Tanh center around zero and has a range $(-1, 1)$. Due to scaling, the gradient of Tanh is stronger and has a wider range than that of the sigmoid (see Fig. 4.2), thus alleviate the vanishing gradient issue that occurs to a single unit. Nevertheless, Tanh still has the vanishing gradient

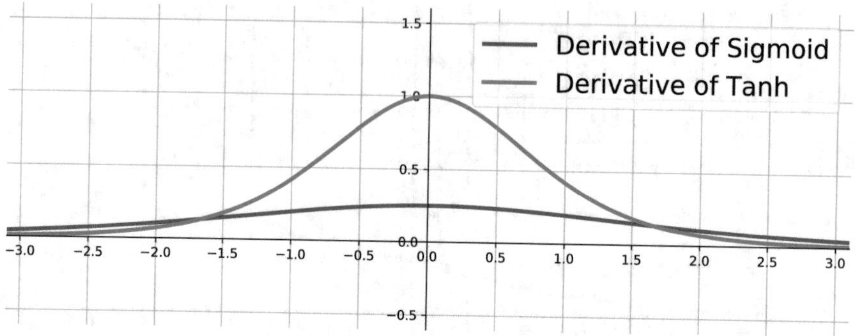

Fig. 4.2 The derivative of Sigmoid (red curve) and the derivative of Tanh (in blue curve) functions

problem at both ends. The gradient of Tanh is given by

$$\begin{aligned}\frac{\partial}{\partial x}\left(\frac{e^x - e^{-x}}{e^x + e^{-x}}\right) &= \frac{(e^x + e^{-x})(e^x + e^{-x}) - (e^x - e^{-x})(e^x - e^{-x})}{(e^x + e^{-x})^2} \\ &= 1 - \frac{(e^x - e^{-x})^2}{(e^x + e^{-x})^2} \\ &= 1 - g^2(x)\end{aligned}$$

using the quotient rule of derivative and knowing $\frac{\partial}{\partial x} e^x = e^x$ and $\frac{\partial}{\partial x} e^{-x} = -e^{-x}$

Softmax extends Sigmoid to handle multi-class classification. Assuming we have K classes, the goal is to estimate the probability of the class label taking on each of the K possible categories, $P(y = k)$ for $k = 1 \cdots, K$. Thus, we can normalize any K-dimensional vector $\boldsymbol{x}$ to a K-dimensional probability vector $\sigma(\boldsymbol{x})$:

$$\sigma(\boldsymbol{x})_i = \frac{e^{x_i}}{\sum_{k=1}^{K} e^{x_k}}$$

Note that $\sigma(\boldsymbol{x})_i$ indicates the i-th element of K-dimensional probability vector.

The Gradient of the Softmax Function is derived as follows. For the $i = j$ case, we have

$$\begin{aligned}\frac{\partial(\sigma(\boldsymbol{x})_i)}{\partial x_j} &= \frac{\partial}{\partial x_j}\left(\frac{e^{x_i}}{\sum_k e^{x_k}}\right) \\ &= \frac{e^{x_i}(\sum_k e^{x_k}) - e^{x_j} e^{x_i}}{(\sum_k e^{x_k})^2}\end{aligned}$$

$$= \frac{e^{x_i}}{\sum_k e^{x_k}} \frac{\sum_k e^{x_k} - e^{x_j}}{\sum_k e^{x_k}}$$
$$= \sigma(\boldsymbol{x})_i (1 - \sigma(\boldsymbol{x})_j)$$

For the $i \neq j$ case, we have

$$\frac{\partial(\sigma(\boldsymbol{x})_i)}{\partial x_j} = \frac{\partial}{\partial x_j}\left(\frac{e^{x_i}}{\sum_k e^{x_k}}\right)$$
$$= \frac{-e^{x_j} e^{x_i}}{(\sum_k e^{x_k})^2}$$
$$= -\sigma(\boldsymbol{x})_j \sigma(\boldsymbol{x})_i$$

Note that the quotient rule is applied in the above derivation, namely given $f(x) = \frac{g(x)}{h(x)}$, $f'(x) = \frac{g'(x)h(x) - h'(x)g(x)}{h(x)^2}$.

In summary, the gradient of the softmax function is

$$\frac{\partial(\sigma(\boldsymbol{x})_i)}{\partial x_j} = \begin{cases} \sigma(\boldsymbol{x})_i (1 - \sigma(\boldsymbol{x})_j), & \text{if } i = j \\ -\sigma(\boldsymbol{x})_j \sigma(\boldsymbol{x})_i, & \text{if } i \neq j \end{cases} \tag{4.3}$$

ReLU The Rectified Linear Unit (ReLU) defined as $g(x) = \max(0, x)$ is half-rectified in the sense that its activation is thresholded at 0. When the input is smaller than 0, the output is always 0. Otherwise, ReLU is the identity function. The major advantages of ReLU are computational efficiency and less prone to vanishing gradient. The gradient is either 1 or 0. It might be surprising why ReLU can lead to a powerful function as it seems to simply zero out negative values. However, despite its simplicity, ReLU is still a nonlinear function which is essential for neural network learning. When multiple ReLU functions stack up, they can produce a complex nonlinear function.

The regular ReLU function may be stuck at zero when x are negative, limiting the learning capacity of the neuron. To solve this issue, the **leaky ReLU** was proposed to introduce a small slope for the negative part instead of strict zero:

$$f(x) = \begin{Bmatrix} ax & \text{for } x < 0 \\ x & \text{for } x \geq 0 \end{Bmatrix}$$

where a is a small constant, e.g., $a = 0.01$.

4.1.2 Loss Function

In contrast to activation functions that perform the transformation of the input data at each unit, a loss function encodes the optimization objective of a neural network and quantifies that gap ("loss") between the predicted output of the neural network as $\hat{\boldsymbol{y}} = f(\boldsymbol{x}; \boldsymbol{W})$ and the ground truth $\boldsymbol{y}$. The choice of loss function depends on data types and tasks (e.g., regression or classification). Different loss functions will yield different loss value for the same prediction and will have a considerable effect on the resulting neural networks. Below are several commonly used loss functions.

Regression For regression tasks, one can use L2 loss such as the mean squared error (MSE) as given by Eq. (3.10). The MSE computes the square of the difference between the actual value and predicted value. Another choice for regression tasks is to use the L1 loss, such as the least absolute deviations as given by

$$L = \frac{1}{N}\sum_{i=1}^{N} |f(\boldsymbol{x}_i) - y_i| \tag{4.4}$$

Compared to L2 loss, the L1 loss is more robust in that it is more resistant to outliers in the data. However, L1 loss is harder to optimize than L2 loss due to the non-smoothness of its gradient.

Binary Classification The negative log-likelihood is a common loss function for binary classification as given by Eq. (4.5).

$$L = -\sum_{i=1}^{N} y_i \log \hat{y}_i + (1 - y_i)\log(1 - \hat{y}_i), \tag{4.5}$$

where y_i is ground truth binary label for observation i and $\hat{y}_i = P(y_i|\boldsymbol{x}_i)$ is the probability estimate of y_i based on data $\boldsymbol{x}_i$.

Multi-Class Classification The **cross-entropy loss** is a common loss function for multi-class classification. Then we can use cross-entropy loss as given by Eq. (4.6) to calculate average performance over all N training data points over all K classes.

$$L = -\sum_{i=1}^{N}\sum_{k=1}^{K} I(y_i = k)\log(P(y_i = k)) \tag{4.6}$$

where $I(y_i = k)$ is binary indicator (0 or 1) if class label k is the correct classification for observation i. And $P(y_i = k)$ is the predicted probability that observation i is of class k. Note that cross-entropy loss and negative log-likelihood loss are essentially equivalent in the binary classification setting.

The Cross-Entropy Loss with Softmax is one of the most common configurations of the output layer of neural networks. Its gradient is fairly simple, but the derivation is a bit involved.

$$\begin{aligned}\frac{\partial \mathcal{L}}{\partial o_i} &= \frac{\partial \mathcal{L}}{\partial L_i}\frac{\partial \mathcal{L}_i}{\partial o_i}\\ &= 1 \cdot \frac{\partial \mathcal{L}_i}{\partial o_i}\end{aligned}$$

where o_i is the softmax output and $L_i = -\sum_{k=1}^{K} I(y_i = k)\log(P(y_i = k))$. Then

$$\begin{aligned}\frac{\partial \mathcal{L}}{\partial o_i} &= -\sum_k I(y_i = k)\frac{\partial \log(P(y_i = k))}{\partial P(y_i = k)}\frac{\partial P(y_i = k)}{\partial o_i}\\ &= -\sum_k I(y_i = k)\frac{1}{P(y_i = k)}\frac{\partial P(y_i = k)}{\partial o_i}\\ &= -\frac{I(y_i = i)}{P(y_i = i)}\frac{\partial P(y_i = i)}{\partial o_i} - \sum_{k \neq i}\frac{I(y_i = k)}{P(y_i = k)}\frac{\partial P(y_i = k)}{\partial o_i}\end{aligned}$$

Now we can plug in the gradient of softmax function from Eq. (4.3) to derive the final gradient:

$$\begin{aligned}\frac{\partial \mathcal{L}}{\partial o_i} &= -I(y_i = i)(1 - P(y_i = i)) + \sum_{k \neq i} I(y_i = k)P(y_i = i)\\ &= -I(y_i = i) + \sum_k I(y_i = k)P(y_i = i)\\ &= P(y_i = i) - I(y_i = i)\\ &= \hat{y}_i - y_i\end{aligned} \tag{4.7}$$

where $\hat{y}_i$ is the probability estimate of class i from the model and y_i is the ground truth binary indicator for class i.

4.1.3 Train a Single Neuron

To train a neural network, we use gradient descent to adjust the weights of the network. Figure 4.3 illustrates the setup of training a single neuron with the sigmoid activation and squared loss function. In particular, we derive the role of each weight

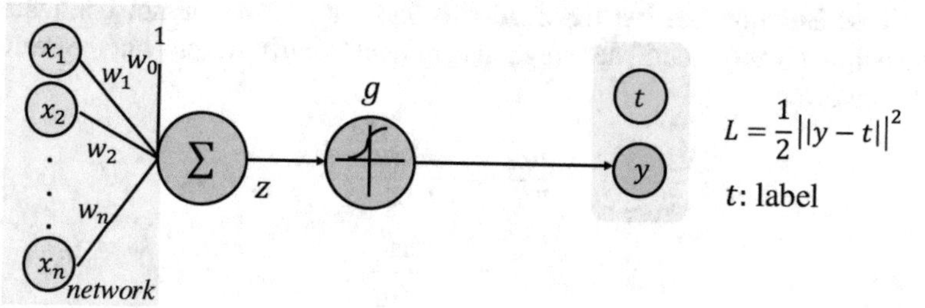

Fig. 4.3 Train a simplest neural network with one neuron. In this case we have sigmoid activation function and squared loss

in the network's overall loss as error gradient $\frac{\partial \mathcal{L}}{\partial w_i}$. Given a data point $(\boldsymbol{x}, t)$ where t is the target label and neural network output $y = f(\boldsymbol{x})$, the error gradient is the following:

$$\begin{aligned}
\frac{\partial \mathcal{L}}{\partial w_i} &= \frac{1}{2}\frac{\partial}{\partial w_i}||y - t||^2 \\
&= (y - t)\,\frac{\partial y}{\partial w_i} \\
&= (y - t)\,\frac{\partial y}{\partial \sum_i w_i x_i}\frac{\partial \sum_i w_i x_i}{\partial w_i} \\
&= (y - t)\,y(1 - y)x_i.
\end{aligned} \tag{4.8}$$

Then we compute $\nabla\mathcal{L} = [\frac{\partial \mathcal{L}}{\partial w_0}, \cdots, \frac{\partial \mathcal{L}}{\partial w_n}]$. Finally, we can update the weight $\boldsymbol{w}$ in the opposite direction of $\nabla\mathcal{L}$ as shown in Algorithm 2.

Algorithm 2 Stochastic gradient descent

Input: training data $(\boldsymbol{x}, t)$, learning rate η
Initialize each w_i to some small random value.
Until convergence
DO

    Initialize each ∇w_i to 0.
    For each $(\boldsymbol{x}, t)$ in training data, **DO**
        Pass $\boldsymbol{x}$ through the neuron to compute output $\boldsymbol{y}$;
        Compute $\mathcal{L}$ for this observation $(\boldsymbol{x}, t)$;
        Compute $\nabla\mathcal{L}$ using Eq. (4.8);
        Update weight $\boldsymbol{w} \leftarrow \boldsymbol{w} - \eta\nabla\mathcal{L}$.

4.2 Multilayer Neural Network

After understanding how to learn a single neuron, next we present the algorithm for learning a general neural network.

4.2.1 Network Representation

Deep neural networks, also called multilayer perceptrons (MLP), feed-forward networks, or fully connected networks, are the most standard neural networks model. The networks contain many neurons organized by multiple layers, and the neurons between consecutive layers are connected.

- The feedforward neural networks define a mapping function $\boldsymbol{y} = f(\boldsymbol{x}; \boldsymbol{W})$ where $\boldsymbol{x}$ are the input feature vectors and $\boldsymbol{W}$ are the parameters of the neural network.
- The parameter set $\boldsymbol{W} = \{\boldsymbol{W}^{(l)}, \boldsymbol{b}^{(l)} | 1 \leq l \leq L\}$ where $\boldsymbol{W}^{(l)}$ and $\boldsymbol{b}^{(l)}$ are the weight matrix and bias vector of the l-th layer, respectively.
- The goal is to determine the values of $\boldsymbol{W}$ such that the neural network can predict correct value $\boldsymbol{y}$ based on input $\boldsymbol{x}$.
- Computation flows from the input vector $\boldsymbol{x}$ to the output vector $\boldsymbol{y}$ via hidden and output layers $\boldsymbol{h}^{(l)} | 1 \leq l \leq L$. The hidden layers are called "hidden" because their values are not observed in the training data.
- For a L-layer neural network, the L is the total number of hidden layers plus the output layer (as a convention, the input layer is not counted). In particular, $\boldsymbol{h}^{(L)}$ is the output layer also denoted as $\boldsymbol{y}$.

The deep neural networks can be leveraged in many predictive tasks such as disease risk prediction using the electronic health records (EHR) data. A common approach is to convert raw EHR data into feature vectors, consisting of various medical codes (e.g., diagnosis and procedure codes). For example, we can transform the raw EHR vectors into binary vectors using multi-hot encoding methods, as illustrated in Fig. 4.4. A **one-hot encoding** vector contains only one "1" at the dimension corresponding to the medical code and "0" otherwise. A **multi-hot encoding** vector has the same number of dimensions as one-hot encoding but can have multiple "1"s, e.g., the "1"s represent multiple medical codes in a single clinical visit. We denote these input vectors as $\boldsymbol{x}$.

For example, a feedforward neural network model can map $\boldsymbol{x}$ to a specific disease prediction such as heart failure onset. Note that the last hidden layer ($(L-1)$-th layer) produces higher-level patient representation from raw EHR data. Some previous studies utilize such learned representation in finding disease subtypes [4, 15, 177].

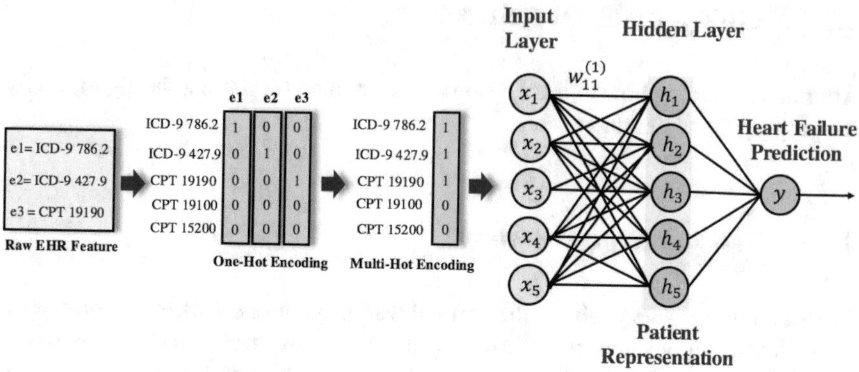

Fig. 4.4 We transform the raw EHR vectors that include multiple medical codes into binary vectors where a dimension with "1" indicates the presence of particular medical codes and "0"s mean the absence of the medical codes. The encoded features are then passed into a Deep Neural Network (DNN) for heart failure prediction

4.2.2 Train a Multilayer Neural Network

We will next walk through the example given by Fig. 4.5 to describe how to train a multilayer neural network. Similar to training a single neuron, we still use gradient descent to adjust the weights $w_{ji}^{(l)}$ and $b_j^{(l)}$ of the network to move its output in the opposite direction of the gradient. The only difference is the expression of the updating rule. The new rule is given by Eq. (4.10).

$$w_{ji}^{(l)} = w_{ji}^{(l)} - \eta \frac{\partial \mathcal{L}}{\partial w_{ji}^{(l)}} \tag{4.9}$$

$$b_j^{(l)} = b_j^{(l)} - \eta \frac{\partial \mathcal{L}}{\partial b_j^{(l)}} \tag{4.10}$$

In this example, we still use sigmoid activations on training data (x, t) to minimize squared error.

Forward Computation

As the name suggests, forward computation is to perform the layer-by-layer computation in a forward manner against an input data point. For better illustration of this process we further define the following variables. We denote $z_j^{(l)}$ as the pre-activation value at the jth node of the lth layer, $g^{(l)}$ as the activation function of the lth layer, and $a_j^{(l)}$ as the output value of the jth node of the lth layer. The $a_j^{(l)}$ is the

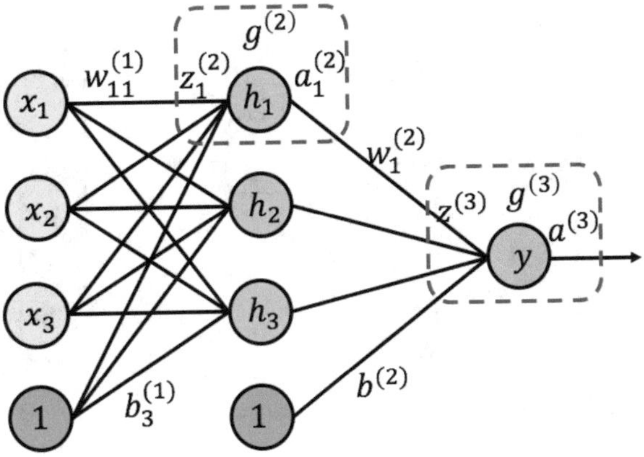

Fig. 4.5 Train a multilayer perceptron. In this case we have sigmoid activation function and squared loss

activation of $z_j^{(l)}$ via $g^{(l)}$. As the first step of the forward computation, each unit in the hidden layer performs a linear combination of the inputs and then transform the linear combination using an activation function:

$$\overbrace{z_1^{(2)}}^{pre\text{-}activation} = \sum_i w_{1i}^{(1)} x_i + b_1^{(1)}, \quad \overbrace{a_1^{(2)}}^{output} = \overbrace{g^{(2)}(z_1^{(2)})}^{activation}$$

$$z_2^{(2)} = \sum_i w_{2i}^{(1)} x_i + b_2^{(1)}, \quad a_2^{(2)} = g^{(2)}(z_2^{(2)})$$

$$z_3^{(2)} = \sum_i w_{3i}^{(1)} x_i + b_3^{(1)}, \quad a_3^{(2)} = g^{(2)}(z_3^{(2)})$$

Similarly each unit in the output layer will take these activation $a_j^{(2)}$ as inputs and perform pre-activation linear combination and activation, respectively:

$$z^{(3)} = \sum_j w_j^{(2)} a_j^{(2)} + b^{(2)}, \quad a^{(3)} = g^{(3)}(z^{(3)}).$$

Note that these computations can be represented via compact vector notations:

$$\begin{aligned} \boldsymbol{z}^{(2)} &= \mathbf{W}^{(1)}\boldsymbol{x} + \boldsymbol{b}^{(1)} \\ \boldsymbol{a}^{(2)} &= g^{(2)}(\boldsymbol{z}^{(2)}) \\ \boldsymbol{z}^{(3)} &= \mathbf{W}^{(2)}\boldsymbol{a}^{(2)} + \boldsymbol{b}^{(2)} \\ a^{(3)} &= g^{(3)}(\boldsymbol{z}^{(3)}) \end{aligned}$$

For a more common case, the forward computation from the lth layer to the $(l+1)$th layer can be expressed as:

$$\boldsymbol{z}^{(l+1)} = \mathbf{W}^{(l)}\boldsymbol{a}^{(l)} + \boldsymbol{b}^{(l)}$$

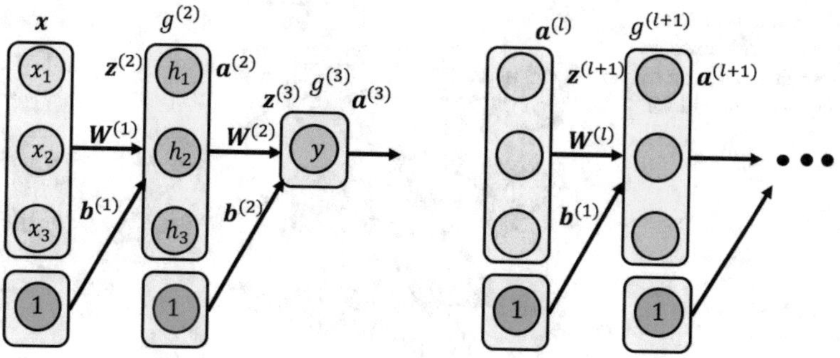

Fig. 4.6 Vector forms of forward computation

$$\boldsymbol{a}^{(l+1)} = g^{(l+1)}(\boldsymbol{z}^{(l+1)}).$$

The vector forms of forward computation for a deep neural network are illustrated in Fig. 4.6.

Backward Propagation

The backpropagation is designed to efficiently compute the partial derivatives $\frac{\partial \mathcal{L}}{\partial w_{ji}^{(l)}}$ and $\frac{\partial \mathcal{L}}{\partial b_j^{(l)}}$ that are needed in the gradient descent optimization procedure. Those derivatives can be computed for neural networks through a backward traversal over the network from the output layer to the input layer. The procedure of backpropagation is described as follows: Given a training data point (x, t), we will first run a forward computation to compute all the activations throughout the network to produce the output value. For example, in Fig. 4.7 the output value is y or $a^{(3)}$. The network output will be used as input $z^{(4)}$ in the computation of loss against target t. Next, we perform the backward error propagation as follows. For each node j in the lth layer, we compute an error term $\delta_j^{(l)}$ that measures how much that node was responsible for the error in the output. The backpropagation update follows the reverse order of the forward computation: $a^{(3)}$,$z^{(3)}$, $\boldsymbol{a}^{(2)}$, and $\boldsymbol{z}^{(2)}$.

First we derive the desired partial derivatives of the weights $\frac{\partial \mathcal{L}}{\partial w_{ji}^{(l)}}$ based on the chain rule.

$$\frac{\partial \mathcal{L}}{\partial w_{ji}^{(l)}} = \frac{\partial \mathcal{L}}{\partial z_j^{(l+1)}} \frac{\partial z_j^{(l+1)}}{\partial w_{ji}^{(l)}}$$

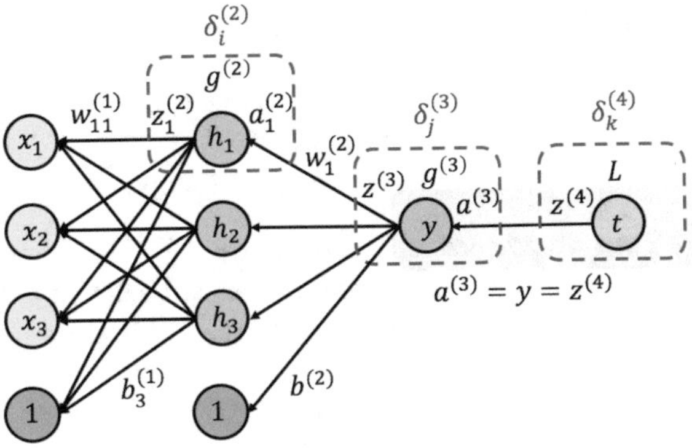

Fig. 4.7 Backpropagation on neural networks

$$
\begin{aligned}
&= \delta_j^{(l+1)} \frac{\partial(\sum_{i'} w_{ji'}^{(l)} a_{i'}^{(l)} + b_{i'}^{(l)})}{\partial w_{ji}^{(l)}} \\
&= \delta_j^{(l+1)} a_i^{(l)}
\end{aligned}
$$

where $\delta_j^{(l+1)} = \frac{\partial \mathcal{L}}{\partial z_j^{(l+1)}}$ defines the error component that measures how much node j of the $l+1$th layer was responsible for the overall error of the output, and $a_i^{(l)}$ is the i-th input from the (l)-th layer. Note that here for $\partial(\sum_{i'} w_{ji'}^{(l)} a_{i'}^{(l)} + b_{i'}^{(l)})$ in the numerator we temporally use i' as the general index, to differentiate it from specific i of $\partial w_{ji}^{(l)}$ in the denominator. There is only one i' that matches i in $\partial w_{ji}^{(l)}$, and other items in the summation will be treated as constant with 0 derivative.

Similarly, we have the partial derivative of the bias weights $\frac{\partial \mathcal{L}}{\partial b_j^{(l)}}$:

$$
\begin{aligned}
\frac{\partial \mathcal{L}}{\partial b_j^{(l)}} &= \frac{\partial \mathcal{L}}{\partial z_j^{(l+1)}} \frac{\partial z_j^{(l+1)}}{\partial b_j^{(l)}} \\
&= \delta_j^{(l+1)} \frac{\partial(\sum_{i'} w_{ji'}^{(l)} a_{i'}^{(l)} + b_{i'}^{(l)})}{\partial b_j^{(l)}} \\
&= \delta_j^{(l+1)}
\end{aligned}
$$

where again $\delta_j^{(l+1)}$ is the error component that measures how much nodes j of the $l+1$th layer was responsible for the overall error of the output.

To compute the partial derivatives, we will need all $\delta_j^{(l)}$. They can be computed from the last layer to the first layer. To start the backpropagation, we first initialize

$\delta^{(4)}$ for the loss computation, which is given by:

$$\delta^{(4)} = \frac{\partial \mathcal{L}}{\partial z_k^{(4)}} = \frac{\partial \frac{1}{2}||y - t||^2}{\partial y} = -(t - y). \tag{4.11}$$

Then we proceed recursively to use $\delta_j^{(l+1)}$ to compute $\delta_j^{(l)}$. In the following, we use the index j to denote both the general index or used as the index for the layers between layers indexed by i and k. The $\delta_j^{(3)}$ is given by:

$$\begin{aligned}
\delta_j^{(3)} &= \frac{\partial \mathcal{L}}{\partial z_j^{(3)}} \\
&= \frac{\partial \mathcal{L}}{\partial z_k^{(4)}} \frac{\partial z_k^{(4)}}{\partial z_j^{(3)}} \\
&= \delta^{(4)} \frac{\partial g^{(3)}(z_j^{(3)})}{\partial z_j^{(3)}} \\
&= \delta^{(4)} (g^{(3)})'(z_j^{(3)}) \\
&= -(t - y)(g^{(3)})'(z^{(3)})
\end{aligned}$$

Next we have $\delta_i^{(2)}$ given by Eq. (4.12).

$$\begin{aligned}
\delta_i^{(2)} &= \frac{\partial \mathcal{L}}{\partial z_i^{(2)}} \\
&= \frac{\partial \mathcal{L}}{\partial z_j^{(3)}} \frac{\partial z_j^{(3)}}{\partial z_i^{(2)}} \\
&= \delta_j^{(3)} \frac{\partial \sum_{i=1}^{d^{(2)}=3} w_{ji}^{(2)} a_i^{(2)}}{\partial z_i^{(2)}} \\
&= \delta_j^{(3)} \frac{\partial \sum_{i=1}^{d^{(2)}=3} w_i^{(2)} a_i^{(2)}}{\partial a_i^{(2)}} \frac{\partial a_i^{(2)}}{\partial z_i^{(2)}} \\
&= \delta_j^{(3)} w_i^{(2)} \frac{\partial a_i^{(2)}}{\partial z_i^{(2)}} \\
&= \delta_j^{(3)} w_i^{(2)} (g^{(2)})'(z_i^{(2)})
\end{aligned}$$

Note that $(g^{(3)})'(\cdot)$ and $(g^{(2)})'(\cdot)$ are the gradients of the activation function $g^{(3)}(\cdot)$ and $g^{(2)}(\cdot)$, respectively. In this specific example, all the $g^{(l)}(\cdot)$ are sigmoid. Thus in computation we need to substitute $g^{(l)}(\cdot)$ and $(g^{(l)}(\cdot))'$ with sigmoid and its derivative. Also in general, we have the following relation between $\delta_j^{(l)}$ and $\delta_k^{(l+1)}$

$$\delta_j^{(l)} = \left[\sum_{k=1}^{d^{(l+1)}} w_{kj}^{(l)} \delta_k^{(l+1)} \right] (g^{(l)})'(z_j^{(l)}). \tag{4.12}$$

Here we summarize the backpropagation algorithm for efficient gradient computation.

Algorithm 3 Backpropagation algorithm

The forward pass
Starting with the input $\boldsymbol{x}$, go forward to output layer, compute and store the variables $z^{(2)}, \boldsymbol{a}^{(2)}, z^{(3)}, \boldsymbol{a}^{(3)}, \cdots, z^{(L)}, \boldsymbol{a}^{(L)}, z^{(L+1)}$.

The backward pass
Initialize $\delta^{(L+1)} = -(t - y) = -(t - z^{(L+1)})$ and compute the derivatives at the output layer as $\frac{\partial L}{\partial w_k^{(L+1)}} = -(t - y)a_j^{(L)}$.
DO
Compute $\delta_j^{(l)} = \left[\sum_{k=1}^{d^{(l+1)}} w_{kj}^{(l)} \delta_k^{(l+1)}\right] (g^{(l)})'(z_j^{(l)})$
compute the derivatives at layer l as $\frac{\partial L}{\partial w_{ji}^{(l)}} = a_i^{(l)} \delta_j^{(l+1)}$ and $\frac{\partial \mathcal{L}}{\partial b_j^{(l)}} = \delta_j^{(l+1)}$

4.2.3 Parameters and Hyper-Parameters

There are several variables in the model for deep neural networks that need to be learned from the data. These variables are called parameters such as the weight matrix $\boldsymbol{W}$ of the neural network. Learning the model parameters is done through a process known as model training. In other words, by training a neural network model with some existing data, we can fit the model parameters. Besides parameters, other parameters cannot be directly learned from the regular training process. These parameters, known as hyperparameters, express higher-level properties of the model and are usually fixed before the actual training process begins. For deep neural networks, hyperparameters include the number of nodes and the number of hidden layers.

To choose hyper-parameters, we can use a randomized search or Bayesian optimization. For randomized search, we can use knowledge of the problem to pre-identify a range of hyperparameters. We randomly select hyperparameters from this region and repeat this process until we find parameters that work well. In [6], the authors showed a randomized search performed better than other methods in their case. For Bayesian optimization, we can use existing experiment information to decide how to adjust the hyper-parameters for the next experiment. An example of this approach can be found in [137].

4.3 Case Study: Readmission Prediction from EHR Data with DNN

Problem Hospital readmissions are a huge problem that affects hospital quality and patient outcomes. A study has shown that 17.6% of hospital admissions resulted in readmissions within 30 days of discharge, with 76% of those are avoidable [158]. Medicare, the national insurance program in the US, has introduced payment penalties for various hospital readmissions within 30 days of discharge. These readmissions used to account for $15 billion in Medicare spending. This kind of penalty has impacted over 2000 hospitals, with $280 million in penalties. To avoid such expensive readmission, the analytic problem is to identify the high-risk individuals who will likely have readmissions before discharge. Therefore, more hospital resources can be used to avoid expensive readmissions such as more proactive follow-up after discharge.

Data The study used the New Zealand National Minimum Dataset, obtained from the New Zealand Ministry of Health. It consists of nearly 3.3 million hospital admissions in the New Zealand hospital system between 2006 and 2012. They have background information on the patient's race, sex, age, and length of stay for each visit. Additionally, they also know the type of facility (public or private), and whether the patient was a transfer. They also have a single Diagnosis Related Group (DRG) code for each visit, selected from a set of 815 unique DRGs that break down admissions into broader diagnoses classes than the particular ICD codes.

Method DNN models are trained to predict readmissions on five patient cohorts for five different phenotypes, respectively [49]. They are pneumonia (PN), chronic obstructive pulmonary disease (COPD), heart failure (HF), acute myocardial infarction (AMI), and total hip arthroplasty or total knee arthroplasty ((THA/TKA). The problem was formalized as five different readmission prediction problems, each is a binary classification task. The features are also multi-hot vectors of 12,045 diagnosis codes (1 indicating the diagnosis and 0 absence). Each data point corresponds to one admission. There are 3,295,775 admissions. The label is 1 if the patient is readmitted within 30 days and 0 otherwise. The entire $3{,}295{,}775 \times 12{,}045$ binary feature matrix is partitioned into 5 matrices, one for each phenotype. The architecture of DNN has an input layer with a binary feature vector corresponding to the diagnosis codes, three hidden layers, and one output, as shown in Fig. 4.8. As a baseline, penalized logistic regression (PLR) is used which a logistic regression with the elastic net regularization (i.e., regularized with $\alpha\|\beta\|_1 + (1-\alpha)\|\beta\|_2$ where α is a hyperparameter between 0 and 1).

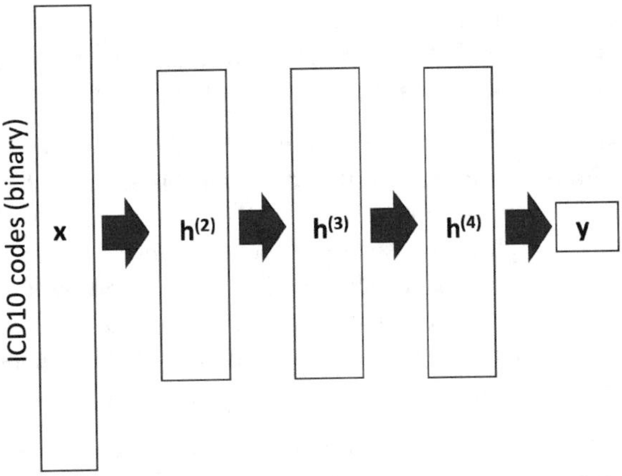

Fig. 4.8 DNN architecture for readmission prediction

Condition	Size	Readmission rate (%)	PLR AUC: mean (SE)	NN AUC: mean (SE)	*p*-Value, one-sided *t*-test
PN	40,442	27.9	0.715 (0.005)	**0.734 (0.004)**	0.01
COPD	31,457	20.4	0.703 (0.003)	**0.711 (0.003)**	0.086
HF	25,941	19.0	0.654 (0.005)	**0.676 (0.005)**	0.004
AMI	29,060	29.5	**0.633 (0.006)**	**0.649 (0.007)**	0.11
THA/TKA	23,128	8.7	**0.629 (0.005)**	**0.638 (0.006)**	0.264

Fig. 4.9 Results from 10-fold cross validation. A penalized logistic regression (PLR) is compared with a deep neural network (NN). *p*-Values for a one-sided t-test showed that DNN has significantly higher AUC than PLR

Results Figure 4.9 shows the resulting AUCs per group for both methods, along with the sample sizes and readmission rates. The deep neural networks consistently had better AUC (3 out of 5 times they were significantly better). But DNN models have a large number of parameters, requiring significantly more computational time to train, which has its limitation.

4.4 Case Study: DNN for Drug Property Prediction

Problem The quantitative structure-activity relationships (QSAR) is a classical problem in the pharmaceutical industry for predicting various activities of a chemical compound. Such predictions help prioritize the experiments during the drug discovery process and reduce the experimental work that needs to be done. However, the QSAR methods are particularly computationally expensive or require the adjustment of many sensitive parameters to achieve good prediction for an individual QSAR data set. In [105], the authors systematically evaluate the performance of DNN models for predicting quantitative structure-activity relationships.

Method This paper compares the performance of a DNN model with ReLU layer with a random forest (RF) classifier. First, the authors want to find out how well DNNs can perform relative to RF. Therefore, over 50 DNNs were trained using different parameter settings. These parameter settings were arbitrarily selected, but they attempted to cover a sufficient range of values of each adjustable parameter. The specific parameter choices can be found in the paper [105]. Then the authors tried the unsupervised pretraining to initialize the DNN parameters. For each data set, the authors trained five different DNN configurations with and without pretraining.

Data The data used in this study was from a 2012 Kaggle competition hosted by Merck. These are in-house Merck data sets, including on-target and ADME (absorption, distribution, metabolism, and excretion) activities. The competition aims to examine how well the state of the art machine learning methods can perform QSAR tasks. In this paper, 15 datasets of various sizes (2000–50,000 molecules), as shown in Fig. 4.10.

data set	type	description	number of molecules	number of unique AP, DP descriptors
		Kaggle Data Sets		
3A4	ADME	CYP P450 3A4 inhibition −log(IC50) M	50000	9491
CB1	target	binding to cannabinoid receptor 1 −log(IC50) M	11640	5877
DPP4	target	inhibition of dipeptidyl peptidase 4 −log(IC50) M	8327	5203
HIVINT	target	inhibition of HIV integrase in a cell based assay −log(IC50) M	2421	4306
HIVPROT	target	inhibition of HIV protease −log(IC50) M	4311	6274
LOGD	ADME	logD measured by HPLC method	50000	8921
METAB	ADME	percent remaining after 30 min microsomal incubation	2092	4595
NK1	target	inhibition of neurokinin1 (substance P) receptor binding −log(IC50) M	13482	5803
OX1	target	inhibition of orexin 1 receptor −log(K_i) M	7135	4730
OX2	target	inhibition of orexin 2 receptor −log(K_i) M	14875	5790
PGP	ADME	transport by *p*-glycoprotein log(BA/AB)	8603	5135
PPB	ADME	human plasma protein binding log(bound/unbound)	11622	5470
RAT_F	ADME	log(rat bioavailability) at 2 mg/kg	7821	5698
TDI	ADME	time dependent 3A4 inhibitions log(IC50 without NADPH/IC50 with NADPH)	5559	5945
THROMBIN	target	human thrombin inhibition −log(IC50) M	6924	5552
		Additional Data Sets		
2C8	ADME	CYP P450 2C8 inhibition −log(IC50) M	29958	8217
2C9	ADME	CYP P450 2C9 inhibition −log(IC50) M	189670	11730
2D6	ADME	CYP P450 2D6 inhibition −log(IC50) M	50000	9729
A-II	target	binding to Angiotensin-II receptor −log(IC50) M	2763	5242
BACE	target	inhibition of beta-secretase −log(IC50) M	17469	6200
CAV	ADME	inhibition of Cav1.2 ion channel	50000	8959
CLINT	ADME	clearance by human microsome log(clearance) μL/min·mg	23292	6782
ERK2	target	inhibition of ERK2 kinase −log(IC50) M	12843	6596
FACTORXIA	target	inhibition of factor Xla −log(IC50) M	9536	6136
FASSIF	ADME	solubility in simulated gut conditions log(solubility) mol/L	89531	9541
HERG	ADME	inhibition of hERG channel −log(IC50) M	50000	9388
HERG (full data set)	ADME	inhibition of hERG ion channel −log(IC50) M	318795	12508
NAV	ADME	inhibition of Nav1.5 ion channel −log(IC50) M	50000	8302
PAPP	ADME	apparent passive permeability in PK1 cells log(permeability) cm/s	30938	7713
PXR	ADME	induction of 3A4 by pregnane X receptor; percentage relative to rifampicin	50000	9282

Fig. 4.10 Datasets used in drug property prediction

To evaluate QSAR methods, each of these data sets was split into two non-overlapping subsets: a training set and a test set. Although a usual way of doing the split is by random selection. QSAR models are applied prospectively. Predictions are made for compounds not yet tested in the appropriate assay, and these compounds may or may not have analogs in the training set. The best way of simulating this is to generate training and test sets by time-split. For each data set, the first 75% of the molecules assayed for the particular activity form the training set, while the remaining 25% of the compounds assayed later form the test set.

As for the features (i.e., molecular descriptors), each molecule is represented by a list of features, that is, the union of the original atom pair descriptor—atom pairs (AP) [11], and donor-acceptor pair descriptors (DP) [85]. Both AP and DP descriptors are of the following form: atom types i-distance in bonds-atom type j. For AP, atom type includes the element, number of nonhydrogen neighbors, and number of pi electrons; it is very specific. For DP, atom type is one of seven (cation, anion, neutral donor, neutral acceptor, polar, hydrophobe, and others).

Various DNN model architectures have been tried with

- different data preprocessing strategies (original value, logarithm transform, binary transform),
- the number of hidden layers (1–4),
- the number of neurons in the hidden layers (varying from 100 to 4500),
- activation functions (Sigmoid vs ReLU),
- dropout rate,
- initialization (random vs. unsupervised pretraining),

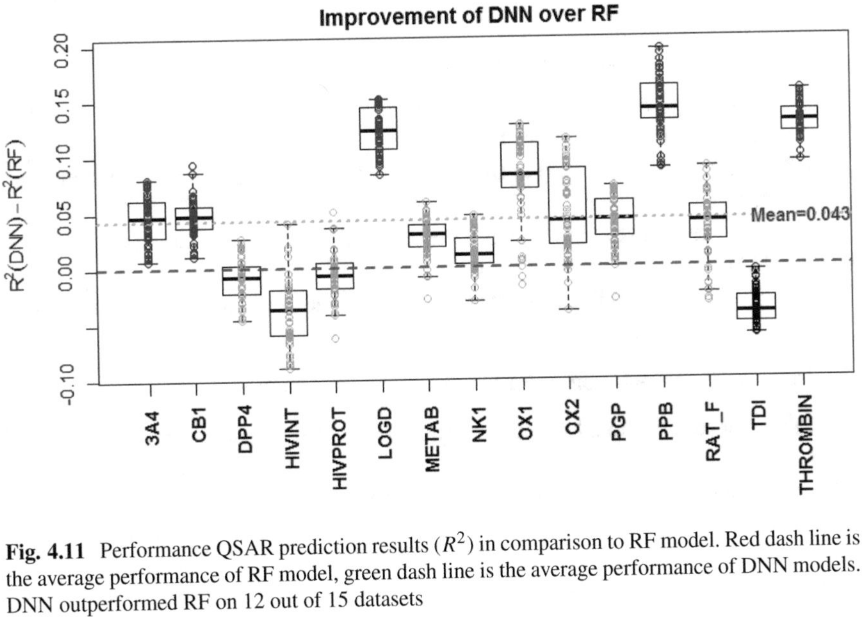

Fig. 4.11 Performance QSAR prediction results (R^2) in comparison to RF model. Red dash line is the average performance of RF model, green dash line is the average performance of DNN models. DNN outperformed RF on 12 out of 15 datasets

- mini-batch sizes and
- the number of epochs.

Results Figure 4.11 demonstrates that DNNs on average outperform RF in 11 out of the 15 data sets. It shows the difference in R^2 between DNNs and RF for each dataset. Each column represents a QSAR dataset, and each circle represents the improvement in R^2 of one DNN model over RF. A positive value means that the corresponding DNN outperforms RF. The average R^2 over all DNNs and all 15 data sets are 0.043 higher than that of RF, or a 10% improvement.

4.5 Exercises

1. Which types of health data do you think can be benefited most by DNN methods? Why?
2. Which types of health data do you think can be benefited least by DNN methods? Why?
3. Which of the following is NOT true about activation functions?
   (a) Activation functions describe non-linear transformation.
   (b) Activation functions are specified by the user when setting up the neural network architectures
   (c) Activation functions are learned directly from the data by neural network models.
   (d) ReLU is able to cope with vanishing gradient problems better than Sigmoid and Tanh.
4. What is NOT true about gradient descent?
   (a) Log-likelihood and likelihood function has the same optimal but log-likelihood is often easier to manipulate.
   (b) Gradient descent is an optimization method for optimizing model parameters.
   (c) Gradient descent is a specific design method for neural network optimization.
   (d) Stochastic gradient descent is a variant of the gradient descent method that is popular for neural networks training.
5. In forward computation, what is the weight $W_{12}^{(1)}$ used for?
   (a) Connect neuron $x1$ from the input layer to output neuron $h2$ in the second layer
   (b) Connect neuron $x2$ from the input layer to output neuron $h1$ in the second layer

(c) Connect neuron $h1$ from the second layer to output neuron $h2$ in the third layer
(d) Connect neuron $h2$ from the second layer to output neuron $h1$ in the second layer

6. In the general form of forward computation, the weight matrix $W^{(l)}$ and bias vector $b^{(l)}$ are used to connect?
7. What is true about back propagation?

(a) Back propagation is an efficient way to compute derivatives on parameters on a neural network.
(b) Back propagation does not require any form of forward pass of the neural network.
(c) Most deep learning packages require users to specify the derivatives of each layer in order to perform back propagation.
(d) Back propagation is a new algorithm invented specifically for training deep learning models.

8. Which is NOT true about Multilayer Neural Networks?

(a) Multilayer neural networks are computed more efficiently on GPU.
(b) There is no bias term in the input layer.
(c) The linear combination of layer 2 is computed as $z_i^{(2)} = \sum_j (w_{ji}^{(1)} x_j + b_j)$

9. Which is NOT true in the readmission study using DNN?

(a) Multiple layers of DNN can help construct better features before the final classification layer.
(b) Separate DNNs are trained for the five different disease cohorts.
(c) DNN models achieved better accuracy than logistic regression models in this study.
(d) DNN can provide a clear interpretation of its prediction.

10. Why do you think DNN is a good model for QSAR applications?

Chapter 5
Embedding

5.1 Overview

The clinically meaningful representations of medical concepts and patients are the key to health analytic applications. Standard machine learning approaches directly construct features mapped from raw data (e.g., ICD or CPT codes) or utilize some ontology mapping such as SNOMED codes. With deep neural networks' successes, people have focused on learning concept representation, namely *embedding vectors*. In this chapter, we present a set of neural network models called *embedding methods* to represent medical concepts (e.g., diagnoses, medications, and procedures) based on co-occurrence patterns in longitudinal electronic health records. The intuition behind the embedding methods is to map medical concepts co-occurring closely in EHR data to similar embedding vectors (i.e., the embedding distance between related medical concepts is small). Depending on how we define the co-occurrence, different embedding methods are proposed:

- Word2Vec [110] is based on the proximity of medical codes appearing in the records;
- GloVe [117] is a unsupervised learning algorithm for word embedding based on word co-occurrence statistics.
- t-SNE embedding [159] is a nonlinear dimensionality reduction method for visualizing high-dimensional data in 2D space.
- Med2Vec [24] leverages two-level hierarchical structures, namely clinical visits over time and co-occurrence within a visit;
- MIME [31] utilizes a three-level hierarchy, namely visits, diagnosis codes, then treatment codes.

Note that Word2Vec, GloVe, and t-SNE are general embedding methods, while Med2Vec and MIME are specifically designed to handle electronic health record data.

C. Xiao, J. Sun, *Introduction to Deep Learning for Healthcare*,
https://doi.org/10.1007/978-3-030-82184-5_5

5.2 Word2Vec

Word2Vec learns real-valued multi-dimensional vectors that capture relations between words by training on the massive text datasets [110]. The trained real-valued vectors will have similar values for similar words such as dog and cat or would and could, but distinct values for words that are not. Like natural language text, electronic health records can be seen as a sequence of "words" (i.e., medical codes such as diagnoses, medications, and procedures). Once the sequences of medical code are formed, we can map raw medical codes (e.g., ICD9, CPT) into embedding vectors using Word2Vec.

5.2.1 *Idea and Formulation of Word2Vec*

Word2Vec or any embedding method aims to learn a vector representation for each word such that closely related words will have similar vector representation. Words in healthcare applications can be medical codes in EHRs. Figure 5.1 depicts a motivating example for using a better representation of medical concepts. Figure 5.1a shows one-hot encoding of N unique diagnoses using N-dimensional vectors. More specifically, each diagnosis's corresponding dimension will be 1, and all the other $N - 1$ dimensions are 0. One-hot encoding is simple but not an effective representation for machine learning. The difference between related diagnoses (like bronchitis and pneumonia) is the same as the difference between unrelated diagnoses (like pneumonia and obesity). In fact, all pairs of different medical diagnoses will have the same distance to each other (i.e., Euclidean distance of $\sqrt{2}$). Figure 5.1b shows a Word2Vec representation in that bronchitis and pneumonia share similar values compared to other diagnoses. Moreover, by

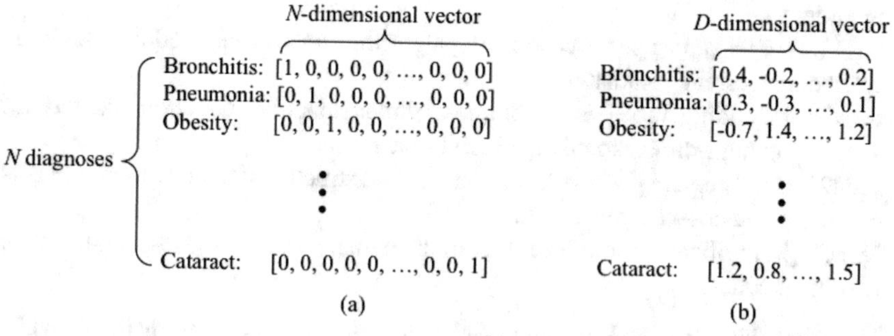

Fig. 5.1 Two different representation of diagnoses. Typically, raw data dimensionality N(>10,000) used in one-hot embedding is much larger than concept dimensionality D(∼100) in Word2Vec. More importantly, Word2Vec will organize similar word embeddings closer to each other in order to capture word relationship while one-hot vector can not. (**a**) One-hot encoding for diagnoses. (**b**) A better representation of diagnoses

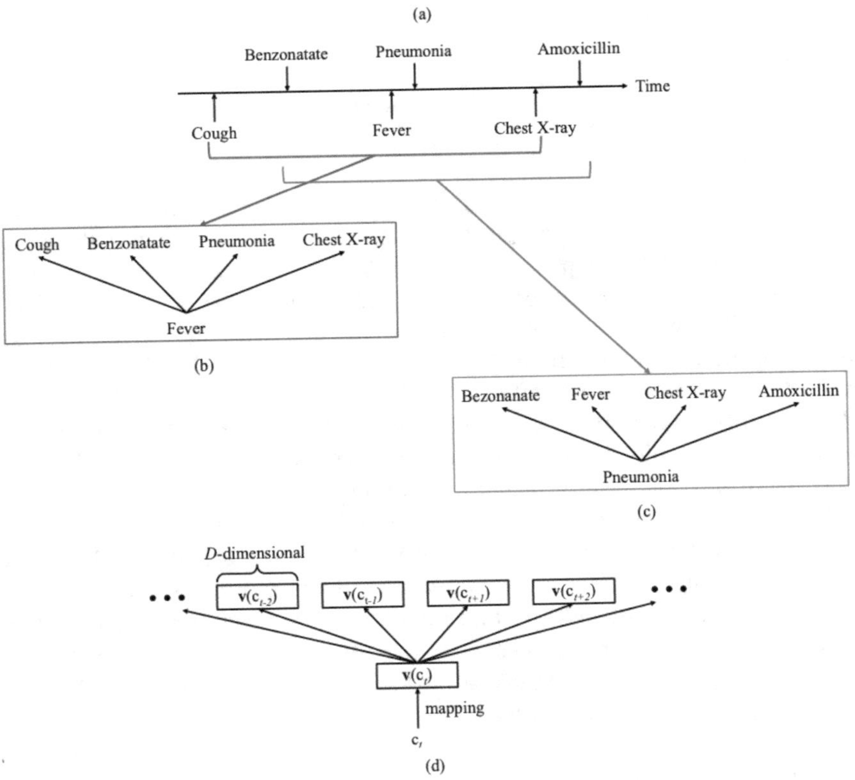

Fig. 5.2 Idea behind Word2Vec and the model architecture. (**a**) Patient medical records on a timeline. (**b**) Predicting neighboring medical concepts given *Fever*. (**c**) Predicting neighboring medical concepts given Pneumonia. (**d**) Model architecture of Skip-gram

using Word2Vec, we will better represent diagnoses and medications and procedures as multi-dimensional real-valued vectors by capturing the latent relations between them.

Next, let us look into the mathematical formulation of Word2Vec. Figure 5.2a is an example of a patient medical record in temporal order. Word2Vec assumes the meaning of a word is determined by its context (i.e., its neighboring words). Therefore, given a sequence of words, Word2Vec picks a target word and tries to predict its neighboring words. Figure 5.2b shows fever as the target word, and the other nearby words are its neighboring words. Then we slide a context window, pick the next target, and make the same context prediction shown by Fig. 5.2c. Since the goal of Word2Vec is to learn the vector representation of words, we need to map words to D-dimensional embedding vectors, where D is a user-defined value (typically between 50 and 1000 for text data). Therefore the actual prediction is conducted with the learned embedding vectors. Formally c_t denotes the word at the t-th timestep, $\boldsymbol{v}(c_t)$ the embedding vector that represents c_t. The goal of Word2Vec is to maximize the following average log probability,

$$\frac{1}{T}\sum_{t=1}^{T}\sum_{-w\leq j\leq w, j\neq 0}\log p(c_{t+j}|c_t)$$

where $p(c_{t+j}|c_t) = \exp[\boldsymbol{v}(c_{t+j})^\top \boldsymbol{v}(c_t)]/\sum_{c=1}^{N}\exp[\boldsymbol{v}(c)^\top \boldsymbol{v}(c_t)]$ and T is the length of the sequence of medical concepts, w the size of the context window, c_t the target medical concept at timestep t, c_{t+j} the neighboring medical concept at timestep $t + j$, $\boldsymbol{v}(c)$ the vector that represents the medical concept c, N the number of unique words. The size of the context window w is typically set to 5, giving us 10 neighboring words surrounding each target word. Note that the conditional probability is expressed as a softmax function. By maximizing the softmax score of the inner product of embeddings between each target word and its neighboring words, By maximizing this softmax function, Word2Vec learns real-valued vectors that capture the co-occurrence relations between words.

To compute Word2Vec, the denominator $\sum_{c=1}^{N}\exp[\boldsymbol{v}(c)^\top \boldsymbol{v}(c_t)]$ can be too expensive to compute as it sums over all words. A practical solution is to use *negative sampling*. The idea is to transform the word embedding problems as a binary classification task. The positive samples are the word pairs in the context window (i.e., c_{t+j}, c_t for $-w \leq j \leq w, j \neq 0$). And the negative samples are randomly sampled (i.e., pairing random words with the target word c_t). Then the objective function can be rewritten as

$$\arg\max \prod_{(c_w,c_t)\in D} p(y=1|c_w,c_t) \prod_{(c_w,c_t)\notin D} p(y=0|c_w,c_t) =$$

$$\arg\max \sum_{(c_w,c_t)\in D} \log \frac{1}{1+e^{-\boldsymbol{v}(c_w)^\top \boldsymbol{v}(c_t)}} + \sum_{(c_w,c_t)\notin D} \log(1 - \frac{1}{1+e^{-\boldsymbol{v}(c_w)^\top \boldsymbol{v}(c_t)}})$$

where $(c_w, c_t) \in D$ indicates the positive samples (i.e., the word pairs in the dataset), $(c_w, c_t) \notin D$ the negative samples (i.e., the word pairs of random word c_w and the target word c_t). The optimization procedure for the new objective function is equivalent to logistic regression classifier, which is more efficient than the original setting of Word2Vec. Note that the word2vec paper [110] present two algorithms for word embeddings, namely *skip gram* and *continuous bag of words*. They are very similar and we presented the skip gram formulation.

5.2.2 *t-Distributed Stochastic Neighbor Embedding (t-SNE)*

Deep learning models often process high-dimensional data (e.g., one-hot vectors of medical codes) and produce high-dimensional data (e.g., hidden states of neural networks). It is desirable to visualize high-dimensional data to understand patterns and relationships of that input and immediate output of neural networks. The t-distributed stochastic neighbor embedding (t-SNE) is a powerful and popular method for visualizing high-dimensional data (e.g., hidden states of a neural network) [159]. More specifically, the input to t-SNE is a high-dimensional data point $\mathbf{x}_i$, and the corresponding output from t-SNE is a low-dimensional (2D) data point $\mathbf{y}_i$. Traditional dimensionality reduction methods such as principal component analysis (PCA) can also produce 2-dimensional embedding for visualization. One major drawback of PCA is that it tries to preserve pairwise distance, dominated by faraway data points, while ignoring the small local variations. However, in real data, the relations of faraway points are often not reliable hence less important. On the other hand, relationships among nearby points are more important and more reliable, which should be the focus of the visualization method.

By highlighting the local relationships, t-SNE becomes a good dimensionality reduction algorithm that can display patterns and clusters in the data in a visually appealing way. Let us define p_{ij} and q_{ij} are the joint probabilities between a pair of points i and j for high-dimensional low-dimensional space, respectively. The objective of t-SNE is to minimize the Kullback–Leibler (KL) divergence between joint probability p_{ij} and q_{ij}:

$$KL(P||Q) = \sum_i \sum_{j \neq i} p_{ij} \log \frac{p_{ij}}{q_{ij}}$$

where the joint probability p_{ij} for the high dimensional data is

$$p_{ij} = \frac{\exp(-\|\mathbf{x}_i - \mathbf{x}_j\|^2/2\sigma^2)}{\sum_{k \neq l} \exp(-\|\mathbf{x}_k - \mathbf{x}_l\|^2/2\sigma^2)}$$

σ is the bandwidth of the Gaussian kernel, and the joint probability q_{ij} for the low dimensional (2D) data uses a Student t-distribution with one degree of freedom

$$q_{ij} = \frac{(1 + \|\mathbf{y}_i - \mathbf{y}_j\|)^{-1}}{\sum_{k \neq l}(1 + \|\mathbf{y}_k - \mathbf{y}_l\|)^{-1}}$$

Additional optimization is introduced to the input joint distribution p_{ij}. Instead of using joint probability, we use a conditional probability

$$p_{j|i} = \frac{\exp(-\|\mathbf{x}_i - \mathbf{x}_j\|^2/2\sigma_i^2)}{\sum_{k \neq i} \exp(-\|\mathbf{x}_i - \mathbf{x}_k\|^2/2\sigma_i^2)}$$

where we can set different bandwidth σ_i for different data point i. This adaptive bandwidth turns out to be important as it can handle different density distribution of input data. The joint distribution p_{ij} is approximated by $p_{ij} = (p_{j|i} + p_{i|j})/2$.

The t-SNE method has been extensively applied to visualize complex structured and high-dimensional health data. For example, in [1], t-SNE was used to visualize

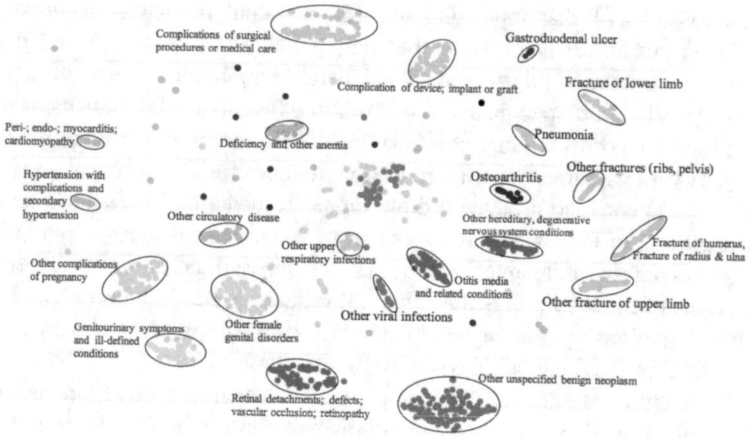

Fig. 5.3 t-SNE scatterplots of medical concepts trained by GRAM [28]

molecularly distinct and clinically relevant prognostic tumor subpopulations from mass spectrometry imaging data. Besides imaging data, t-SNE has been used to visualize genomic data. A particular example given by Taskesen et al. [151] shows when projecting tissue samples in a 2D-map (tSNE-map) using the gene expression profiles, t-SNE could retain local similarities between samples at the cost of retaining the similarities between dissimilar samples. As a result, t-SNE better preserves local (dis)similarities as they are not condensed due to the large dissimilarities in the data set. Moreover, t-SNE was also used to visualize learned phenotypes from EHR data. For example, in [94], t-SNE was used to project learned features into two-dimensional embeddings. It is easy to visually identify subpopulations of gout and leukemia that might have pathophysiologic differences.

The following examples show how researchers used t-SNE to evaluate the performance of their phenotyping algorithm visually. Figure 5.3 used t-SNE to represent the final representations of 2000 randomly chosen diseases learned by GRAM [28] for sequential diagnoses prediction using EHR data. Here t-SNE provides an intuitive way to qualitatively assess the interpretability of the learned representations of the medical codes. The color of the dots represents the highest disease categories, and the text annotations represent the detailed disease categories in CCS multi-level hierarchy. The figure shows how learned disease representations align with domain knowledge. Another demonstration in Fig. 5.4 shows how learned medical concepts from [24] could form distinct groups.

5.2.3 Healthcare Application of Word2Vec

Next, we present a study using Word2Vec for heart failure prediction [26].

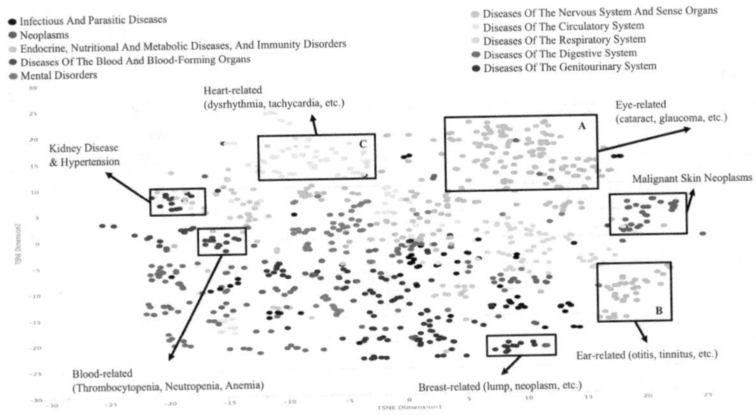

Fig. 5.4 t-SNE scatterplots of medical concepts trained by Med2vec [27]

Data Data in this study were from Sutter Palo Alto Medical Foundation (Sutter-PAMF) primary care patients. Sutter-PAMF is large primary care and multispecialty group practice that has used an EHR for more than a decade. The study dataset was extracted with cases and controls identified within the interval from 2000 to 2013. The EHR data included demographics, smoking and alcohol consumptions, clinical and laboratory values, International Classification of Disease version 9 (ICD-9) codes associated with encounters, order, and referrals, procedure information in Current Procedural Terminology (CPT) codes, and medication prescription information in medical names. The dataset contained 265,336 patients with 555,609 unique clinical events in total.

Configuration of Word2Vec To apply Word2Vec to longitudinal EHR data, the authors processed medication orders, procedure orders, and problem list records of all 265,336 patients and extracted diagnosis, medication, and procedure codes assigned to each patient in a temporal order. If a patient received multiple diagnoses, medications, or procedures at a single visit, those medical codes were ordered randomly within the same timestamp. The respective number of unique diagnoses, medications, and procedures was 11,460, 17,769, and 9,370, totaling 38,599 unique medical concepts. 100-dimensional medical concept embedding vectors are used (i.e., D=100 in Fig. 5.1b).

Qualitative Assessment Figure 5.5a shows the Word2Vec diagnosis embedding vectors, where a t-SNE [109] is produced to visualize high-dimensional data in 2D space. One Thousand randomly chosen diagnoses (ICD-9 codes) are displayed in Fig. 5.5a. In it, diagnoses are generally well grouped by their disease categories. However, if some diagnoses from the same category are still quite different, they should be apart. This is shown by the red box and the blue box in Fig. 5.5a. Even though they are from the same neoplasms category, the red box indicates malignant skin neoplasms (172.X, 173.X) while the blue box indicates a benign

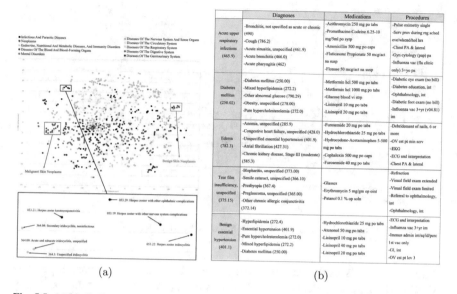

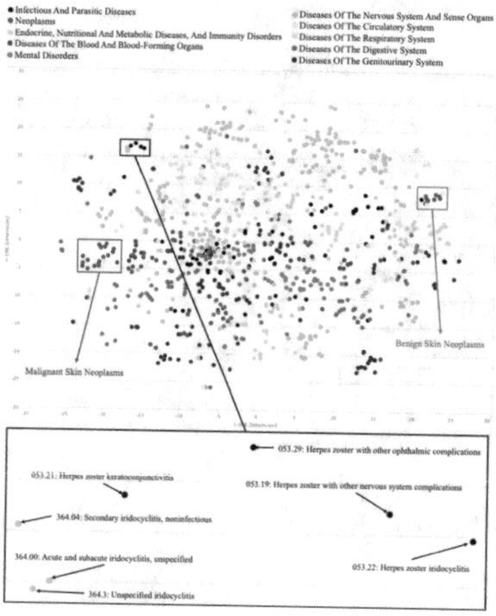

(a)

	Diagnoses	Medications	Procedures
Acute upper respiratory infections (465.9)	-Bronchitis, not specified as acute or chronic (490) -Cough (786.2) -Acute sinusitis, unspecified (461.9) -Acute bronchitis (466.0) -Acute pharyngitis (462)	-Azithromycin 250 mg po tabs -Promethazine-Codeine 6.25-10 mg/5ml po syrp -Amoxicillin 500 mg po caps -Fluticasone Propionate 50 mcg/act na susp -Flonase 50 mcg/act na susp	-Pulse oximetry single -Serv prov during reg sched eve/wkend/hol hrs -Chest PA & lateral -Gyn cytology (pap) pa -Influenza vac (flu clinic only) 3+yo pa
Diabetes mellitus (250.02)	-Diabetes mellitus (250.00) -Mixed hyperlipidemia (272.2) -Other abnormal glucose (790.29) -Obesity, unspecified (278.00) -Pure hypercholesterolemia (272.0)	-Metformin hcl 500 mg po tabs -Metformin hcl 1000 mg po tabs -Glucose blood vi strp -Lisinopril 10 mg po tabs -Lisinopril 20 mg po tabs	-Diabetic eye exam (no bill) -Diabetes education, int -Ophthalmology, int -Diabetic foot exam (no bill) -Influenza vac 3+yr (v04.81) im
Edema (782.3)	-Anemia, unspecified (285.9) -Congestive heart failure, unspecified (428.0) -Unspecified essential hypertension (401.9) -Atrial fibrillation (427.31) -Chronic kidney disease, Stage III (moderate) (585.3)	-Furosemide 20 mg po tabs -Hydrochlorothiazide 25 mg po tabs -Hydrocodone-Acetaminophen 5-500 mg po tabs -Cephalexin 500 mg po caps -Furosemide 40 mg po tabs	-Debridement of nails, 6 or more -OV est pt min serv -EKG -ECG and interpretation -Chest PA & lateral
Tear film insufficiency, unspecified (375.15)	-Blepharitis, unspecified (373.00) -Senile cataract, unspecified (366.10) -Presbyopia (367.4) -Preglaucoma, unspecified (365.00) -Other chronic allergic conjunctivitis (372.14)	-Glasses -Erythromycin 5 mg/gm op oint -Patanol 0.1 % op soln	-Refraction -Visual field exam extended -Visual field exam limited -Referral to ophthalmology, int -Ophthalmology, int
Benign essential hypertension (401.1)	-Hyperlipidemia (272.4) -Essential hypertension (401.9) -Pure hypercholesterolemia (272.0) -Mixed hyperlipidemia (272.2) -Diabetes mellitus (250.00)	-Hydrochlorothiazide 25 mg po tabs -Atenonol 50 mg po tabs -Lisinopril 10 mg po tabs -Lisinopril 40 mg po tabs -Lisinopril 20 mg po tabs	-ECG and interpretation -Influenza vac 3+yr im -Immun admin im/sq/id/perc 1st vac only -GI, int -OV est pt lev 3

(b)

Fig. 5.5 (**a**) Medical concept embedding vectors projected to 2D space; (**b**) Examples of diagnoses and their closest medical concepts

skin group neoplasms (216.X). The detailed figure of the red and blue boxes are in the supplementary section. As the black box shows, diagnoses from different groups are located close to one another if they are actually co-occurred often. In the black box, iridocyclitis and eye infections related to herpes zoster are closely located, which corresponds to approximately 43% of herpes zoster ophthalmicus (HZO), commonly known as shingles, patients develop iridocyclitis [154].

One important benefit of Word2Vec is that it can map different types of medical codes (e.g., diagnosis codes and procedure codes) into a common embedding space so that related medical codes of different types will be closer to each other. Figure (5.5b) shows examples of top-5 nearest neighbors from different types of medical codes to a diagnosis code. For example, embedding for the diagnosis code of "Acute upper respiratory infections" is close to "Bronchitis" (diagnosis), "Azithromycin" (antibiotic medication), "Influenza vac" (procedure), which are clinically meaningful.

Quantitative Assessment The ultimate value of embedding vectors is to generate better features for prediction or classification tasks. In this study, the task is to predict whether patients will develop heart failure (HF) based on various patient representations.

Figure 5.6 shows the AUC of various models and input feature vectors. The colors indicate the prediction results using different **patient representations**:

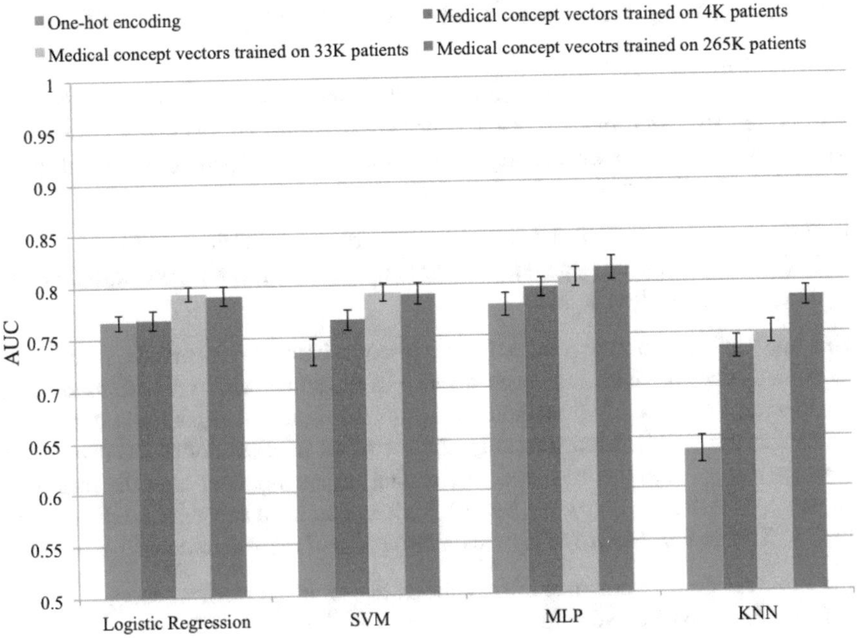

Fig. 5.6 Heart failure prediction performance of various embedding vectors

- **One-hot encoding** is to represent medical codes using one-hot encoding and then to sum over the one-hot encodings of the patient's medical codes.
- **Medical concept vectors** are simply the summation of all Word2Vec embeddings of her medical codes, where Word2Vec vectors are trained on various patient cohorts.

The error bars indicate the standard deviation derived from the six-fold cross evaluation. The power of medical concept representation learning is evident as all models show significant improvement in the HF prediction performance. Interestingly, KNN benefits the most from using the medical concept vectors, even those trained on the smallest dataset. Considering that KNN classification is based on the distances between data points, it is clear that medical concept representation using Word2Vec provides much better representations than the simple one-hot encoding. Figure 5.6 also tells us that medical concept representation is best learned with a large dataset. However, in most models, straightforward algorithms like KNN, even the medical concept vectors trained with the smallest number of patients improve prediction performance.

5.3 Med2Vec: Two-Level Embedding for EHR

Word2Vec assumes a global ordering of the input medical codes to create the embedding. However, many medical codes are documented together within a visit without any specific order, making it hard to use Word2Vec directly. In fact, EHR data of a patient follow a two-level hierarchy:

1. **Visit level:** Patient EHR data consists of a sequence of visits over time.
2. **Code level:** Each visit includes multiple medical codes, e.g., diagnosis, procedure, and medication codes.

This hierarchical structure provides two types of relational information, namely the sequential order of visits and co-occurrence of the codes within a visit. `Med2Vec` is a hierarchical embedding method that learns the representations for both medical codes and visits [24]. More formally, the set of all medical codes are denoted as $\mathcal{C} = \{c_1, c_2, \ldots, c_{|\mathcal{C}|}\}$ with size $|\mathcal{C}|$. EHR data for each patient is in the form of a sequence of visits $V_1, \ldots, V_T$ where each visit contains a subset of medical codes $V_t \subseteq \mathcal{C}$. The goal of Med2Vec is to learn two types of representations:

- **Code representations** map every code in the set of all medical codes $\mathcal{C}$ to non-negative real-valued vectors.
- **Visit representations** learn another embedding that maps every visit (a set of medical codes) to a real-valued vector of dimension n.

5.3.1 Med2Vec Method

Med2Vec first learns embedding vectors for individual medical codes such as diagnosis and procedure codes. Using the code embedding, we can map the visit binary vectors into intermediate embedding vectors, where each dimension corresponds to a binary variable for a specific medical code. Then through another nonlinear transformation, the final visit embedding is computed. The figurerefembed-fig:Med2Vec depicts the architecture of the Med2Vec model (Fig. 5.7).

Learning Code Representation A natural choice to capture the code co-occurrence information is to modify Word2Vec. In particular, we can train $\boldsymbol{W}_c \in \mathbb{R}^{m\times|\mathcal{C}|}$ (which can be used to produce intermediate visit level representations) so that the i-th column of $\boldsymbol{W}_c$ will be the representation for the i-th medical code among the total $|\mathcal{C}|$ codes. Note that given the unordered nature of the codes inside a visit, unlike the original Word2Vec, there is no ordering among medical codes within a visit.

From a set of visits $V_1, V_2, \ldots, V_T$, the code-level representations can be learned by maximizing the following log-likelihood,

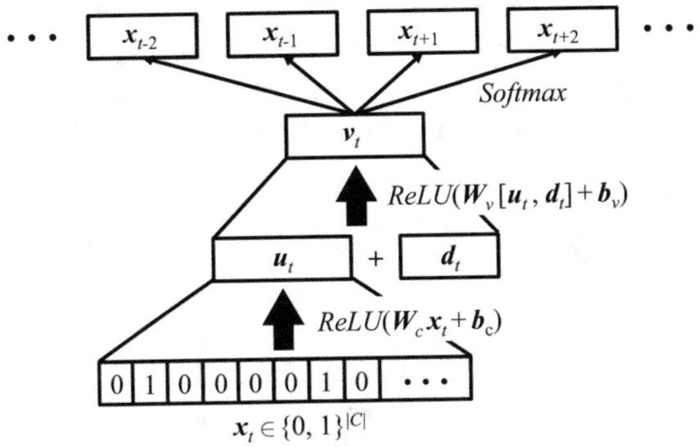

Fig. 5.7 Med2Vec model: a visit comprised of several medical codes is converted to a binary vector (i.e., the summation of one-hot embeddings of all medical codes within the visit). The binary vector is then converted to an intermediate visit representation, which is concatenated with a vector of demographic information to learn the final visit representation $\boldsymbol{v}_t$. Similar to Word2Vec, each visit from Med2Vec is trained to predict medical codes in the neighboring visits

$$\max_{\boldsymbol{W}_c} \quad \frac{1}{T}\sum_{t=1}^{T}\sum_{c_i \in V_t}\sum_{c_j \in V_t, j \neq i} \log p(c_j|c_i),$$

$$\text{where} \quad p(c_j|c_i) = \frac{\exp\left(\boldsymbol{W}_c[:, j]^\top \boldsymbol{W}_c[:, i]\right)}{\sum_{k=1}^{|\mathcal{C}|} \exp\left(\boldsymbol{W}_c[:, k]^\top \boldsymbol{W}_c[:, i]\right)}.$$

Learning Visit Representation Given a visit V_t, a multi-layer perceptron (MLP) is used to generate the corresponding visit representation $\boldsymbol{v}_t$. First, visit V_t is represented by a binary vector $\boldsymbol{x}_t \in \{0, 1\}^{|\mathcal{C}|}$ where the i-th entry is 1 only if code $c_i \in V_t$. Then $\boldsymbol{x}_t$ is converted to an intermediate visit representation $\boldsymbol{u}_t \in \mathbb{R}^m$ as follows,

$$\boldsymbol{u}_t = ReLU(\boldsymbol{W}_c \boldsymbol{x}_t + \boldsymbol{b}_c)$$

using the code weight matrix $\boldsymbol{W}_c \in \mathbb{R}^{m \times |\mathcal{C}|}$ and the bias vector $\boldsymbol{b}_c \in \mathbb{R}^m$. The ReLU unit ensures the nonnegative output for intuitive interpretation as negative values are typically hard to interpret and the ReLU unit eliminates them. Demographic information $\boldsymbol{d}_t \in \mathbb{R}^d$ including age and gender is concatenated with $\boldsymbol{u}_t$, where d is the size of the demographic information vector. Then the visit embedding $\boldsymbol{v}_t \in \mathbb{R}^n$ is computed as follows,

$$\boldsymbol{v}_t = ReLU(\boldsymbol{W}_v[\boldsymbol{u}_t, \boldsymbol{d}_t] + \boldsymbol{b}_v)$$

using the visit weight matrix $\boldsymbol{W}_v \in \mathbb{R}^{n \times (m+d)}$ and the bias vector $\boldsymbol{b}_v \in \mathbb{R}^n$, where n is the predefined size of the visit representation.

Similar to Word2Vec, given a visit representation one should be able to predict what has happened in the past, and what will happen in the future. Specifically, given a visit representation $\boldsymbol{v}_t$, we train a softmax classifier that predicts the medical codes of the visits within a context window. The cross-entropy loss is as follows,

$$\min_{\boldsymbol{W}_s, \boldsymbol{b}_s} \frac{1}{T} \sum_{t=1}^{T} \sum_{-w \le i \le w, i \ne 0} -\boldsymbol{x}_{t+i}^{\top} \log \hat{\boldsymbol{y}}_t - (\boldsymbol{1} - \boldsymbol{x}_{t+i})^{\top} \log(\boldsymbol{1} - \hat{\boldsymbol{y}}_t),$$

where $\hat{\boldsymbol{y}}_t = \text{Softmax}(\boldsymbol{W}_s \boldsymbol{v}_t + \boldsymbol{b}_s)$ are the predicted labels, $\boldsymbol{W}_s \in \mathbb{R}^{|\mathcal{C}| \times n}$ and $\boldsymbol{b}_s \in \mathbb{R}^{|\mathcal{C}|}$ are the weight matrix and bias vector for the softmax classifier, w the predefined context window size.

Clinical Use Case of Med2Vec Similar to Word2Vec, Med2Vec is mainly used as an alternative embedding method for longitudinal EHR data. In the papers [24], the authors have demonstrated the benefit of predictive performance and interpretability of the embedding vectors themselves. Here we present one result from [24] where the prediction performance of Med2Vec and other baselines are compared. The first row of Fig. 5.8 shows the Recall@30 for predicting the future medical codes. First, in all of the experiments, Med2Vec achieves the highest performance, although it is constrained to be positive and interpretable. The second observation is that Med2Vec's performance is robust to the hyperparameters' choice in a wide range of values. Compared to Skip-gram's more volatile performance, we can see that including the visit information in training improves the performance and stabilizes it.

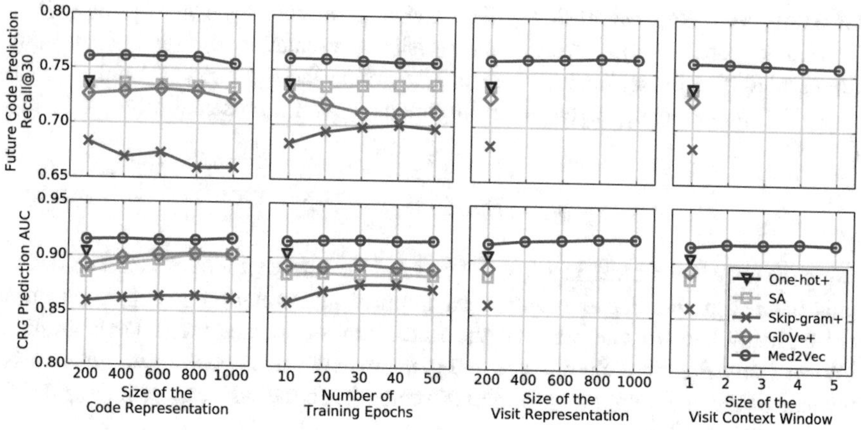

Fig. 5.8 Multiple baselines are compared, including one-hot encoding, stacked autoencoder (SA), Skip-gram, a version of Word2Vec, and GloVe, another efficient variant of embedding based on matrix factorization. The top row and the bottom row respectively show the Recall@30 for predicting the future medical codes and the AUC for predicting the CRG class when changing different hyperparameters

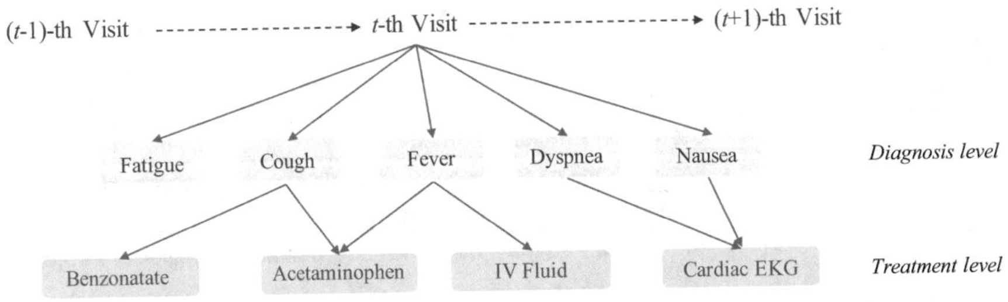

Fig. 5.9 Illustration of a single visit. Red denotes diagnosis codes, and blue denotes medication/procedure codes. A visit encompasses a set of codes and a hierarchical structure and heterogeneous relations among these codes. For example, while both *Acetaminophen* and *IV fluid* form an explicit relationship with *Fever*, they also are correlated with each other as descendants of *Fever*

5.4 MiME: Embed Internal Structure

Med2Vec utilizes the two-level structure of longitudinal EHR, namely, visits and codes within a visit. However, there is more nuance within a visit. The relationships between diagnoses and treatments, such as medication and procedures (see Fig. 5.9). MiME is another embedding method that leverages the inherent multilevel structure of EHR data and, in particular, the encoded relationships among medical codes [31]. This work also jointly performs auxiliary prediction tasks that rely on this inherent EHR structure without the need for external labels. Their overall objective is to learn robust embedding vectors even when the EHR dataset is small.

5.4.1 *Notations of MIME*

Assume a patient has a sequence of visits $\mathcal{V}^{(1)}, \ldots, \mathcal{V}^{(t)}$ over time, where each visit $\mathcal{V}^{(t)}$ contains a varying number of diagnosis objects $\mathcal{O}_1^{(t)}, \ldots, \mathcal{O}_{|\mathcal{V}^{(t)}|}^{(t)}$. Each $\mathcal{O}_i^{(t)}$ consists of a single diagnosis code $d_i^{(t)} \in \mathcal{A}$ and a set of associated treatments (medications or procedures) $\mathcal{M}_i^{(t)}$. Similarly, each $\mathcal{M}_i^{(t)}$ consists of varying number of treatment codes $m_{i,1}^{(t)}, \ldots, m_{i,|\mathcal{M}_i^{(t)}|}^{(t)} \in \mathcal{B}$. We omit the superscript (t) indicating the t-th visit to reduce clutter when we are discussing a single visit.

In Fig. 5.9, there are five diagnosis codes, hence five diagnosis objects $\mathcal{O}_1^{(t)}, \ldots, \mathcal{O}_5^{(t)}$. More specifically, the first diagnosis object $\mathcal{O}_1$ has $d_1^{(t)} = \textit{Fatigue}$ as the diagnosis code, but no treatment codes. $\mathcal{O}_2$, on the other hand, has diagnosis code $d_2^{(t)} = \textit{Cough}$ and two associated treatment codes $m_{2,1}^{(t)} = \textit{Benzonatate}$ and $m_{2,2}^{(t)} = \textit{Acetaminophen}$. In this case, we can use $g(d_2^{(t)}, m_{2,1}^{(t)})$ to capture the interaction between diagnosis code *Cough* and treatment code *Benzonatate*, which will be fed to $f(d_2^{(t)}, \mathcal{M}_2^{(t)})$ to obtain the vector representation of diagnosis object

Table 5.1 Notations for MIME. Note that the same dimensionality z is used in many places due to the use of skip-connections

Notation	Definition
$\mathcal{A}$	Set of unique diagnosis codes
$\mathcal{B}$	Set of unique treatment codes (medications and procedures)
$\mathbf{h}$	A vector representation of a patient
$\mathcal{V}^{(t)}$	A patient's t-th visit, which contains diagnosis objects $\mathcal{O}_1^{(t)}, \ldots, \mathcal{O}_{\lvert\mathcal{V}^{(t)}\rvert}^{(t)}$
$\mathbf{v}^{(t)} \in \mathbb{R}^z$	A vector representation of $\mathcal{V}^{(t)}$
$\mathcal{O}_i^{(t)}$	i-th diagnosis object of t-th visit consisting of diagnosis code $d_i^{(t)}$ and treatment codes $\mathcal{M}_i^{(t)}$
$\mathbf{o}_i^{(t)} \in \mathbb{R}^z$	A vector representation of $\mathcal{O}_i^{(t)}$
$p(d_i^{(t)}\lvert\mathbf{o}_i^{(t)}), p(m_{i,j}^{(t)}\lvert\mathbf{o}_i^{(t)})$	Auxiliary predictions, respectively for a diagnosis code and a treatment code based on $\mathbf{o}_i^{(t)}$
$d_i^{(t)} \in \mathcal{A}$	diagnosis code of diagnosis object $\mathcal{O}_i^{(t)}$
$\mathcal{M}_i^{(t)}$	a set of treatment codes associated with i-th diagnosis code $d_i^{(t)}$ in visit t
$m_{i,j}^{(t)} \in \mathcal{B}$	j-th treatment code of $\mathcal{M}_i^{(t)}$
$g(d_i^{(t)}, m_{i,j}^{(t)})$	A function that captures the interaction between $d_i^{(t)}$ and $m_{i,j}^{(t)}$
$f(d_i^{(t)}, \mathcal{M}_i^{(t)})$	A function that computes embedding of diagnosis object $\mathbf{o}_i^{(t)}$
$r(\cdot) \in \mathbb{R}^z$	A helper notation for extracting $d_i^{(t)}$ or $m_{i,j}^{(t)}$'s embedding vector

$\mathbf{o}_2^{(t)}$. Using the five diagnosis object embeddings $\mathbf{o}_1^{(t)}, \ldots, \mathbf{o}_5^{(t)}$, we can obtain a visit embedding $\mathbf{v}^{(t)}$. Also, some treatment codes (*e.g., Acetaminophen*) can be shared by two or more diagnosis codes (*e.g., Cough, Fever*) if the doctor ordered a single medication for more than one diagnosis. Then each diagnosis object will have its own copy of the treatment code attached to it, in this case, denoted, $m_{2,2}^{(t)}$ and $m_{3,1}^{(t)}$, respectively. Table 5.1 provides all the notations of MIME.

5.4.2 *Description of MIME*

Multilevel Embedding MIME explicitly captures the hierarchy between diagnosis codes and treatment codes depicted in Fig. 5.9. Figure 5.10 illustrates how MIME builds the representation of $\mathcal{V}$ (omitting the superscript (t)) in a bottom-up fashion via multilevel embedding. In a single diagnosis object $\mathcal{O}_i$, a diagnosis code d_i and its associated treatment codes $\mathcal{M}_i$ are used to obtain a vector representation of $\mathcal{O}_i$, $\mathbf{o}_i$. Then multiple diagnosis object embeddings $\mathbf{o}_0, \ldots, \mathbf{o}_{\lvert\mathcal{V}\rvert}$ in a single visit are used to obtain a visit embedding $\mathbf{v}$, which in turn forms a patient embedding $\mathbf{h}$ with other visit embeddings. The formulation of MIME is as follows:

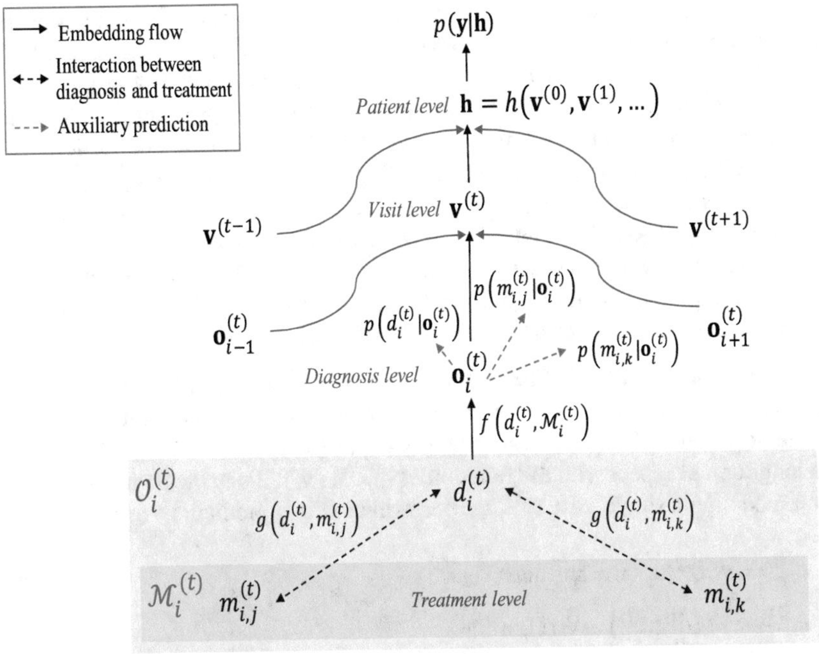

Fig. 5.10 Prediction model using MIME. Codes are embedded into multiple levels: diagnosis-level, visit-level, and patient-level. Final prediction $p(\mathbf{y}|\mathbf{h})$ is based on the patient representation $\mathbf{h}$, which is derived from visit representations $\mathbf{v}^{(0)}, \mathbf{v}^{(1)}, \ldots$, where each $\mathbf{v}^{(t)}$ is generated using MIME framework

$$\mathbf{v} = \sigma\Big(\mathbf{W}_v\Big(\underbrace{\sum_i^{|\mathcal{V}|} f(d_i, \mathcal{M}_i)}_{\text{F: used for skip-connection}}\Big)\Big) + F \tag{5.1}$$

$$f(d_i, \mathcal{M}_i) = \mathbf{o}_i = \sigma\Big(\mathbf{W}_o\Big(\underbrace{r(d_i) + \sum_j^{|\mathcal{M}_i|} g(d_i, m_{i,j})}_{\text{G: used for skip-connection}}\Big)\Big) + G \tag{5.2}$$

$$g(d_i, m_{i,j}) = \sigma\big(\mathbf{W}_m r(d_i)\big) \odot r(m_{i,j}) \tag{5.3}$$

where Eqs. (5.1), (5.2), and (5.3) describe MIME in a top-down fashion, respectively corresponding to *Visit level*, *Diagnosis level* and *Treatment level* in Fig. 5.10 and $\odot$ denotes the element-wise multiplication. In Eq. (5.1), a visit embedding $\mathbf{v}$ is obtained by summing diagnosis object embeddings $\mathbf{o}_1, \ldots, \mathbf{o}_{|\mathcal{V}|}$, which are then transformed with $\mathbf{W}_v \in \mathbb{R}^{z \times z}$, and σ is a non-linear activation function such as sigmoid or rectified linear unit (ReLU). In Eq. (5.2), $\mathbf{o}_i$ is obtained by summing $r(d_i) \in \mathbb{R}^z$, the vector representation of the diagnosis code d_i, and the effect of the interactions between d_i and its associated treatments $\mathcal{M}_i$, which are then transformed with $\mathbf{W}_o \in \mathbb{R}^{z\times z}$. The interactions captured by $g(d_i, m_{i,j})$ are added to the $r(d_i)$, which can be interpreted as adjusting the diagnosis representation according to its associated treatments (medications and procedures). Note that in both Eqs. (5.1) and (5.2), the term F and G denote skip-connections [67]. In Eq. (5.3), the interaction between a diagnosis code embedding $r(d_i)$ and a treatment code embedding $r(m_{i,j})$ is captured by element-wise multiplication $\odot$. Weight matrix $\mathbf{W}_m \in \mathbb{R}^{z\times z}$ sends the diagnosis code embedding $r(d_i)$ into another latent space, where the interaction between d_i and the corresponding $m_{i,j}$ can be effectively captured. With Eq. (5.3) in mind, G in Eq. (5.2) can also be interpreted as $r(d_i)$ being skip-connected to the sum of interactions $g(d_i, m_{i,j})$.

Joint Training with Auxiliary Tasks Patient embedding $\mathbf{h}$ is often used for specific prediction tasks, such as heart failure prediction or mortality. The representation power of $\mathbf{h}$ comes from properly capturing each visit $\mathcal{V}^{(t)}$, and modeling the longitudinal aspect with the function $h(\mathbf{v}_0, \ldots, \mathbf{v}_t)$. Since the focus of this work is on modeling a single visit $\mathcal{V}^{(t)}$, we perform auxiliary predictions as follows:

$$\hat{d}_i^{(t)} = p(d_i^{(t)}|\mathbf{o}_i^{(t)}) = \text{softmax}(\mathbf{U}_d\mathbf{o}_i^{(t)}) \tag{5.4}$$

$$\hat{m}_{i,j}^{(t)} = p(m_{i,j}^{(t)}|\mathbf{o}_i^{(t)}) = \sigma(\mathbf{U}_m\mathbf{o}_i^{(t)}) \tag{5.5}$$

$$L_{aux} = -\lambda_{aux}\sum_t^T\Bigg(\sum_i^{|\mathcal{V}^{(t)}|}\bigg(CE(d_i^{(t)}, \hat{d}_i^{(t)}) + \sum_j^{|\mathcal{M}_i^{(t)}|} CE(m_{i,j}^{(t)}, \hat{m}_{i,j}^{(t)})\bigg)\Bigg) \tag{5.6}$$

Given diagnosis object embeddings $\mathbf{o}_1^{(t)}, \ldots, \mathbf{o}_{|\mathcal{V}^{(t)}|}^{(t)}$, while aggregating them to obtain $\mathbf{v}^{(t)}$ as in Eq. (5.1), MIME predicts the diagnosis code $d_i^{(t)}$, and the associated treatment code $m_{i,j}^{(t)}$ as depicted by Fig. 5.10. In Eqs. (5.4) and (5.5), $\mathbf{U}_d \in \mathbb{R}^{|\mathcal{A}|\times z}$ and $\mathbf{U}_m \in \mathbb{R}^{|\mathcal{B}|\times z}$ are weight matrices used to compute the prediction of diagnosis code $\hat{d}_i^{(t)}$ and the prediction of the treatment code $\hat{m}_{i,j}^{(t)}$, respectively. In Eq. (5.6), T denotes the total number of visits the patient made, $CE(\cdot,\cdot)$ the cross-entropy function and λ_{aux} the coefficient for the auxiliary loss term. We used the softmax function for predicting $d_i^{(t)}$ since in a single diagnosis object $\mathcal{O}_i^{(t)}$, there is only one diagnosis code involved. However, there could be multiple treatment codes associated with $\mathcal{O}_i^{(t)}$, and therefore we used $|\mathcal{B}|$ number of sigmoid functions for predicting each treatment code.

5.4.3 Experiment Results of MIME

This section highlights some experiment evaluation of MIME. More detailed evaluation can be seen at [31].

Baseline Models First, we use Gated Recurrent Units (GRU) described in Chap. 7 with different embedding strategies to map visit embedding sequence $\mathbf{v}^{(1)}, \ldots, \mathbf{v}^{(T)}$ to a patient representation $\mathbf{h}$:

- **raw**: A single visit $\mathcal{V}^{(t)}$ is represented by a binary vector $\mathbf{x}^{(t)} \in \{0, 1\}^{|\mathcal{A}|+|\mathcal{B}|}$. Only the dimensions corresponding to the codes occurring in that visit is set to 1, and the rest are 0.
- **linear**: The binary vector $\mathbf{x}^{(t)}$ is linearly transformed to a lower-dimensional vector $\mathbf{v}^{(t)} = \mathbf{W}_c\mathbf{x}^{(t)}$ where $\mathbf{W}_c \in \mathbb{R}^{b\times(|\mathcal{A}|+|\mathcal{B}|)}$ is the code embedding matrix. This is equivalent to taking the vector representations of the codes (i.e. columns of the embedding matrix $\mathbf{W}_c$) in the visit $\mathcal{V}^{(t)}$, and summing them up to derive a single vector $\mathbf{v}^{(t)} \in \mathbb{R}^b$.
- **sigmoid, tanh, relu**: The binary vector $\mathbf{x}^{(t)}$ is transformed to a lower-dimensional vector $\mathbf{v}^{(t)} = \sigma(\mathbf{W}_c\mathbf{x}^{(t)})$ where we use either *sigmoid*, *tanh*, or *ReLU* for $\sigma(\cdot)$ to add non-linearity to **linear**.
- **sigmoid**$_{mlp}$, **tanh**$_{mlp}$, **relu**$_{mlp}$: We add one more layer to **sigmoid**, **tanh** and **relu** to increase their expressivity. The visit embedding is now $\mathbf{v}^{(t)} = \sigma(\mathbf{W}_{c_2}\sigma(\mathbf{W}_{c_1}\mathbf{x}^{(t)}))$ where σ is either sigmoid, tanh or ReLU. We do not test **linear**$_{mlp}$ since two consecutive linear layers can be collapsed to a single linear layer.

Second, two EHR embedding methods Med2Vec [24] and GRAM [28] are also compared.

Heart Failure Prediction The objective is to predict the first diagnosis of heart failure (HF), given the 18-months observation records discussed. Among 30,764 patients, 3,414 were case patients diagnosed with HF within a 1-year window after the 18-months observation. The remaining 27,350 patients were controls. The logistic regression is scored against the patient representation $\mathbf{h}$ to obtain a probability score between 0 (no HF onset) and 1 (HF onset).

To evaluate MIME's performance from another perspective, we created four datasets E_1, E_2, E_3, E_4 from the original data. Each dataset consisted of patients with varying maximum sequence length T_{max} (i.e., the maximum number of visits). In order to simulate a new hospital collecting patient records over time, we increased T_{max} for each dataset such that 10, 20, 30, 150 for E_1, E_2, E_3, E_4 respectively. Each dataset had 6299 (414 cases), 15794 (1177 cases), 21128 (1848 cases), 27428 (3173 cases) patients respectively. For MIME$_{aux}$, we used the same 0.015 for the auxiliary loss coefficient λ_{aux}.

Figure 5.11 shows the test PR-AUC for HF prediction across all datasets. We can readily see that MIME outperforms all baseline models across all datasets. However, the performance gap between MIME and the baselines are larger in datasets E_1, E_2 than in datasets E_3, E_4, confirming our assumption that exploiting the inherent structure of EHR can alleviate the data insufficiency problem. Especially for the smallest dataset E_1, MIME$_{aux}$ (0.2831 PR-AUC) demonstrated significantly better performance than the best baseline **tanh**$_{mlp}$ (0.2462 PR-AUC), showing 15% relative improvement.

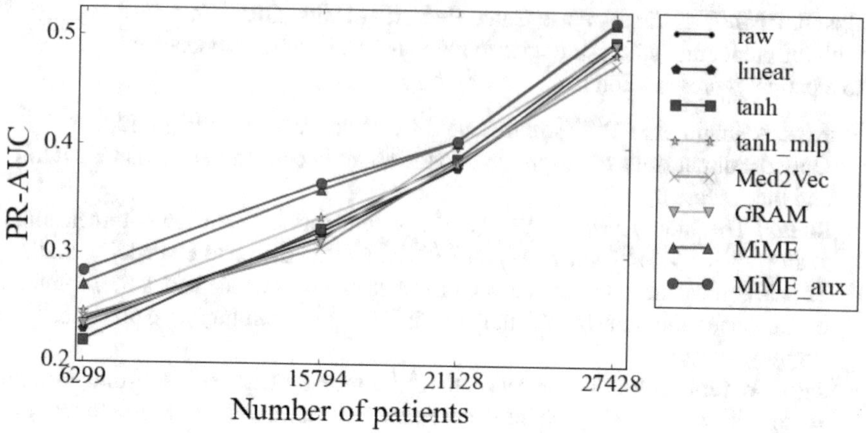

Fig. 5.11 Test PR-AUC of HF prediction for increasing data size

5.5 Exercises

1. What is the key difference between Med2Vec and Word2Vec?
2. What is the key difference between Med2Vec and MiME?
3. What is NOT true about one-hot encoding?

   (a) One-hot encoding vector is a multi-dimensional vectors of all 0s except for one dimension of 1.
   (b) One-hot encoding will group vectors of similar concepts together.
   (c) Distance between any two one-hot encoding vectors is always the same.
   (d) One-hot encoding is commonly used to encode categorical data.

4. What is NOT true about Word2vec?

   (a) One-hot encoding vector is a multi-dimensional vectors of all 0s except for one dimension of 1.
   (b) Larger context window means words that are farther apart will be considered similar in the skip gram calculation.
   (c) The denominator $\sum_{\text{all words}(w)} \exp(v_w \top v_t)$ in $p(c|t)$ can be easily computed for Skip-gram.
   (d) Negative sampling treats the pairs of context words and the target word as positive examples, and pairs of random words and the input target word as negative examples.

5. Which of the following is NOT a suitable medical applications of Word2vec?

   (a) Similarity search: To find similar medical concepts based on the Euclidian distance of the word2vec embeddings of those medical concepts.
   (b) Algebra operation: To perform summation and subtraction of word2vec embeddings in order to better understand a combination of medical concepts.

(c) Features for predictive modeling: To utilize word2vec embeddings as input feature vectors to support downstream classification or regression models.
(d) Visualization: to directly visualize the word2vec embeddings of medical concepts in order to understand the relationship among medical concepts.

6. What are the challenges in visualizing high-dimensional data? (multiple correct answers)

   (a) To preserve the relationship of original data when visualizing in 2D space.
   (b) To ensure similar data points mapped to nearby location in 2D space.
   (c) To provide computationally efficient methods to produce the visualization.
   (d) To produce aesthetically pleasing effects when visualizing the data.

7. Which statement is NOT true comparing PCA and t-SNE?

   (a) PCA is a dimensionality reduction algorithm that tries to preserve global distance between all pairs of data points.
   (b) t-SNE tries to project high-dimensional data into 2D space while preserving local distance.
   (c) t-SNE is more appropriate for visualization high-dimensional data.
   (d) t-SNE is computationally more efficient than PCA.

8. Which is NOT true about Med2Vec method?

   (a) It models two level hierarchy of medical data namely visit level and patient level.
   (b) Med2Vec is most suitable to model clinical notes
   (c) Med2Vec is designed to model sequences of clinical codes.
   (d) Mec2Vec is a generalization of word2vec for electronic health record data.

9. Which is NOT true about MiME: Multilevel medical embedding method?

   (a) It leverages the dependency from diagnosis to treatments.
   (b) It models EHR data with multi-level hierarchy (treatment -> diagnosis -> visit—patient).
   (c) It introduces auxiliary prediction task to predict diagnosis and treatment within a visit.
   (d) It provides a direct and intuitive interpretation for each prediction.

Chapter 6
Convolutional Neural Networks (CNN)

Convolutional neural networks (CNN or ConvNet) are a specific type of neural networks for processing grid-like data such as images and time series. In healthcare applications, the CNN models are widely used in automatic feature learning and disease classification from medical images, for example, automatic classification of skin lesions [45], detection of diabetic retinopathy [61], and COVID X-ray classification [120]. In addition, CNN demonstrated great performance in disease detection using biosignals such as Electrocardiography (ECG) [155] and electroencephalogram (EEG) [7]. More recently, researchers also applied CNN models on structured EHR data [18, 177] and clinical text [3, 114].

6.1 CNN Intuition

CNN are neural networks comprised of layers of **convolutions** often with additional nonlinear activation and **pooling** layers, followed by fully connected layers. Unlike DNN models that connect each neuron to all neurons in the next layer, CNN models focus on local properties. In particular, they use convolutions over the input layer to create **local connections** such that each region in the input is connected to a unit in the next layer. The convolution outputs are called **feature maps**, which will be discussed in more detail in the next section. After convolution, the **pooling** layers progressively reduce the size of the feature map.

The design of convolution and pooling layers leverages the local properties of grid-like data (e.g., images or time-series signals), namely **translational invariance** and **compositionality**.

- Translational invariance means statistics of one local region (e.g., a section in the image or a fragment of ECG series) are similar to the other local regions. Thus features learned from a local region can be used in all regions.

C. Xiao, J. Sun, *Introduction to Deep Learning for Healthcare*,
https://doi.org/10.1007/978-3-030-82184-5_6

- Compositionality refers to the intrinsic hierarchical structure within image or signal data: lower-level features such as a pixel in an image or a beat in ECG signals can be composed into higher-level representation such as a scene or a rhythm pattern.

CNNs often repeat convolution and pooling layers multiple times and later employ fully connected layers to fuse all local features to produce more abstract features for classification tasks. Different layers can be stacked as deep networks.

6.2 Architecture of CNN

This section describes the components of the CNN architecture, namely, convolution layers, pooling layers, and fully connected layers. The related notations are defined in Table 6.1.

6.2.1 Convolution Layer: 1D

Intuition A convolution layer is the building block that distinguishes CNNs from other deep learning models. For a 1D convolution, the idea is to extract various local patterns over 1D signals such as EEG. The way to do that is to define those patterns with *filters* (also called kernels) and then to repeatedly apply those filters over the signals to generate features called a *feature map*. Then multiple convolution operations can be applied in sequence to generate more and more sophisticated features.

Notations The input and output of a convolution layer are called *feature maps*, which are denoted by $\boldsymbol{F}^{(l)}$. In particular, the feature map from layer-l $\boldsymbol{F}^{(l)}$ will be the input to the convolution operation at layer-l to generate the output feature map $\boldsymbol{F}^{(l+1)}$. The convolution operation itself is specified by a set of m *filters* each

Table 6.1 Notations for convolutional neural networks

Notation	Definition
$\boldsymbol{F}^{(l)} \in \mathbb{R}^{T \times n}$	1D feature map at layer l
$\boldsymbol{F}^{(l)} \in \mathbb{R}^{T_1 \times T_2 \times n}$	2D feature map at layer l
T, $T_1 \times T_2$	Size of 1D signals or 2D images
n	The number of input channels or depth
m	The number of filters or output channels
k_1, $k_1 \times k_2$	1D or 2D filter size
$\boldsymbol{W} \in \mathbb{R}^{k_1 \times m \times n}$	Weight tensor in 1D convolution
$\boldsymbol{W} \in \mathbb{R}^{k_1 \times k_2 \times m \times n}$	Weight tensor in 2D convolution
$\boldsymbol{b}^{(l)} \in \mathbb{R}^{m}$	Bias vector

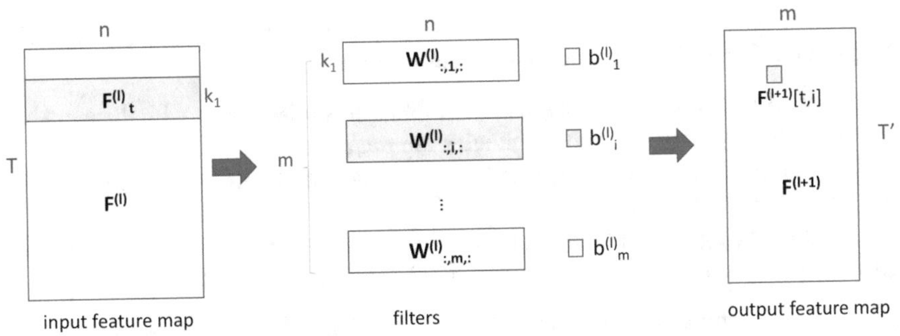

Fig. 6.1 Illustration of general 1D convolution of m filters over input feature map $\boldsymbol{F}^{(l)} \in \mathbb{R}^{T\times n}$ to generate output feature map $\boldsymbol{F}^{(l+1)}$. Filter i is specified by the weight matrix $\boldsymbol{W}_{:,i,:} \in \mathbb{R}^{k_1\times n}$. The entire set of filters is specified by a 3D tensor $\boldsymbol{W} \in \mathbb{R}^{k_1\times m\times n}$. $\boldsymbol{F}_t^{(l)} \in \mathbb{R}^{k_1\times n}$ is the t-th patch of the input feature map

parameterized by a weight matrix $\boldsymbol{W}_{:,i,:} \in \mathbb{R}^{k_1\times n}$ and a bias term $b_i^{(l)}$ (i.e., a scalar) where filter index $i = 1$ to m. The entire convolution is specified by a 3D weight tensor $\boldsymbol{W} \in \mathbb{R}^{k_1\times m\times n}$ and a bias vector $\boldsymbol{b}^{(l)} \in \mathbb{R}^m$. Here k_1 is the filter size, m the number of filters (also the number of output channels), n is the number of input channels, For example, if we apply 50 filters of size 100 on a 6-channel EEG data, we have $k_1 = 100$ (filter size), $m = 50$ (number of filters) and $n = 6$ (number of channels) (Fig. 6.1).

Convolution Each element of the output feature map is computed as the following.

$$\boldsymbol{F}^{(l+1)}[t,i] = \boldsymbol{W}^{(l)}_{:,i,:} \otimes \boldsymbol{F}^{(l)}_t + b^{(l)}_i$$

where i is the filter index and $\boldsymbol{F}_t^{(l)} \in \mathbb{R}^{k_1\times n}$ is the t-th patch when we slide a filter over the input, and $\boldsymbol{F}^{(l+1)}[t,i]$ is the (t,i) element of the output. Here $\otimes$ refers to the element-wise multiplication followed by summation: $\boldsymbol{W}^{(l)}_{:,i,:} \otimes \boldsymbol{F}_t^{(l)} = \sum_{a=1}^{k}\sum_{b=1}^{n} \boldsymbol{W}^{(l)}_{a,i,b} \cdot \boldsymbol{F}_t^{(l)}[a,b]$. This is analogous of the inner product but generalized to an operation between two matrices. Furthermore, it is quite common to apply a nonlinear activation such as ReLU on the output feature map. In this case, we will have

$$\boldsymbol{F}^{(l+1)}[t,i] = \sigma(\boldsymbol{W}^{(l)}_{:,i,:} \otimes \boldsymbol{F}^{(l)}_t + b^{(l)}_i)$$

where σ is the activation function.

Stride One important parameter is the *stride size* S, which determines how often we apply the filter operations over the input. When $S = 1$, it means we slide the filter one element at a time. When $S = 2$, we will slide the filter two elements at time, which means we will apply the filter every other element over the input. The large stride size leads to smaller output and vice versa.

Padding Another important detail for convolution is how to deal with the elements on the boundary. Two common strategies are *padding* or no padding. The idea of padding is to add extra values (usually zeroes) outside the input data boundary to ensure convolution can be applied to elements near the boundary. For example, if the input is of length T and the filter is of size $2P + 1$, we can pad P zeroes on each side of the input to have an output of length T (assuming stride 1).

Now we summarize the convolution layer of CNN with its parameters and hyperparameters. A convolution layer accepts input data of size $T \times n$. The convolution layer has the following hyperparameters, including the number of filters m, filter size k_1, stride size S, and padding size P. Then the layer will produce an output whose size is given by $T' \times m$ where $T' = (T - k_1 + 2P)/S + 1$.

6.2.2 *Convolution Layer: 2D*

Intuition When we process images, a 2D convolution becomes essential. The intuition is to construct various local pattern extractors (*filters*) and then apply them everywhere on an image to generate meaningful features. Again convolution layers can be stacked to generate more and more sophisticated features. For example, the lower level filters detect simple patterns such as edges and dots, while higher-level filters find different objects such as faces. For 2D convolution, we consider a simple example shown in Fig. 6.2 where in the middle is a 5×5 binary input matrix. On the left is a 3×3 filter. We will perform a convolution of the filter matrix over the input matrix. It is more common to have multiple input channels and multiple filters (hence multiple output channels) when applying the convolution operation.

Notations The input and output feature maps are denoted by $\boldsymbol{F}^{(l)}$ and $\boldsymbol{F}^{(l+1)}$, respectively. The 2D convolution operation is also specified by a set of m *filters*

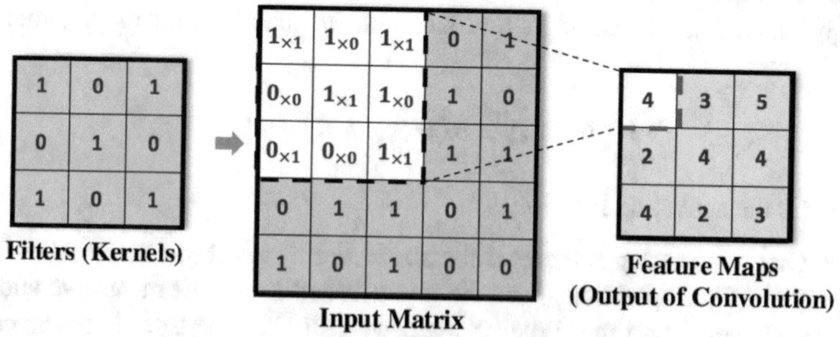

Fig. 6.2 Filters slide over an input image to produce feature maps

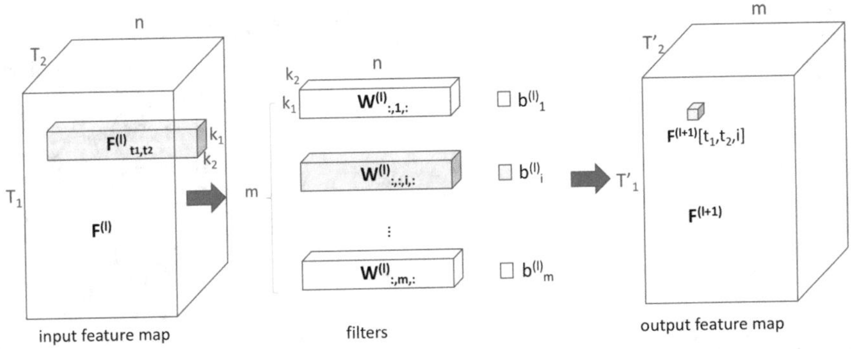

Fig. 6.3 Illustration of general 2D convolution of m filters over input feature map $\boldsymbol{F}^{(l)} \in \mathbb{R}^{T_1 \times T_2 \times n}$ to generate output feature map $\boldsymbol{F}^{(l+1)}$. A patch $\boldsymbol{F}^{(l)}_{t_1,t_2} \in \mathbb{R}^{k_1 \times k_2 \times n}$ performs element-wise multiplication followed by summation with each filter. The filter i is specified by the weight tensor $\boldsymbol{W}_{:,:,i,:} \in \mathbb{R}^{k_1 \times k_2 \times n}$ with the filter size $k_1 \times k_2$. The entire set of filters is specified by a 4D tensor $\boldsymbol{W} \in \mathbb{R}^{k_1 \times k_2 \times m \times n}$

each parameterized by a 3D weight tensor $\boldsymbol{W}_{:,:,i,:} \in \mathbb{R}^{k_1 \times k_2 \times n}$ and a bias term $b_i^{(l)}$ where filter index $i = 1$ to m. The entire convolution is specified by a 4D weight tensor $\boldsymbol{W} \in \mathbb{R}^{k_1 \times k_2 \times m \times n}$ and a bias vector $\boldsymbol{b}^{(l)} \in \mathbb{R}^m$. Here $k_1 \times k_2$ is the filter size, m the number of filters (also the number of output channels), n is the number of input channels, For example, if we apply 50 filters of size 3×3 on a 3-channel RGB image, we have $k_1 = k_2 = 3$, $m = 50$ and $n = 3$ (Fig. 6.3).

Convolution The convolution operation for 2D input is similar the 1D case but with one more index:

$$\boldsymbol{F}^{(l+1)}[t_1, t_2, i] = \sigma(\boldsymbol{W}^{(l)}_{:,:,i,:} \otimes \boldsymbol{F}^{(l)}_{t_1,t_2} + b_i^{(l)})$$

where $\boldsymbol{F}^{(l)}_{t_1,t_2} \in \mathbb{R}^{k_1 \times k_2 \times n}$ is a patch that operates with filter i via element-wise multiplication followed by summation, $\boldsymbol{W}^{(l)}_{:,:,i,:} \in \mathbb{R}^{k_1 \times k_2 \times n}$ and $b_i^{(l)}$) are the weight tensor and the bias term for filter i, respectively. And $\boldsymbol{F}^{(l+1)}[t_1, t_2, i]$ is an element of the output feature map and σ is the activation function.

In summary, a 2D convolution layer accepts input data of size $T_1 \times T_2 \times n$ where $T_1 \times T_2$ is the image size and n is the number of input channels or its depth. For example, a color medical image of size 1024×1024 is a 3D tensor of size $1024 \times 1024 \times 3$ (given RGB color channels). The convolution layer has the following hyperparameters including number of filters m, filter size $k_1 \times k_2$, stride S and number of paddings P. Then the layer will produce an output feature map of size $T_1' \times T_2' \times m$ where $T_1' = (T_1 - k_1 + 2P)/S + 1$ and $T_2' = (T_2 - k_2 + 2P)/S + 1$.

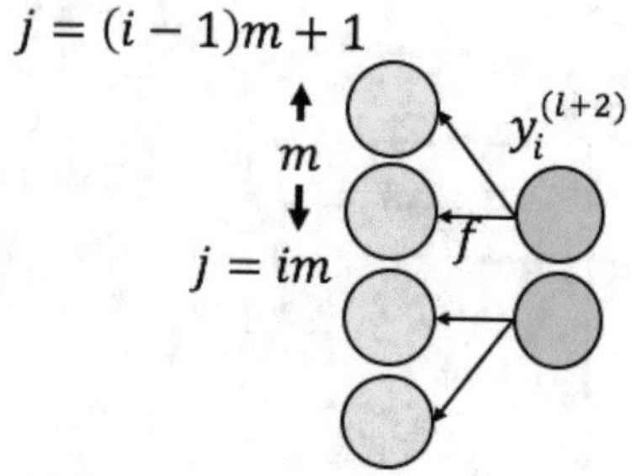

Fig. 6.4 Pooling layers of the CNN

6.2.3 *Pooling Layer*

Pooling is to subsample a feature map by aggregation. The pooling layer often follows after the convolution or activation step to produce translational invariance local features, called a pooled feature map. For example, as illustrated in Fig. 6.4, to produce one unit $y_i^{(l+2)}$ in the pooled feature map, the pooling operation focuses on one pooling region with size m in $(l+1)$th layer, indexed from $(i-1)m+1$ to im. Let $f(\cdot)$ be the pooling function such that $y_i^{(l+2)} = f([o_{(i-1)m+1}^{(l+1)}, \ldots, o_{im}^{(l+1)}])$, where $o_j^{(l+1)}$ are the output from the convolution layer. Here are several common pool functions:

- **Mean pooling** computes average values from the pooling region:

$$f([o_{(i-1)m+1}^{(l+1)}, \ldots, o_{im}^{(l+1)}]) = \frac{1}{m}(\sum_{j=(i-1)m+1}^{im} o_j^{(l+1)})$$

- **Max pooling** picks the maximum value from the pooling region:

$$f([o_{(i-1)m+1}^{(l+1)}, \ldots, o_{im}^{(l+1)}]) = \max_{(j=(i-1)m+1):(j=im)} o_j^{(l+1)}$$

- **Sum pooling** sums up all values from the pooling region:

$$f([o_{(i-1)m+1}^{(l+1)}, \ldots, o_{im}^{(l+1)}]) = \sum_{j=(i-1)m+1}^{im} o_j^{(l+1)} \tag{6.1}$$

Regardless of the pooling function we use, pooling layers will reduce the size of the feature map. The local connections and tied weights followed by pooling will result in translation-invariant local features. We can repeat convolution and pooling multiple times and later employ fully connected layers to fuse all local features and output more abstract features for classification tasks.

To summarize the pooling layer of 2D CNN has the following parameters and hyperparameters: A pooling layer accepts input data of size is $T_1 \times T_2 \times n$. A pooling layer has the following hyperparameters, including size $F \times F$ and stride S. Then it will produce an output of size $T_1' \times T_2' \times m$ where $T_1' = (T_1 - F)/S + 1$, $T_2' = (T_1 - F)/S + 1$. And the number of output channels remains the same as the number of input channels.

6.2.4 *Fully Connected Layer*

The fully connected layers are often added after all convolution and pooling layers. The reasons for adding the fully connected layers are.

- First, after a series of convolutional and pooling layers, we now have high-level features of the input data. And the fully connected layers work as classifiers to use these features for mapping the input image into various classes based on the training dataset.
- Second, the fully connected layers can perform flexible nonlinear combination to integrate features to provide better classification results.

A softmax activation function is often used in the final output layer for multiclass classification tasks, e.g., classifying whether a chest X-ray corresponds to COVID-19, viral pneumonia, bacteria pneumonia, or healthy cases like in [120].

6.3 Backpropagation Algorithm in CNN*

In the following, we will describe forward computation and backward propagation of CNN models for 1D signals. The generalization of 2D images is straightforward. The idea is very similar to DNN, but more complicated due to the convolutional and pooling operations.

6.3.1 *Forward and Backward Computation for 1D Data*

To present the forward computation and backward propagation, we consider a simplified 1D CNN shown in Fig. 6.5. The 1D CNN has an input feature map $\boldsymbol{x}^{(l-1)}$. We first transform the input feature map using a convolution filter $\boldsymbol{w}^{(l)}$ to produce the output feature map $\boldsymbol{x}^{(l)}$. We then apply a nonlinear activation function such as ReLU over $\boldsymbol{x}^{(l)}$ to output $\boldsymbol{o}^{(l+1)}$. Next we apply a pooling function $f()$ on the output $\boldsymbol{o}^{(l+1)}$ to produce a pooled feature map $\boldsymbol{y}^{(l+2)}$. Fully connected layers can follow these steps to generate final predictions. In the following, we omit the fully connected layers since their computations as they have been described in Chap. 4.

Forward Computation For this simple CNN, the forward computation is given by the following equations.

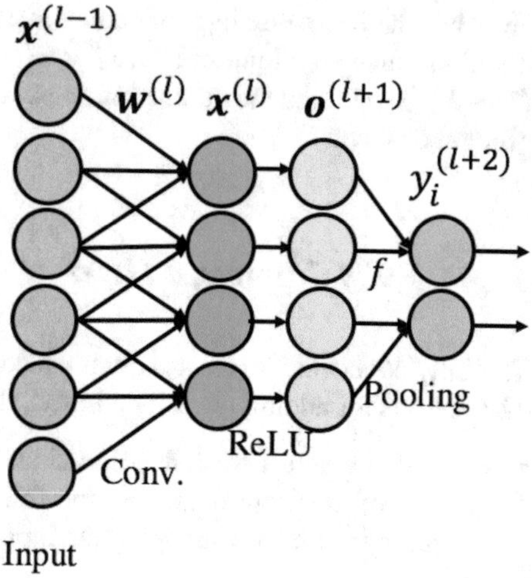

Fig. 6.5 Forward computation of a simple 1D CNN

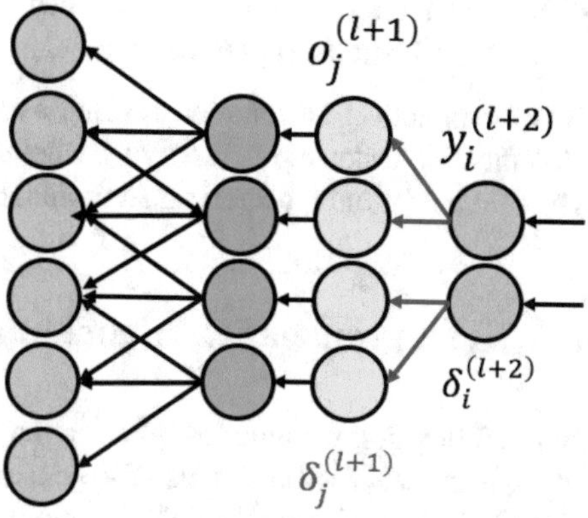

Fig. 6.6 Backward propagation for a pooling layer

$$x_i^{(l)} = \sum_m w_m^{(l)} x_{i+m}^{(l-1)} + b^{(l)}$$

$$\boldsymbol{o}^{(l+1)} = ReLU(\boldsymbol{x}^{(l)})$$

$$y_i^{(l+2)} = f([o_j^{(l+1)}]|j \in (i-1)m+1 : im)$$

where $f()$ is the pooling function.

Backpropagation for Pooling Layers For the backward propagation, we start from the pooling layer, illustrated in Fig. 6.6. We define $\delta_j^{(l+1)} = \frac{\partial L}{\partial o_j^{(l+1)}}$ to measure how much node j that is corresponding to the ith pooling region of $(l+1)$th layer (e.g., the region from $(i-1)m+1$ to im) was responsible for errors in the output of that region. Likewise, we also let $\delta_i^{(l+2)} = \frac{\partial L}{\partial y_j^{(l+2)}}$ measure how much node i of $(l+2)$th layer was responsible for errors. Then the gradient descent updating rule for the units of the layer before pooling layer, denoted as $o_j^{(l+1)}$, can be expressed as

$$o_j^{(l+1)} = o_j^{(l+1)} - \eta \frac{\partial L}{\partial o_j^{(l+1)}}$$

where η is the learning rule. For updating this formula we will need to estimate $\delta_j^{(l+1)} = \frac{\partial L}{\partial o_j^{(l+1)}}$. By chain rule, we have the following derivation.

$$\begin{aligned}
\delta_j^{(l+1)} &= \frac{\partial L}{\partial o_j^{(l+1)}} \\
&= \frac{\partial L}{\partial y_i^{(l+2)}} \frac{\partial y_i^{(l+2)}}{\partial o_j^{(l+1)}} \\
&= \delta_i^{(l+2)} \frac{\partial y_i^{(l+2)}}{\partial o_j^{(l+1)}}
\end{aligned}$$

where $\frac{\partial y_i^{(l+2)}}{\partial o_j^{(l+1)}}$ has different formulation depends on the pooling function. They are summarized as follows:

- For mean pooling, we have $\frac{\partial y_i^{(l+2)}}{\partial o_j^{(l+1)}} = \frac{1}{m}$;
- For sum pooling we have $\frac{\partial y_i^{(l+2)}}{\partial o_j^{(l+1)}} = 1$;
- For max pooling, for the unit $j = \arg\max(o_j^{(l+1)})$, we have $\frac{\partial y_i^{(l+2)}}{\partial o_j^{(l+1)}} = 1$, otherwise 0. That is the gradient passed back from layer $l+2$ is only towards that neuron which achieved the max. All other neurons have zero gradient.

Backpropagation for Convolution Layers Next we will describe how to perform backpropagation of a convolution layer. For the example in Fig. 6.7, we define $\delta_j^{(l-1)} = \frac{\partial L}{\partial x_j^{(l-1)}}$ to measure how much node j in the $(l-1)$th layer (the feature map) was responsible for errors in the output. By chain rule, we have the equations below.

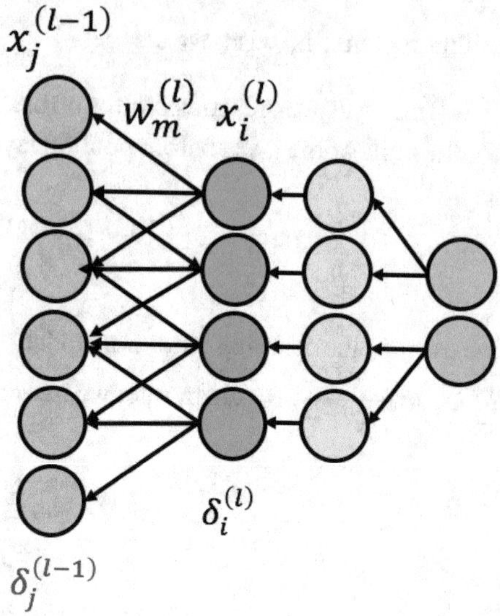

Fig. 6.7 Backward propagation for a convolution layer

$$\begin{aligned}
\delta_j^{(l-1)} &= \frac{\partial L}{\partial x_j^{(l-1)}} \\
&= \frac{\partial L}{\partial x_i^{(l)}} \frac{\partial x_i^{(l)}}{\partial x_j^{(l-1)}} \\
&= \delta_i^{(l)} \frac{\partial x_i^{(l)}}{\partial x_j^{(l-1)}} \\
&= \delta_i^{(l)} \frac{\partial (\sum_m w_m^{(l)} x_{i+m}^{(l-1)} + b^{(l)})}{\partial x_j^{(l-1)}} \\
&= \delta_i^{(l)} \sum_m w_m^{(l)}
\end{aligned}$$

Next we analyze the gradient of the weight vector $\frac{\partial L}{\partial w_m^{(l)}}$. By the chain rule, we have the equations below.

$$\begin{aligned}
\frac{\partial L}{\partial w_m^{(l)}} &= \frac{\partial L}{\partial x_i^{(l)}} \frac{\partial x_i^{(l)}}{\partial w_m^{(l)}} \\
&= \delta_i^{(l)} \frac{\partial x_i^{(l)}}{\partial w_m^{(l)}}
\end{aligned}$$

$$= \delta_i^{(l)} \frac{\partial(\sum_k w_k^{(l)} x_{i+k}^{(l-1)} + b^{(l)})}{\partial w_m^{(l)}}$$

$$= \delta_i^{(l)} \sum_m x_{i+m}^{(l-1)}.$$

Similarly, we can find the gradient of the bias term $\frac{\partial L}{\partial b^{(l)}}$:

$$\frac{\partial L}{\partial b^{(l)}} = \frac{\partial L}{\partial x_i^{(l)}} \frac{\partial x_i^{(l)}}{\partial b^{(l)}}$$

$$= \delta_i^{(l)} \frac{\partial x_i^{(l)}}{\partial b^{(l)}}$$

$$= \delta_i^{(l)} \frac{\partial(\sum_k w_k^{(l)} x_{i+k}^{(l-1)} + b^{(l)})}{\partial b^{(l)}}$$

$$= \delta_i^{(l)}.$$

Once the gradients are identified, the update rules are simply

$$w_m^{(l)} = w_m^{(l)} - \eta \frac{\partial L}{\partial w_m^{(l)}}$$

and

$$b^{(l)} = b^{(l)} - \eta \frac{\partial L}{\partial b^{(l)}}.$$

where η is the learning rate.

6.3.2 *Special CNN Architectures*

Many different CNN architectures have been proposed over the years. Next, we introduce a few popular CNN architectures. Most of them have been compared on the ILSVRC ImageNet challenge.[1] Different architectures are compared based on the top 5 classification error for the competition, which is the percentage of mistakes in the model's top 5 predictions. The ImageNet dataset has 1000 classes and includes many images that are hard to be distinguished from others. From Fig. 6.8, we

[1] http://image-net.org.

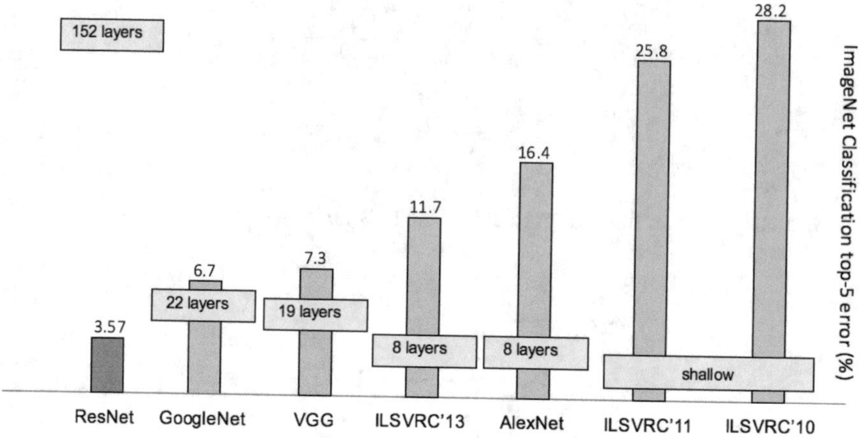

Fig. 6.8 The trend of CNN model performance on the ImageNet challenge

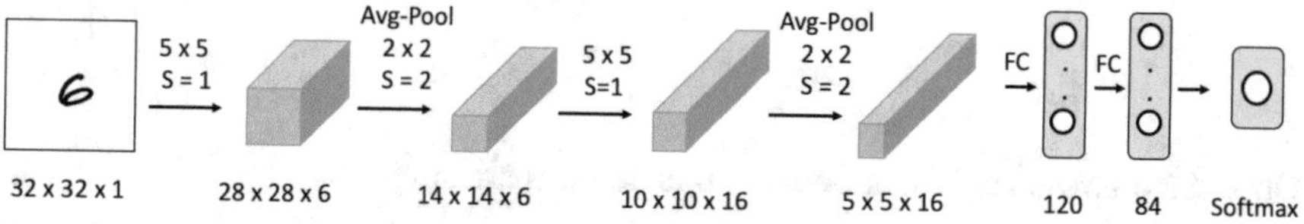

Fig. 6.9 The LeNet architecture

observe CNN variants become more and more accurate in image classification. Meanwhile, architectures become much larger and deeper.

LeNet

LeNet [96] is an earlier CNN structure that contains seven levels of a convolutional network and classifies digits. In the original work, it was applied to recognize handwritten numbers on checks. As shown in Fig. 6.9, LeNet takes 32-by-32 grayscale images as input and first apply six 5×5 convolutional filters with stride 1 and no padding to produce a feature map of $28 \times 28 \times 6$. A 2×2 average pooling filter with stride 2 is applied to produce a feature map of $14 \times 14 \times 6$. After that, another 16 5×5 convolutional filters with stride 1 and no padding are applied to generate a feature map of $10 \times 10 \times 16$. Then another average pooling layer is introduced, followed by two fully connected layers to generate the final softmax classification.

LeNet has about 60k parameters. To process higher resolution images, LeNet needs more and larger convolutional layers. Given that LeNet was proposed before the popularity of GPU, the available computation hardware limited its architecture.

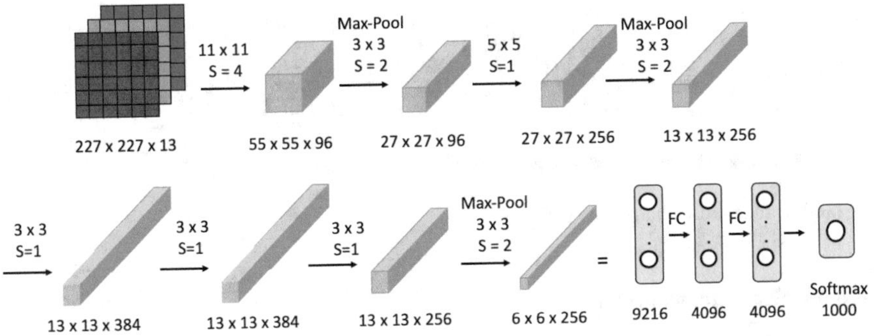

Fig. 6.10 The AlexNet architecture

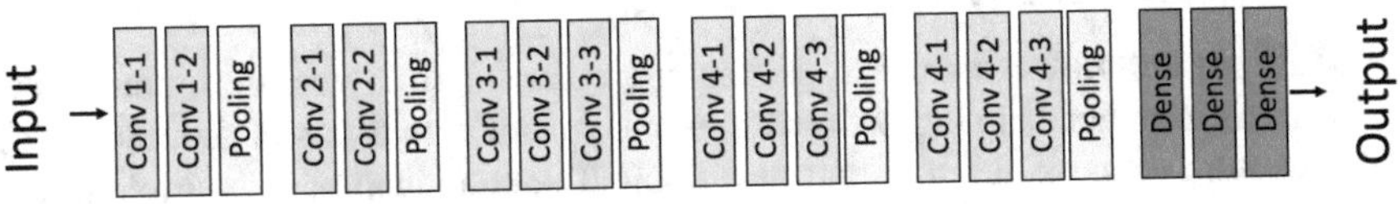

Fig. 6.11 The VGG16 architecture

AlexNet

The AlexNet was architecturally similar to LeNet [90] but is deeper and has more filters per layer, and has stacked convolutional layers. AlexNet introduces the ReLU activation following convolution layers. It has about 60 million parameters. AlexNet is the first deep learning model that won the ImageNet challenge in 2012 with a top-5 error rate of 15.3%, compared to the second place top-5 error rate of 26.2%. After that, all the winning models of the ImageNet challenge are deep learning models (Fig. 6.10).

VGG

VGG16 is a convolutional neural network model proposed in [136]. VGG16 improved AlexNet by replacing large filters (e.g., 11×11 and 5×5) with multiple small filters one after another. Figure 6.11 shows the detailed architecture of VGG16. VGG16 also introduces the 1×1 filter, which performs a linear combination of input channels followed by a nonlinear activation (ReLU function). It has 138 million parameters. For example, the VGG16 model takes over 533MB storage, which can be prohibitively expensive for training and inference.

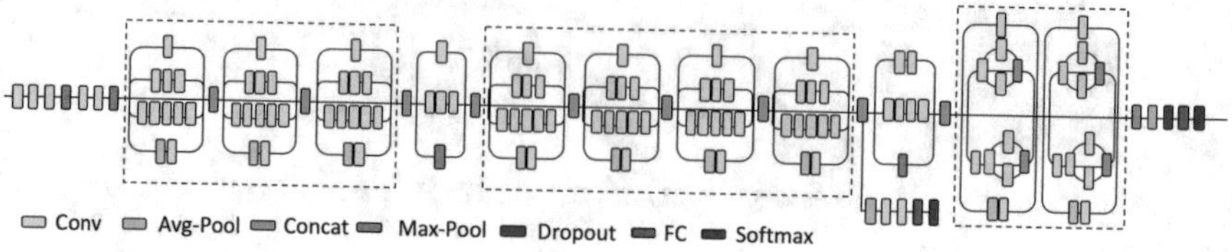

Fig. 6.12 Inception V3 architecture

GoogLeNet Inception Net

GoogleLeNet Inception architecture is another popular CNN architecture with several important ideas [146] as shown in Fig. 6.12:

- **Multiple resolutions:** Instead of stacking convolution layers, inception architectures introduce parallel paths of multiple convolution filters of different sizes to capture patterns at a different resolution. The combination of multiple filters together serves as the building blocks called *inception cells*, which will be stack up to form the CNN architecture.
- **Stacking up smaller filters:** To reduce computational cost and the number of parameters, it is more efficient to stack multiple smaller filters to approximate a larger filter. For example, a 5×5 filter can be approximated by connecting two 3 filters. Similarly, a 3×3 filter can be approximated by a 3×1 filter followed by 1×3 filter. Like VGG16, 1×1 filters are also used to adjust the number of output channels by combining the input channels.
- **Auxiliary loss:** Adding auxiliary loss in the middle of the network improves the model performance. This idea will be significantly enhanced in ResNet via the notion of skipped connection.

The number of parameters of Inception architecture is about 5 million for V1 and 23 million for V3.

ResNet

Residual Neural Network (ResNet) [66] overcomes a troubling phenomenon when training a very deep neural network called *degradation problem*. That is, when the depth of the neural network increases the performance of the network decreases. The intuitive explanation of why degradation happens is that each layer has to construct a brand new set of features without reusing the features learned from previous layers. To use features from previous layers, ResNet proposes "skip connections." that allows input directly passing through without any transformation. As a result, the new features learned at any layer model the residual that the input features have not already captured. Formally, this effect is modeled by a residual block as shown in Fig. 6.13.

Fig. 6.13 Residual block

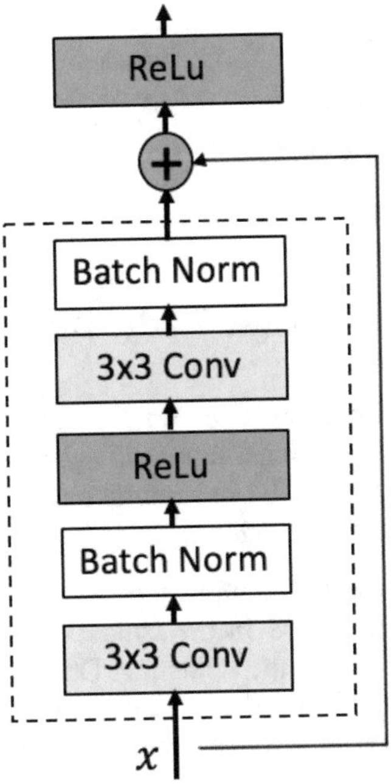

The residual learning has analogous effects on auxiliary loss or gated units. Thanks to this technique, ResNet can train a very deep neural network (e.g., 152 layers) while still achieving high accuracy. The number of parameters of a ResNet model is actually moderate. For example, the popular architecture ResNet-50 has 25 million parameters.

DenseNet

Densely connected convolutional network (DenseNet) [75] generalizes the idea of skipped connections by connecting the output of a layer as input to all later layers. In this way, DenseNet can maximally reuse features from all layers. Thanks to the feature reuse, DenseNet can perform well with a small number of filters (e.g., 12 filters per layer). As a result, it leads to fewer parameters than ResNet. DenseNet also repeats computational units called dense blocks to construct deeper networks, as shown Fig. 6.14. Thanks to dense connections, the gradient can flow more easily through the deep network.

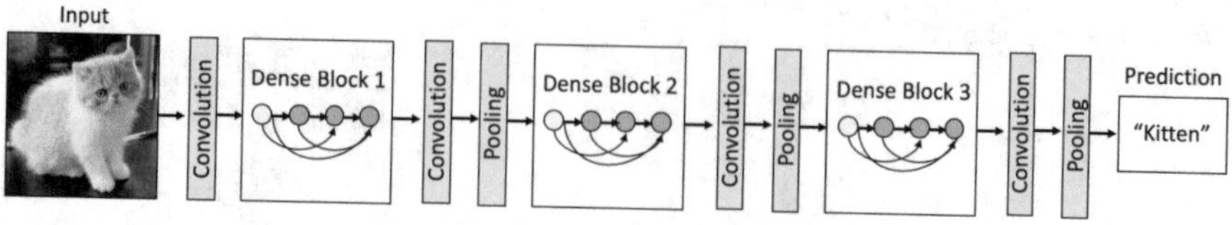

Fig. 6.14 DenseNet architecture

6.4 Case Study: Diabetic Retinopathy Detection

Problem How do the CNN models perform on detecting diabetic retinopathy from retinal fundus images? How does the model performance compare to manual grading by ophthalmologists? A systematic study is presented in [61] to address these questions.

Data The training data were macula-centered retinal fundus images obtained from EyePACS in the United States and India among patients who received diabetic retinopathy screening. Ophthalmologists graded all images in the development and clinical validation sets for the presence of diabetic retinopathy. Diabetic retinopathy severity (none, mild, moderate, severe, or proliferative) was graded according to the International Clinical Diabetic Retinopathy scale. The data are summarized in Table 6.2. Note that the labeled training/development set is very large, over 128K, which gives the edge for training a complex CNN model.

Method To make classification, a convolutional neural network was adopted to compute diabetic retinopathy severity from the intensities of the pixels in a fundus image. It first combines nearby pixels into local features, then aggregates those into global features. Although the network does not explicitly detect lesions (e.g., hemorrhages, microaneurysms), it likely learns to recognize them using the local features. The specific neural network used in this work is the Inception v3 architecture [147].

Results CNN models showed high sensitivity and specificity on the tasks. In 2 validation sets of 9963 images and 1748 images, at the operating point selected for high specificity, the algorithm had 90.3 and 87.0% sensitivity and 98.1 and 98.5% specificity for detecting referable diabetic retinopathy, defined as moderate or worse diabetic retinopathy or referable macular edema by the majority decision of a panel of at least 7 US board-certified ophthalmologists. At the operating point selected for high sensitivity, the algorithm had 97.5 and 96.1% sensitivity and 93.4 and 93.9% specificity in the two validation sets. Another important result in this work is to illustrate the importance of training sample size and labels' reliability. Figure 6.15a shows the increasing trend of model performance as the size of training data. In this task, 50k training images seem to be sufficient. Figure 6.15b shows the increasing performance trend as more grades per image are assigned. More grades per image lead to more reliable labels, which in turn can improve the model performance.

Table 6.2 Data set summary of diabetic retinopathy detection study

Characteristics	Dev set	EyePACS-1 validation data	Messidor-2 validation data
No. of images	128,175	9963	1748
No. of ophthalmologists	54	8	7
No. of grades per image	3–7	8	7
Grades per ophthalmologists, medium	2021 (304–8366)	8906 (8744–9360)	1745 (1742–1748)
No. of unique patients	69,573	4997	874
Age (mean)	55.1 (11.2)	54.4 (11.3)	57.6 (15.9)
% of female	59.9	62.2	42.6
% of fully gradable images	75.1	88.4	99.8
# images for both diabetic retinopathy and macular edema	118,419	8788	1745
No diabetic retinopathy	53,759	7252	1217
Mild diabetic retinopathy	30,637	842	264
Severe diabetic retinopathy	5298	54	28
Proliferative diabetic retinopathy	4359	95	25
Referable diabetic macular edema	18,224	272	125
Referable diabetic retinopathy	33,246	683	254

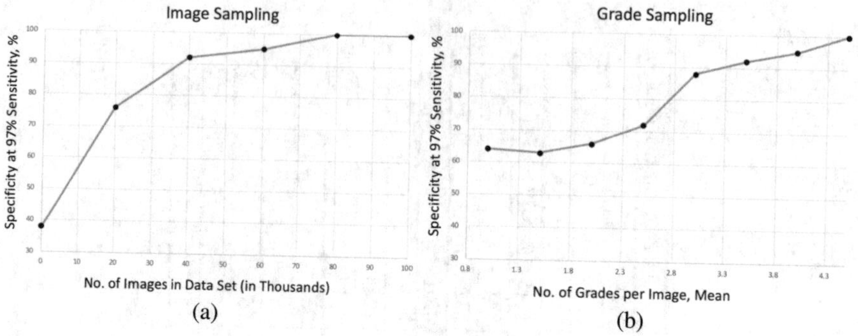

Fig. 6.15 Model performance for diabetic retinopathy detection as the training data size and number of grades per image vary

6.5 Case Study: Skin Cancer Detection

Problem Another famous example is to use CNN to assist skin cancer detection.

Data and Method In [44], researchers trained a CNN using a dataset of 129,450 clinical skin images. In particular, the dataset is composed of dermatologist-labeled images organized in a tree-structured taxonomy of 2032 diseases, in which the individual diseases form the leaf nodes. The images come from 18 different clinician-curated, open-access online repositories, and clinical data from Stanford University Medical Center. The dataset is split into 127,463 training and validation images and 1942 biopsy-labeled test images. CNNs were applied for two diagnosis tasks: classification of keratinocyte carcinomas versus benign seborrheic keratoses; and malignant melanomas versus benign nevi. The first case represents the identification of the most common cancers. The second represents the identification of the deadliest skin cancer. An Inception V3 model was pretrained on approximately 1.28 million images (1000 object categories) from the 2014 ImageNet Large Scale Visual Recognition Challenge. To initialize with the pretrained model, the CNN model was further trained (i.e., finetuning) on the skin images. The CNN model is trained using 757 disease classes.

Results The performance was compared against 21 board-certified dermatologists. The CNN achieves performance on par with all tested experts across both tasks, demonstrating an artificial intelligence capable of classifying skin cancer with a level of competence comparable to dermatologists. The detailed results are shown in Fig. 6.16, where the CNN model outperforms the average dermatologists. Figure 6.17 shows the t-SNE plot of the last layer of the CNN model, where a clear separation of images from different classes can be observed.

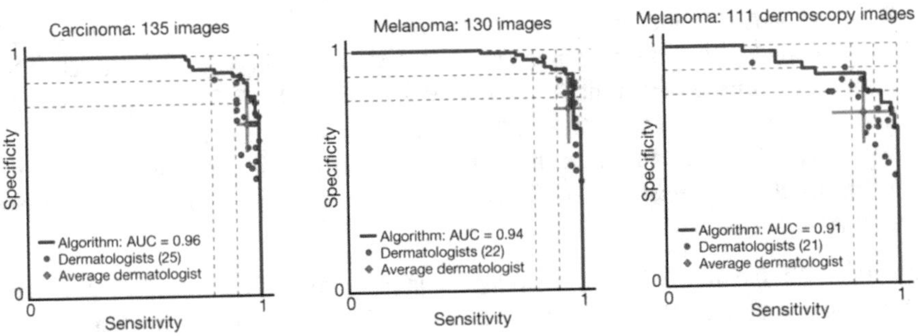

Fig. 6.16 Performance of skin cancer detection: These figures show the performance comparison on 3 test tests where 21–25 dermatologists also scored the same test set. The red dots indicate the individual doctors' performance, and green cross is the average performance of the dermatologists. The blue curve is the ROC curve of the CNN model, which is higher than the performance of the average dermatologists

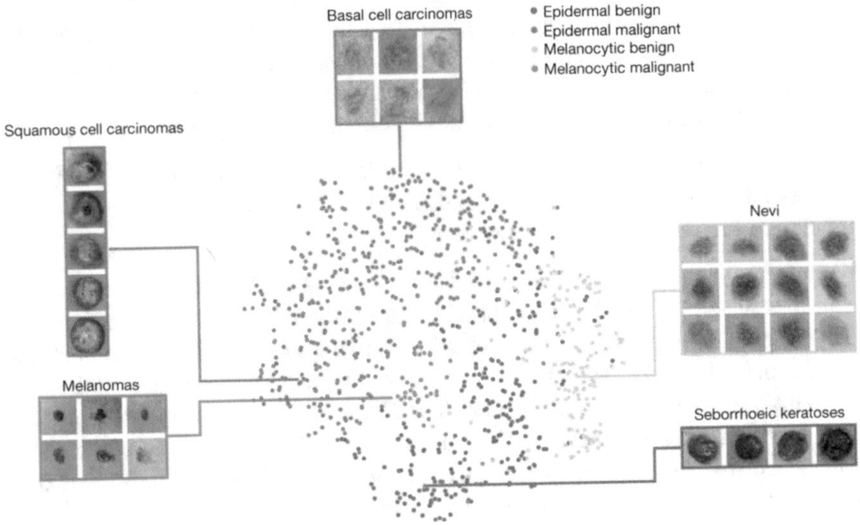

Fig. 6.17 The t-SNE plot of the last layer of CNN model can clearly cluster the images based on different types of skin cancers

6.6 Case Study: Automated Surveillance of Cranial Images for Acute Neurologic Events

Problem How to perform accurate and efficient screen head CT images for acute neurologic events? Authors of [156] introduce a 3D-CNN model trained with weak supervision provided by the NLP program.

Data The data used in this work includes 37,236 imaging studies and 96,303 radiology reports from the Icahn School of Medicine AI Consortium (AISINAI).

All imaging studies and radiology reports were annotated with silver labels based on diagnostic terms derived from the Universal Medical Language System (UMLS) concept of universal identifiers. The NLP labels for UMLS concept universal identifiers were aggregated into higher-level disease types. A small number of images (180) are used to create the test set, manually reviewed, and labeled. The rest are used as training and validation, which are labeled using the silver labels based on extracted UMLS identifiers.

Method To identify whether an image contained acute neurological illnesses, ResNet-50 architecture followed by a 3D-CNN was trained to predict disease acuity. In their simulation, the studies were marked as critical or non-critical by the deep learning model. Then images are ordered in a work queue according to the probability of a critical finding. A random order was used as the baseline for comparison. For the test data, 180 images were randomly queried from the dataset of silver-standard labels to achieve an approximately 1:1 split of noncritical to critical studies. Gold-standard labels were obtained through manual review, where radiologists manually assigned each disease's acuity as critical or non-critical. The remaining studies with silver labels were split into training and validation sets with an 80 : 20 ratio. The prevalence of critical findings of the silver labels is 7.6, 0.8, and 0.7% at thresholds of 4, 8, and 10 UMLS critical findings per note, respectively.

Result There are two sets of results. One set is on model prediction performance such as AUC, accuracy, sensitivity, and specificity. The other set is about a trial simulation for triage based on image interpretation.

Model Performance Since the model is trained with silver labels, their performance is tested on silver label data and, ultimately, the small gold standard test set. For predicting the silver labels of critical findings on the training set, the 3D-CNN achieved a high AUC of 0.88. However, the model performance on the gold standard test set is significantly lower. The DL model achieved an AUC of 0.73. The sensitivity and specificity of the model were 0.79 and 0.48. In comparison, the physicians' average sensitivity and specificity are 0.79 (s.d. 0.04) and 0.85 (s.d. 0.07), which is much higher, especially in specificity. This result suggests that human physicians are still significantly better in this task than DL models, probably because of the limited quality of silver labels used for model training.

Trial Simulation Authors simulated a randomized control trial (RCT) of image interpretation. In the simulation, both the DL model and radiologists were assessed regarding how quickly they recognized and provided notification of a critical finding. Since queue prioritization and rapid assessment are the focus, the model was assessed for its runtime. The average time for the DL model to score an image and potentially raise the alarm was 1.2 s versus 177 s for humans. The triaged queue constructed by the DL model had a significantly lower distribution of queue positions for critical studies compared with noncritical studies (two-sided Wilcoxon rank-sum test, $P = 0.01$, $n = 180$). This seems to confirm the DL model's potential utilization in triage, even with limited prediction accuracy.

6.7 Case Study: Detection of Lymph Node Metastases from Pathology Images

Problem Accurately detecting metastases in whole-slide pathology images is an important task for diagnosing breast cancer. Currently, the task was performed by pathologists, who are expensive and time-consuming. In [42] the authors reported a research competition (CAMELYON16) to develop automated solutions for detecting lymph node metastases.

Data The training data used in the analysis was a dataset of whole-slide images from 2 centers in the Netherlands (110 with nodal metastases, 160 without nodal metastases). Algorithm performance was evaluated in an independent test set of 129 whole-slide images (49 with and 80 without metastases). A panel of 11 pathologists also evaluated the same test set with time constraint (WTC—2 h to evaluate 129 test images) from the Netherlands to ascertain the likelihood of nodal metastases for each slide in a flexible 2-h session, simulating routine pathology workflow, and also by 1 pathologist without time constraint (WOTC).

Method Many methods are proposed in the context of the CAMELYON16 competition. Several CNN architectures were used to analyze whole-slide pathology images. There are two tasks in this competition:

- **Task 1 Tumor localization** identifies the locations of individual metastases on the images. The algorithms were evaluated for their ability to identify specific metastatic foci in a whole-slide image. The metric for task 1 is specialized. In particular, a set of locations need to be scored based on a true-positive fraction, which is from 6 predefined false-positive rates: $1/4$ (meaning 1 false-positive result in every 4 images), $1/2$, 1, 2, 4, and 8 false-positive findings per whole-slide image;
- **Task 2 Image classification** classifies the whole images without the need to specify the locations of metastases. The evaluation metric for task 2 is the standard metric of the area under the receiver operating curve (AUC). Task 2 evaluated the algorithms' ability to discriminate between 49 whole-slide images with SLN metastases vs. 80 without SLN metastases (control). In this case, identification of specific foci within images was not required. Participants provided a confidence score, using the same rating schema as task 1, indicating the probability that each whole-slide image contained any evidence of SLN metastasis from breast cancer.

Next, we describe the winning method from MGH and MIT [42]. First, a threshold-based algorithm is used to differentiate the tissue regions and the background. Then CNN models are only trained on the tissue regions. Millions of 256×256 patches are sampled from both positive and negative regions to construct large samples to train the CNN models. Various CNN architectures are used with different accuracy. Similarly, different magnification levels (40x, 20x, and 10x) are tested. GoogLeNet and 40x magnification led to the best performance for patch level classification. Based on the patch level classification, a set of false-positive patches are added into the training set as the "hard negative" patches. Data augmentation such as rotation, random cropping, and addition of color noise are also added to enrich the training data's diversity.

Result The best performing algorithm [42] used a GoogLeNet architecture, which outperformed all with a score of 0.807 (95%CI, 0.732–0.889) for task 1, and an AUC of 0.994 (95%CI, 0.983–0.999) for task 2. This AUC exceeded the pathologists' mean performance with the time constraint (mean AUC, 0.810 [$range, 0.738 -$ 0.884]) in the diagnostic simulation exercise.

6.8 Case Study: Cardiologist-Level Arrhythmia Detection and Classification in Ambulatory ECG

Problem Computerized electrocardiogram (ECG) interpretation is an important problem. Authors in [65] propose a deep learning model for detecting 12 rhythm classes from ECG data.

Data One major reason that limits deep learning in ECG analysis is the lack of appropriate training data. In this work, a large ECG dataset was constructed with expert annotation with a broad range of ECG rhythm classes. The training dataset consists of a single lead EEG with 91,232 ECG records from 53,549 patients.
The ECG data were recorded by a single-lead, patch-based ambulatory ECG monitor that continuously records data from a single vector (modified Lead II) at 200Hz. The mean and median wear time was 10.6 and 13.0 days, respectively. Mean age was 69 ± 16 years, and 43% were women. The model was evaluated on a test dataset that consisted of 328 ECG records collected from 328 unique patients, which was annotated by a consensus committee of expert cardiologists. Annotations are done by certified ECG technicians, which specified the start time and the end time of all rhythms. Rare rhythms such as AVB are oversampled in the training set. The ground truth labels are assigned with the consensus from the cardiologist committees of 3 members each.

Method This work develops a deep neural network (DNN) to classify 12 rhythm classes using 91,232 single-lead ECGs from 53,549 patients who used a single-lead ambulatory ECG monitoring device. A CNN model is developed, as shown in Fig. 6.18. The model takes a 30 s ECG record of 200 Hz (6000-dimensional vectors) and outputs probability score distribution over 12 classes: (1) Atrial Fibrillation, (2) Atrio-ventricular Block, (3) Bigeminy, (4) Ectopic Atrial Rhythm, (5) Idioventricular Rhythm, (6) Junctional Rhythm, (7) Noise, (8) Sinus Rhythm, (9) Supraventricular Tachycardia, (10) Trigeminy, (11) Ventricular Tachycardia, and (12) Wenckebach. The model is trained and applied in a sliding window fashion and outputs the 12-dimensional prediction every 256 elements (every 1.28 s). The architecture is based on ResNet.

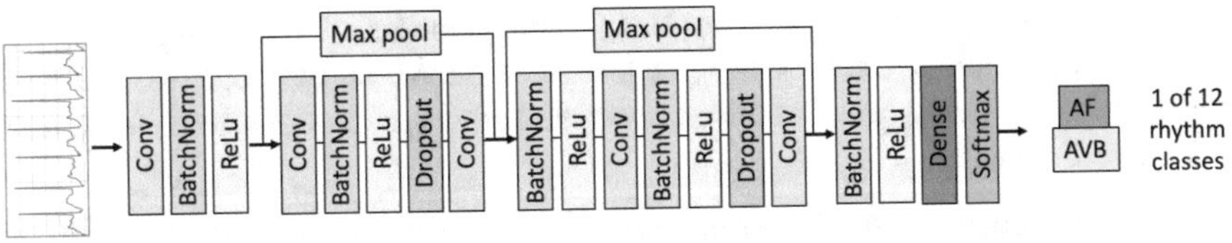

Fig. 6.18 Thirty seconds ECG record of 200 Hz is processed through this CNN model for 12 class classification

Results The proposed model was validated against an independent test dataset annotated by a consensus committee of board-certified practicing cardiologists. The DNN achieved an average area under the receiver operating characteristic curve (ROC) of 0.97. The average F1 score, which is the harmonic mean of the positive predictive value and sensitivity, for the DNN (0.837) exceeded that of average cardiologists (0.780). With specificity fixed at the average specificity achieved by cardiologists, the sensitivity of the DNN exceeded the average cardiologist sensitivity for all rhythm classes.

6.9 Case Study: COVID X-Ray Image Classification

Problem Nothing is probably more surprising and devastating to the whole world than the COVID-19 pandemic in 2020. Accurate and efficient diagnosis and triaging of COVID-19 can be of great value for hospitals to fight the pandemic. Researchers of [120] studied the possibility of differentiating chest x-ray images of COVID-19 against other pneumonia and healthy patients using deep neural networks. Our main task is to differentiate between chest x-ray images of COVID-19 and other pneumonia and healthy patients, which can be considered multiple classification tasks.

Data We combined two publicly available datasets:

- **COVID Chest X-ray (CCX) dataset:** We obtain the COVID-19 pneumonia images from the CCX dataset, which contains a few X-ray images from the other classes.
- **Kaggle Chest X-ray (KCX) dataset:** This dataset contains three types of X-ray images: normal, bacterial pneumonia, and non-COVID-19 viral pneumonia.

All KCX images and most CCX images are based on an anteroposterior (AP) or posteroanterior (PA) view. We only included images with both AP and PA view for consistency purposes in our final experimental dataset. The dataset comprises a total of 5508 chest radiography images across 2874 independent patient cases. All images in KCX data are all in AP/PA view. CCX data has 131 images, of which 119 are AP/PA images. We only selected the 119 AP/PA images in our experiments, including 100 covid-related pneumonia, 11 viral pneumonia, 7 bacterial pneumonia, and 1 normal patient Chest X-ray images. Because AP and PA are two different types of X-ray views, we introduced horizontal flips and random noise to convert PA into AP view.

Method We construct the X-ray imaging data from two publicly available sources including include 5508 chest x-ray images across 2874 patients with four classes: normal, bacterial, non-COVID-19 viral pneumonia, and COVID-19. To identify COVID-19, we propose a Focal Loss Based Neural Ensemble Network (FLANNEL), a flexible module to ensemble several convolutional neural networks (CNN) models and fuse with a focal loss for accurate COVID-19 detection on class imbalance data.

Stage-1 Base Learner Training The convolutional neural networks (CNNs) have been widely used in image classification and get huge successes. Here, we choose 5 popular and state-of-the-art CNN classification models as base learners to model the COVID-19 identification task. The following models were chosen due to their flexibility and high performance with general image classification.

- Inception v3: It is the third edition of Google's Inception Convolutional Neural Network[146].
- VGG19: The model architecture is from the VGG group with batch normalization and consists of 19 layers, where 16 Convolutional layers and 3 Fully Connected layers [136].
- ResNeXt101: This 101-layer architecture is designed by the ResNeXt group [168].
- Resnet152: This is a 152-layer Deep Residual Neural Network that learns the residual representation functions instead of directly learning the signal representations [66].
- Densenet161: This is a Densely Connected Convolutional Network with 161 layers [75].

Stage-2 Ensemble Model Learning We take the linear combination of the base learner predictions using the resulting base learner weights (denoted as $\boldsymbol{w}$) to obtain the final prediction $\hat{y} = \text{Softmax}(\sum_i w_i P_i)$.

However, heavy class imbalances in the data during training will overwhelm and dominate the gradient, making optimal parameter updates difficult. To overcome this class imbalance challenge, we adapt *focal loss*. Originally, focal Loss is a loss function proposed for binary classification tasks, where the well-classified examples are down-weighted and can focus on learning the hard imbalanced examples [16]. Here, we extend focal loss to multiclass classification in our model to address these imbalance issues. For each image, we define the focal loss as:

$$L(\hat{y}, y) = \sum_{m=1}^{M} -\alpha_m y_m (1 - \hat{y}_m)^{\gamma} \log(\hat{y}_m)$$

Table 6.3 Performance comparison on F1-score: class-specific F1-score is calculated using one class vs. the rest strategy

	COVID	Viral pneumonia	Bacterial pneumonia	Normal	Macro-F1
InceptionV3	0.5904(0.27)	0.5864(0.05)	0.8056(0.01)	0.8771(0.04)	0.7149(0.09)
VGG19	0.6160(0.06)	0.5349(0.04)	0.7967(0.02)	0.8691(0.03)	0.7042(0.02)
ResNeXt101	0.6378(0.12)	0.5649(0.03)	0.7959(0.01)	0.8537(0.02)	0.7140(0.03)
Resnet152	0.6277(0.11)	0.5506(0.02)	0.7988(0.01)	0.8700(0.01)	0.7110(0.03)
Densenet161	0.6880(0.07)	0.5930(0.02)	0.8017(0.01)	0.8953(0.01)	0.7445(0.02)
Voting	0.7684(0.04)	0.6005(0.03)	0.8214(0.03)	0.9079(0.01)	0.7745(0.01)
FLANNEL	0.8168(0.03)	0.6063(0.02)	0.8267(0.00)	0.9144(0.01)	0.7910(0.01)

where M is the number of classes, $(1-\hat{y}_m)^\gamma$ is the modulating factor with a focusing parameter γ, and α_m represents a weight parameter for class m.

Results FLANNEL consistently outperforms baseline models on the COVID-19 identification task in all metrics. Compared with the best baseline, FLANNEL shows a higher macro-F1 score with a 6% relative increase on the Covid-19 identification task where it achieves 0.7833±0.07 in Precision, 0.8609±0.03 in Recall, and 0.8168±0.03 F1 score (Table 6.3). Ensemble learning that combines multiple independent basis classifiers can increase robustness and accuracy. In summary, FLANNEL effectively combines state-of-the-art CNN classification models and tackle class imbalance with Focal loss to achieve better performance on Covid-19 detection from X-rays.

6.10 Exercises

1. If you are given a dataset of 100 X-ray images, would you still use CNN models? If so, which architecture would you try? And why?
2. What about you are given 10,000 images, which CNN models would you try?
3. Question 1 Which of the following is NOT true about convolutional neural networks (CNN)?

   (a) Compared to fully connected neural network, CNN has more local connections.
   (b) CNN enables weight sharing through filters.
   (c) CNN utilizes pooling to try to address the translation invariance challenge.
   (d) CNN usually has much more parameters than fully connected neural networks.

4. Given input sequence = [1, 2, 3, 4, 5, 6] and a filter [1 2 1], what is the output of the convolution operation with stride 2 with no padding?

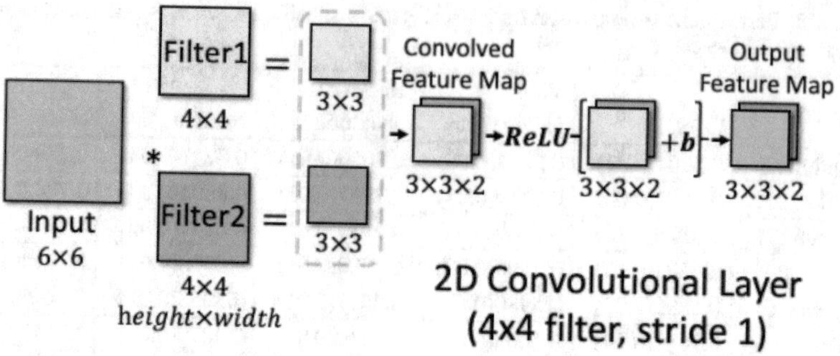

Fig. 6.19 CNN exercise

5. What is the size of the output feature map given 6x6 input and two filters of 4x4 with stride 1 and no padding as illustrated in Fig. 6.19?
6. What is the number of parameters for a convolutional layer given 6x6 input and two filters of 4x4 with stride 1 and no padding as illustrated in Fig. 6.19?
7. What is the output of 1D max pooling over input [1, 2, 3, 2, 3, 5] with filter of size 2 and stride 2?
8. What is NOT true about AlexNet?

   (a) The first deep neural network that won the ImageNet classification challenge.
   (b) AlexNet uses larger filter of 11x11 which is computationally more efficient than the subsequent CNN models such as VGG and ResNet.
   (c) It has parameters in feedforward layers than the convolution layers.
   (d) It uses more computational power in the convolution operations than feedforward computation in fully connected layers.

9. What is NOT true about CNN architectures?

   (a) VGG introduces the idea of stacking smaller filters instead of a larger filter
   (b) Inception Net introduces the parallel paths.
   (c) Inception Net uses 1x1 filters to adjust the output size so that the dimensions across different parallel paths are the same
   (d) ResNet introduces skip connections to allow learning networks of variable depths.

10. Which of the following is true about CNN models?

    (a) CNN is a single model for imaging classification.
    (b) ResNet has more parameters than both VGG and Inception net.
    (c) CNN can be applied to both images and text data.
    (d) The size of a CNN model (number of model parameters) is proportional to the amount of computation (FLOPS).

11. Why did the CNN model succeed in diabetic retinopathy detection application?
    (a) Many standardized retina images exist.
    (b) Many labeled images exist.
    (c) Multiple labels are collected to generate gold standard labels.
    (d) This is a simple task.
12. What neural network architecture was used to detect skin cancer in [44]?

Chapter 7
Recurrent Neural Networks (RNN)

Recurrent Neural Networks (RNN) are a family of deep learning models for sequential data such as longitudinal patient records and time-series data. Two prominent RNN models, namely long short-term memory (LSTM) [71], and gated recurrent unit (GRU) [22] have gained popularity since they alleviate technical challenges related to capturing long-term dependencies and addressing vanishing gradient problems.

Why RNN? RNN is very natural to model variable-length sequences such as longitudinal EHR data, time-series like Electroencephalogram (EEG) and Electrocardiogram (ECG), and text sequences like clinical notes. In healthcare applications, RNN models were used in modeling longitudinal electronic health record (EHR) data [30], clinical notes [77], or continuous monitoring data [102]. RNN has been applied for various tasks, including medical concept embedding [4, 15, 144], diagnostic classification [3, 25, 28, 59, 83, 102, 106], and sequential prediction [23, 28, 30, 76, 77, 116, 118, 119, 162].

In this chapter, we will first define basic concepts and notations related to RNN. Then we will talk about how to train RNN models using Backpropagation Through Time (BPTT) algorithm. After that, we will introduce two RNN variants: the LSTM and GRU units designed to address the vanishing gradient problem to capture long-term dependencies. After that, we will describe the bidirectional RNN models and the sequence-to-sequence models. Last we present several healthcare applications of RNN models.

7.1 RNN Fundamentals

Input and Output The input to RNN models are a sequence of vectors $\boldsymbol{x}^{(1)}, \boldsymbol{x}^{(2)}, \ldots, \boldsymbol{x}^{(T)}$. We denote $\boldsymbol{x}^{(t)}$ as the input vector of time t. Each input vector $\boldsymbol{x}^{(t)}$ maps to a corresponding hidden layer $\boldsymbol{h}^{(t)}$. Then the hidden representation $\boldsymbol{h}^{(t)}$

C. Xiao, J. Sun, *Introduction to Deep Learning for Healthcare*,
https://doi.org/10.1007/978-3-030-82184-5_7

produces the output layer as $\boldsymbol{o}^{(t)}$ for time t. We can apply an activation function $g(\cdot)$ such as the softmax function over $\boldsymbol{o}^{(t)}$ to obtain prediction $\hat{\boldsymbol{y}}^{(t)}$ which will be used to compare with the target label $\boldsymbol{y}^{(t)}$ at time t. For example, the target label $\boldsymbol{y}^{(t)}$ can be an indicator of heart failure diagnosis at next time step $t+1$ and $\hat{\boldsymbol{y}}^{(t)}$ is the prediction of the target based on the input up to time t. Note that for a prediction task, the target label of time t actually comes from information at the future time e.g., $t+1$.

Parameters of RNN Let $\boldsymbol{U}$ be the weight matrix that maps the input $\boldsymbol{x}^{(t)}$ to the hidden layer $\boldsymbol{h}^{(t)}$, $\boldsymbol{W}$ be the weight matrix between hidden $\boldsymbol{h}^{(t-1)}$ and $\boldsymbol{h}^{(t)}$, and $\boldsymbol{V}$ be the weight matrix between the hidden layer $\boldsymbol{h}^{(t)}$ and the output layer $\boldsymbol{o}^{(t)}$. Finally, we have $\hat{\boldsymbol{y}}^{(t)} = g(\boldsymbol{o}^{(t)})$. The notations are summarized in Table 7.1 and the architecture diagram is shown in Fig. 7.1.

Table 7.1 Notations for recurrent neural networks

Notation	Definition
$\boldsymbol{x}^{(t)}$	Input at time t
$\boldsymbol{h}^{(t)}$	Hidden state at time t
$\boldsymbol{h}^{(t-1)}$	Hidden state at time $t-1$
$\boldsymbol{o}^{(t)}$	Output vector at time t
$\hat{\boldsymbol{y}}^{(t)}$	Prediction at time t
$\boldsymbol{y}^{(t)}$	Target label at time t
$\boldsymbol{U}$	Weight matrix between hidden layers
$\boldsymbol{V}$	Weight matrix from input to hidden layer
$\boldsymbol{W}$	Weight matrix from hidden layer to output layer
$\boldsymbol{b}_1$	Bias term at the hidden layer
$\boldsymbol{b}_2$	Bias term at output layer
$f(\cdot)$	Activation function at the hidden layer
$g(\cdot)$	Activation function at the output layer
$\mathcal{L}$	Loss function
$\boldsymbol{c}^{(t)}$	Cell state of LSTM at time t
$\boldsymbol{U}^i, \boldsymbol{U}^f, \boldsymbol{U}^c, \boldsymbol{U}^o$	Weight matrices connecting input to input gate, forget gate, cell state, and output gate
$\boldsymbol{W}^i, \boldsymbol{W}^f, \boldsymbol{W}^c, \boldsymbol{W}^o$	Weight matrices connecting hidden state to input gate, forget gate, cell state, and output gate
$\boldsymbol{V}^o$	Weight matrix connecting hidden state to output
$\boldsymbol{b}^i, \boldsymbol{b}^f, \boldsymbol{b}^c, \boldsymbol{b}^o$	Bias vectors of input gate, forget gate, cell state, and output gate in LSTM
$\boldsymbol{U}^r, \boldsymbol{U}^z, \boldsymbol{U}^h$	Weight matrices connecting input to reset gate, update gate, memory content
$\boldsymbol{W}^r, \boldsymbol{W}^z, \boldsymbol{W}^h$	Weight matrices connecting hidden state to reset gate, update gate, memory content
$\boldsymbol{b}^r, \boldsymbol{b}^z, \boldsymbol{b}^h$	Bias vectors of reset gate, update gate and memory content
$\overrightarrow{\boldsymbol{h}}^{(t)}$	Forward hidden layer of bidirectional RNN at time t
$\overleftarrow{\boldsymbol{h}}^{(t)}$	Backward hidden layer of bidirectional RNN at time t

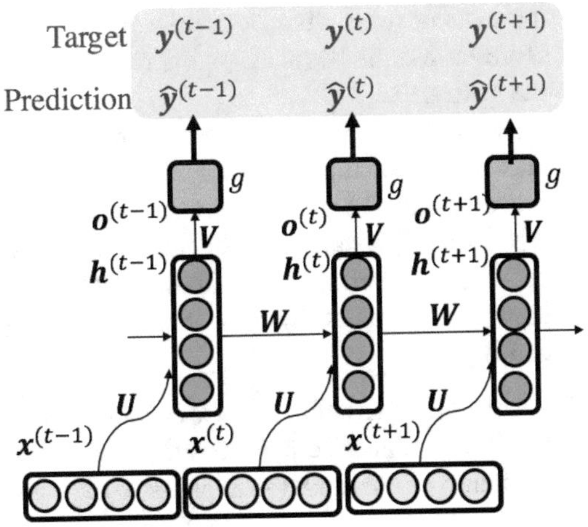

Fig. 7.1 The architecture diagram of RNN with an unrolled representation for an input sequence of length three, three hidden units. Each input time step is combined with the previous hidden state of the RNN to produce the current hidden state, demonstrating the memory effect of the RNN model

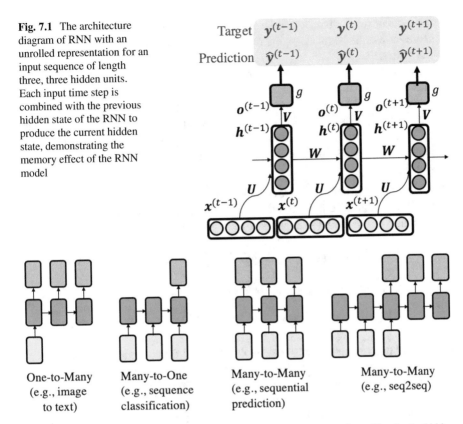

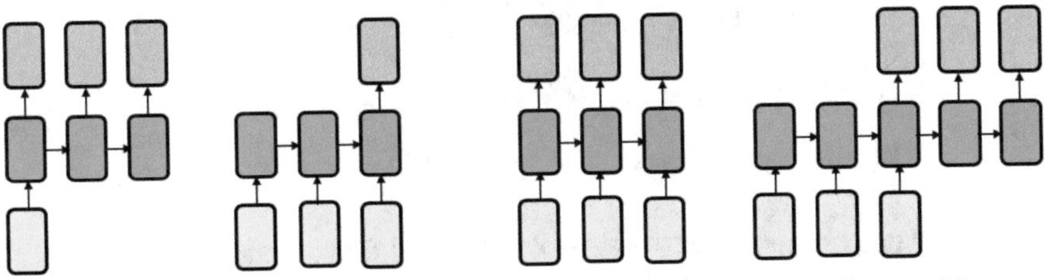

Fig. 7.2 Four types of RNN structure, where yellow box represents input layer, blue for the hidden layer, and green for output and prediction layers

At each time step t, RNN models take current time input $\boldsymbol{x}^{(t)}$ along with previous hidden layer $\boldsymbol{h}^{(t-1)}$ to compute the current hidden state $\boldsymbol{h}^{(t)}$, which serves as the memory of the network at time t. Then an output $\boldsymbol{o}^{(t)}$ and prediction $\hat{y}^{(t)}$ will be made solely based on the memory at time t i.e., $\boldsymbol{h}^{(t)}$. Below we list different types of RNN structures, which are visualized in Fig. 7.2.

1. *One-to-Many* receives one initial input but makes predictions at every time step to produce an output sequence. This model can generate a text description from other types of data, such as an X-ray image.
2. *Many-to-One* receives inputs at each time but makes a single prediction at the last time step. This type can be applied to mortality prediction given the longitudinal EHR of a patient [14].
3. *Many-to-Many sequential prediction* receives new inputs and makes predictions at each time step, thus the length of the output sequence is the same as the input sequence. In this case, the input and output are aligned along time. This structure is suitable for sequential prediction tasks such as predicting clinical events of

the next hospital visit over time. Here the input at each time step is a vector representing the hospital visit at that time, while the output is the prediction for the next visit.

4. *Many-to-Many seq2seq:* Sometimes the input and output are not aligned. In particular, the input sequence will be consumed first through an encoding process; then, the output sequence will be generated via a decoding process. This type of RNN is called a sequence-to-sequence model or seq2seq in short. It has been used for machine translation traditionally. In healthcare, researchers have used such a model for recommending a list of medications based on diagnosis codes [174].

The choice of a particular RNN architecture should be based on the application. The mathematics behind them is the same. The following equations define the sequential computation of the model from input to the final prediction.

$$\begin{aligned}\textbf{Input to hidden}: \quad & \boldsymbol{h}^{(t)} = f\left(\boldsymbol{U}\boldsymbol{x}^{(t)} + \boldsymbol{W}\boldsymbol{h}^{(t-1)} + \boldsymbol{b}_1\right) \\ \textbf{Hidden to output}: \quad & \boldsymbol{o}^{(t)} = \boldsymbol{V}\boldsymbol{h}^{(t)} + \boldsymbol{b}_2 \\ \textbf{Output to prediction}: \quad & \hat{\boldsymbol{y}}^{(t)} = g\left(\boldsymbol{o}^{(t)}\right).\end{aligned}$$

Most other deep neural networks such as DNN and CNN models have a different set of parameters at each layer. However, for RNN the parameters $\boldsymbol{U}, \boldsymbol{V}, \boldsymbol{W}, \boldsymbol{b}_1, \boldsymbol{b}_2$ are shared across all time steps (hence the name "recurrent" neural network). Such parameter sharing also greatly reduces the model size.

The hidden layer activation function f is usually nonlinear functions such as **tanh** or **ReLU**. The output activation function g can be **softmax**. For example in sequential disease prediction, RNN will output a vector of probabilities of different disease risks at each clinical visit. These parameters $\boldsymbol{U}, \boldsymbol{V}, \boldsymbol{W}$ can be intuitively understood with the following special cases.

- When the input to hidden weight $\boldsymbol{U}$ is **1**, it means the input directly gets added to the hidden activation in every time step.
- When the hidden to hidden weight $\boldsymbol{W}$ is **1**, it means without any new input, the hidden unit remembers its previous value.
- When the hidden to output weight $\boldsymbol{V}$ is **1**, it means the output unit copies the hidden activation.

Fortunately, these weights and biases are not set by hands but learned directly from the training data. In particular, we will unroll the RNN model across multiple time steps (e.g., Fig. 7.1 is unrolled by 3 time steps). This particular backpropagation algorithm is called *Backpropagation Through Time (BPTT)*.

7.2 Backpropagation Through Time (BPTT) Algorithm

The backpropagation through time (BPTT) [127] algorithm is a learning algorithm often used for training recurrent neural networks. It extends the original backpropagation algorithm to suit the need of RNNs for modeling multiple time steps. In this section, we will describe how to compute both forward and backward passes.

7.2.1 *Forward Pass*

Consider the unrolled aligned many-to-many RNN, as shown in Fig. 7.1. The computation procedure of the forward pass is given below. For better illustration, we also elaborate on the intermediate steps.

$$\begin{aligned}
z^{(t)} &= \boldsymbol{U}\boldsymbol{x}^{(t)} + \boldsymbol{W}\boldsymbol{h}^{(t-1)} + \boldsymbol{b}_1 \\
\boldsymbol{h}^{(t)} &= f\left(z^{(t)}\right) \\
\boldsymbol{o}^{(t)} &= \boldsymbol{V}\boldsymbol{h}^{(t)} + \boldsymbol{b}_2 \\
\hat{\boldsymbol{y}}^{(t)} &= g\left(\boldsymbol{o}^{(t)}\right)
\end{aligned}$$

Here the activation function $f(\cdot)$ can be tanh and $g(\cdot)$ can be softmax. And the total loss for a given sequence $\{\boldsymbol{x}^{(1)}, \cdots, \boldsymbol{x}^{(T)}\}$ is the sum of losses over all time steps. For example, let loss $L^{(t)}$ at time t be the negative log-likelihood of prediction $\hat{\boldsymbol{y}}^{(t)}$ given $\{\boldsymbol{x}^{(1)}, \cdots, \boldsymbol{x}^{(t)}\}$. Then we have the total loss $\mathcal{L} = \sum_{t=1}^{T} L^{(t)} = -\sum_{t=1}^{T} \log p(\boldsymbol{y}^{(t)} | \{\boldsymbol{x}^{(1)}, \cdots, \boldsymbol{x}^{(t)}\})$.

7.2.2 *Backward Pass*

During the backward pass, we will update all parameters $\boldsymbol{U}, \boldsymbol{V}, \boldsymbol{W}, \boldsymbol{b}_1, \boldsymbol{b}_2$, and the sequences of nodes indexed by time t such as $\boldsymbol{x}^{(t)}$, $\boldsymbol{h}^{(t)}$, $\boldsymbol{o}^{(t)}$ and $L^{(t)}$. For each node we need to compute the gradient recursively, starting with the nodes immediately preceding the final loss we have $\nabla_{L^{(t)}}\mathcal{L} = 1$. For more concrete illustration, we have hidden layer activation $f(\cdot) = tanh(\cdot)$ and output activation $g(\cdot)$ as the softmax function and adopt negative log-likelihood loss to compute $L^{(t)}$. In this setting, the gradient on output node is given by

$$(\nabla_{\boldsymbol{o}^{(t)}}\mathcal{L})_i = \frac{\partial \mathcal{L}}{\partial \boldsymbol{o}_i^{(t)}} = \frac{\partial \mathcal{L}}{\partial \mathcal{L}^{(t)}} \frac{\mathcal{L}^{(t)}}{\partial \boldsymbol{o}_i^{(t)}} = \hat{\boldsymbol{y}}_i^{(t)} - \boldsymbol{y}_i^{(t)}. \tag{7.1}$$

The derivation of Eq. (7.1) is based on Eq. (4.7). Next, we take gradient starting from the final time step of the hidden state $\boldsymbol{h}^T$. Since it does not have a hidden node as a descendant, the gradient can be computed by Eq. (7.2).

$$\nabla_{\boldsymbol{h}^{(T)}}\mathcal{L} = \boldsymbol{V}^T \nabla_{\boldsymbol{o}^{(T)}}\mathcal{L} \tag{7.2}$$

We then iterate backward in time from $t = T - 1$ to 1, which all have descendants in both hidden and output layers. The gradient to $\boldsymbol{h}^T$ for $T \in \{1, \cdots, T-1\}$ is then given by Eq. (7.4).

$$\nabla_{\boldsymbol{h}^{(t)}}\mathcal{L} = \left(\frac{\partial \boldsymbol{h}^{(t+1)}}{\boldsymbol{h}^{(t)}}\right)^T (\nabla_{\boldsymbol{h}^{(t+1)}}\mathcal{L}) + \left(\frac{\partial \boldsymbol{o}^{(t)}}{\boldsymbol{h}^{(t)}}\right)^T (\nabla_{\boldsymbol{o}^{(t)}}\mathcal{L}) \tag{7.3}$$

$$= \boldsymbol{W}^T (\nabla_{\boldsymbol{h}^{(t+1)}}\mathcal{L}) diag\left(1 - (\boldsymbol{h}^{(t+1)})^2\right) + \boldsymbol{V}^T (\nabla_{\boldsymbol{o}^{(t)}}\mathcal{L}) \tag{7.4}$$

where $diag\left(1 - (\boldsymbol{h}^{(t+1)})^2\right)$ indicates the diagonal matrix containing the elements $1 - (h_j^{(t+1)})^2$. This is the Jacobian of the tanh function associated with the hidden unit j at time t.

After obtaining the gradients on all hidden and output nodes, we now obtain the gradients on the parameters as given by Eq. (7.5).

$$\begin{aligned}
\nabla_{\boldsymbol{V}}\mathcal{L} &= \sum_t \sum_k \left(\frac{\partial \mathcal{L}}{\partial o_k^{(t)}}\right) \nabla_{\boldsymbol{V}} o_k^{(t)} = \sum_t (\nabla_{\boldsymbol{o}^{(t)}}\mathcal{L}) \boldsymbol{h}^{(t)^T} \\
\nabla_{\boldsymbol{W}}\mathcal{L} &= \sum_t \sum_j \left(\frac{\partial \mathcal{L}}{\partial h_j^{(t)}}\right) \nabla_{\boldsymbol{W}} h_j^{(t)} = \sum_t diag(1 - (\boldsymbol{h}^{(t)})^2)(\nabla_{\boldsymbol{h}^{(t)}}\mathcal{L}) \boldsymbol{h}^{(t-1)^T} \\
\nabla_{\boldsymbol{U}}\mathcal{L} &= \sum_t \sum_j \left(\frac{\partial \mathcal{L}}{\partial h_j^{(t)}}\right) \nabla_{\boldsymbol{U}} h_j^{(t)} = \sum_t diag(1 - (\boldsymbol{h}^{(t)})^2)(\nabla_{\boldsymbol{h}^{(t)}}\mathcal{L}) \boldsymbol{x}^{(t)^T} \\
\nabla_{\boldsymbol{b}_1}\mathcal{L} &= \sum_t \left(\frac{\partial \boldsymbol{h}^{(t)}}{\partial \boldsymbol{b}^{(t)}}\right)^T \nabla_{\boldsymbol{h}^{(t)}}\mathcal{L} = \sum_t diag(1 - (\boldsymbol{h}^{(t)})^2) \nabla_{\boldsymbol{h}^{(t)}}\mathcal{L} \\
\nabla_{\boldsymbol{b}_2}\mathcal{L} &= \sum_t \left(\frac{\partial \boldsymbol{o}^{(t)}}{\partial \boldsymbol{b}_2}\right)^T \nabla_{\boldsymbol{o}^{(t)}}\mathcal{L} = \sum_t \nabla_{\boldsymbol{o}^{(t)}}\mathcal{L}
\end{aligned} \tag{7.5}$$

These updated rules are similar to those of DNN, except that the weight updates need to be summed over all time steps.

Vanishing Gradient Problem For each layer, the gradient is backpropagated and can become smaller and smaller, leading to the vanishing gradient problem. Next, we will introduce different RNN variants that address the vanishing gradient problem.

7.3 RNN Variants

There are many different variants of RNN: Some aim at overcoming the vanishing gradient problem, such as the Long Short-Term Memory model (LSTM) and Gated Recurrent Unit (GRU). Some extend the one-directional sequential structure to bi-directional, like bi-directional RNN. Other introduces the encoding and decoding stages for an RNN to handle different input and output lengths, such as sequence-to-sequence models.

7.3.1 *Long Short-Term Memory (LSTM)*

Overcoming the vanishing gradient problem is the main motivation behind the LSTM model [72]. LSTM introduces a new structure called the *cell state*, which is designed to remember useful information and forget unnecessary information over time.

The key idea to control what information to remember or forget is through various gates. Specifically, a gate is a sigmoid function $\sigma(\cdot)$ over the linear combination of the input. Intuitively, if the sigmoid is close to 1, the gate is open. If the sigmoid is close to 0, the gate is closed. LSTM comprises of three gates: *input gate, forget gate* and *output gate*, which are visualized in Fig. 7.3. Here are some notations used in the LSTM model:

- Input unit to the LSTM cell at time t: $\boldsymbol{x}^{(t)} \in \mathbb{R}^m$;
- Hidden unit to the LSTM cell from time $t-1$: $\boldsymbol{h}^{(t-1)} \in \mathbb{R}^n$;
- Weight matrices connecting input $\boldsymbol{x}^{(t)}$ to input gate, forget gate, cell state, and output gate: $\boldsymbol{U}^i, \boldsymbol{U}^f, \boldsymbol{U}^c, \boldsymbol{U}^o$, all $\in \mathbb{R}^{k\times m}$;
- Weight matrices connecting previous hidden state to input gate, forget gate, cell state, and output gate: $\boldsymbol{W}^i, \boldsymbol{W}^f, \boldsymbol{W}^c, \boldsymbol{W}^o$, all $\in \mathbb{R}^{k\times n}$;
- Weight matrix connecting hidden state to the output $\boldsymbol{V}^o \in \mathbb{R}^{k\times k}$;
- Bias vectors of input gate, forget gate, cell state, and output gate: $\boldsymbol{b}^i, \boldsymbol{b}^f, \boldsymbol{b}^c, \boldsymbol{b}^o$, all $\in \mathbb{R}^k$.

Cell State LSTM introduce a cell state at each time t as $\boldsymbol{c}^{(t)}$, which is a vector representation of the internal state of LSTM over time. Depending on the current input $\boldsymbol{x}^{(t)}$ and the previous hidden state $\boldsymbol{h}^{(t-1)}$, LSTM will update the cell state. Before we describe the cell state update, we first need to introduce *forget gate* and *input gate*.

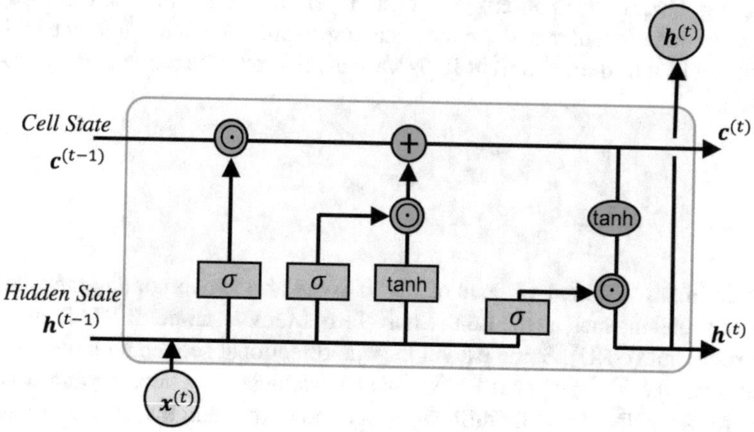

Fig. 7.3 LSTM structure. The LSTM model has a cell state $\boldsymbol{c}^{(t)}$ that is a vector representing the current state of the LSTM. The LSTM model has an input gate, an output gate, and a forget gate that regulates the cell state's interactions with RNN's input, hidden state, and output

Forget Gate As illustrated in Fig. 7.4 controls how much of the previous cell state should be kept based on the previous hidden state. To be specific, it computes a linear combination of hidden state $\boldsymbol{h}^{(t)}$ and then followed by a sigmoid activation function to produce an output between 0 and 1. If the forget gate generates a value close to 1, it will remember the previous cell state; if the value is close to 0, it will forget the previous cell state.

More specifically, we denote $f^{(t)}$ as the activation function of the forget gate at time t.

$$f^{(t)} = \sigma(\boldsymbol{U}^f \boldsymbol{x}^{(t)} + \boldsymbol{W}^f \boldsymbol{h}^{(t-1)} + \boldsymbol{b}^f) \tag{7.6}$$

Input Gate As illustrated in Fig. 7.5 decides what new information will be added into the cell state. Formally, we denote $\tilde{c}^{(t)} \in \mathbb{R}^k$ as the new information and $i^{(t)} \in \mathbb{R}^k$ as the input gate that controls how much this new information to add into the cell state.

$$\tilde{c}^{(t)} = tanh(\boldsymbol{U}^c \boldsymbol{x}^{(t)} + \boldsymbol{W}^c \boldsymbol{h}^{(t-1)} + \boldsymbol{b}^c) \tag{7.7}$$

$$i^{(t)} = \sigma(\boldsymbol{U}^i \boldsymbol{x}^{(t)} + \boldsymbol{W}^i \boldsymbol{h}^{(t-1)} + \boldsymbol{b}^i) \tag{7.8}$$

Cell State Update Now we have all the necessary components for updating cell state: the forget gate activation $f^{(t)}$, the input gate activation $i^{(t)}$, and the new information $\tilde{c}^{(t)}$. The new cell state $c^{(t)}$ at time t can be updated with the following equation:

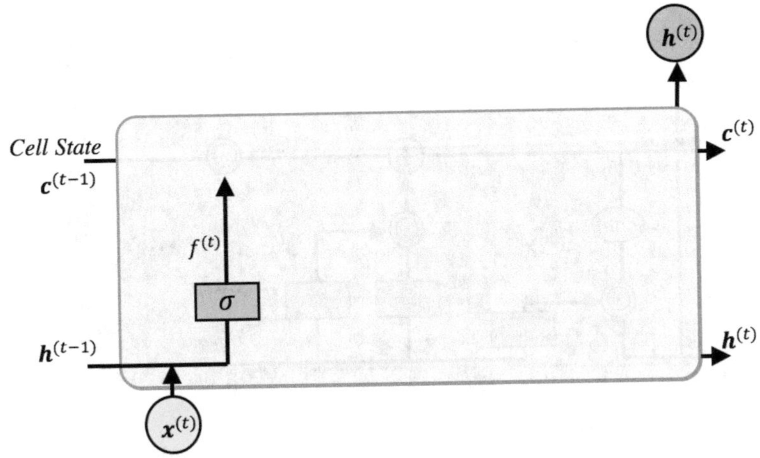

Fig. 7.4 The forget gate controls how much of previous cell state should be kept

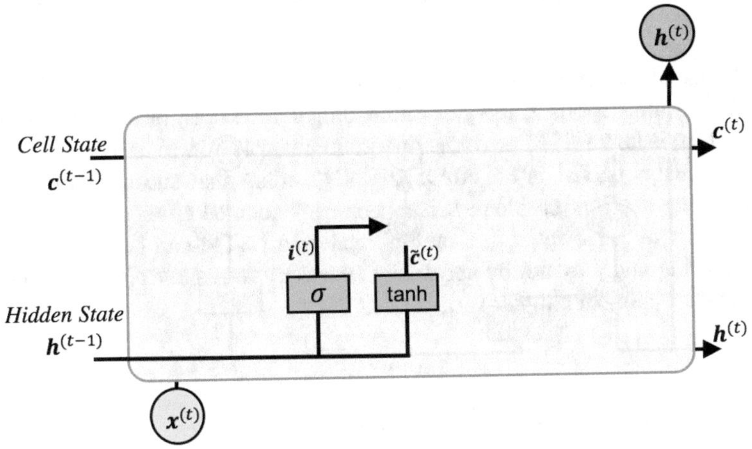

Fig. 7.5 The input gate adds the new information to the cell state

$$c^{(t)} = i^{(t)} \odot \tilde{c}^{(t)} + f^{(t)} \odot c^{(t-1)} \tag{7.9}$$

where $\odot$ is element-wise multiplication.

Output Gate As illustrated in Fig. 7.6 determines which part of the cell state becomes output as the next hidden state $\boldsymbol{h}^{(t)}$. Specifically, the new cell state $c^{(t)}$ is passed through nonlinearity and multiplied by the output gate (the sigmoid activation of the input and previous hidden state).

$$o^{(t)} = \sigma(\boldsymbol{U}^{o}\boldsymbol{x}^{(t)} + \boldsymbol{W}^{o}\boldsymbol{h}^{(t-1)} + \boldsymbol{b}^{o}) \tag{7.10}$$

$$\boldsymbol{h}^{(t)} = o^{(t)} \odot tanh(c^{(t)}) \tag{7.11}$$

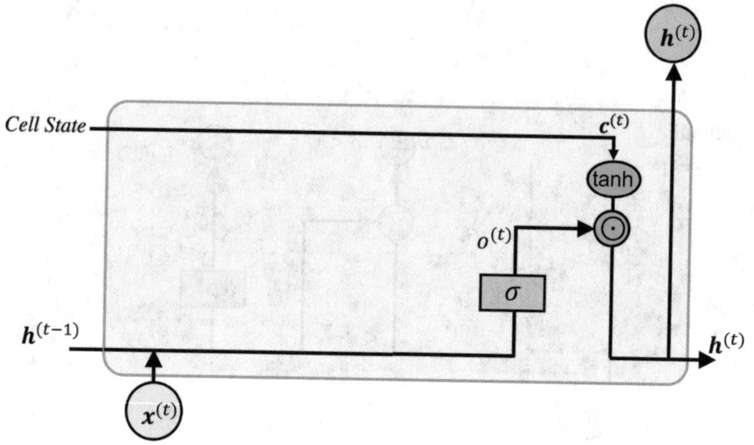

Fig. 7.6 The output gate decides which part of the cell state to output. Specifically, the cell state $c^{(t)}$ is passed through nonlinearity and multiplied by the sigmoid activation of the input

Note that all the gates (and the cell state) are all embedding vectors, which means for different dimensions in the gate embedding can be open or close to a different degree. That is how LSTM provides fine-grain controls how to update.

In summary, LSTM is an effective RNN variant that successfully alleviates the vanishing gradient problem. It has been implemented efficiently in most deep learning software. However, the multiple gates in LSTM can be complicated for understanding and may not be absolutely necessary to make RNN work. Next we will introduce another simpler variant of RNN.

7.3.2 Gated Recurrent Unit (GRU)

Gated recurrent unit (GRU) is another popular variant of RNN models [21]. Compared with LSTM, the GRU uses a similar gating mechanism to learn long-term dependencies and alleviate the vanishing gradient problem. GRU removes the cell state in LSTM and uses the hidden state $\boldsymbol{h}^{(t)}$ serve as both the cell state and output state. GRU has only two gates: a *reset gate* r, and an *update gate* z. Intuitively, the reset gate determines how to combine the new input with the previous memory, and the update gate defines how much of the previous memory to keep. The GRU model is illustrated in Fig. 7.7.

For updating a GRU model, we are given the following variables.

- Input unit to the GRU at time t: $\boldsymbol{x}^{(t)}$;
- Weight matrices connecting input to the hidden state for update gate $\boldsymbol{U}^z$, for the reset gate $\boldsymbol{U}^r$, and for hidden state itself $\boldsymbol{U}^h$;

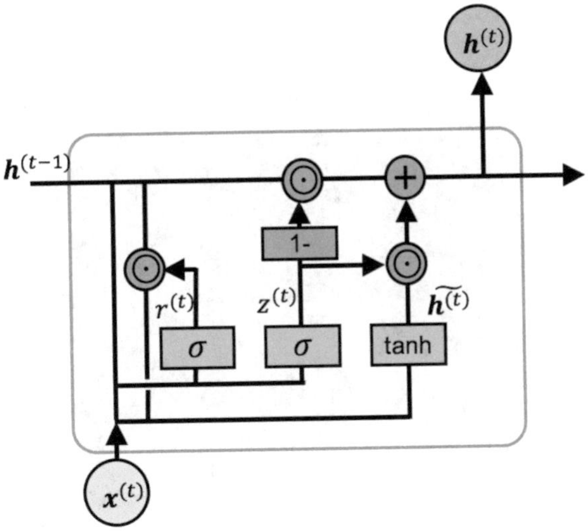

Fig. 7.7 The GRU structure. The GRU model has with only two gates: a reset gate r, and an update gate z. Intuitively, the reset gate determines how to combine the new input with the previous hidden state, and the update gate defines how much of the previous hidden state to keep

- Weight matrices connecting previous hidden state to the new hidden state for the reset gate $\boldsymbol{W}^r$, update gate $\boldsymbol{W}^z$, and for hidden state itself $\boldsymbol{W}^h$;
- Bias vectors of the reset gate, update gate and hidden state: $\boldsymbol{b}^r$, $\boldsymbol{b}^z$, $\boldsymbol{b}^h$.

Update Gate One important simplication from GRU is to combine the forget gate and input gate of LSTM into one update gate. Visually, the update gate is illustrated in Fig. 7.8a. The update gate helps determine how much of the previous hidden state $\boldsymbol{h}^{(t-1)}$ to remove and how much new information to add to the current hidden state $\boldsymbol{h}^{(t)}$. In particular, the update gate is computed as the following:

$$z^{(t)} = \sigma(\boldsymbol{U}^z \boldsymbol{x}^{(t)} + \boldsymbol{W}^z \boldsymbol{h}^{(t-1)} + \boldsymbol{b}^z) \tag{7.12}$$

Reset Gate As shown in Fig. 7.8b determines how much of the past information to forget (or remember). Similar to the update gate, the reset gate is computed via Eq. (7.13).

$$r^{(t)} = \sigma(\boldsymbol{U}^r \boldsymbol{x}^{(t)} + \boldsymbol{W}^r \boldsymbol{h}^{(t-1)} + \boldsymbol{b}^r) \tag{7.13}$$

Then we add new information to the current hidden state $\boldsymbol{h}^{(t)}$, which uses the reset gate to store the relevant information from the past. It is shown in Fig. 7.8c and given by Eq. (7.14).

$$\tilde{\boldsymbol{h}}^{(t)} = tanh(\boldsymbol{U}^h \boldsymbol{x}^{(t)} + r^{(t)} \odot \boldsymbol{W}^h \boldsymbol{h}^{(t-1)} + \boldsymbol{b}^h) \tag{7.14}$$

Note that $\odot$ is the elementwise multiplication.

Last we calculate $\boldsymbol{h}^{(t)}$, a vector that contains the current information. This information will be passed down to the network. This is given by Eq. (7.15).

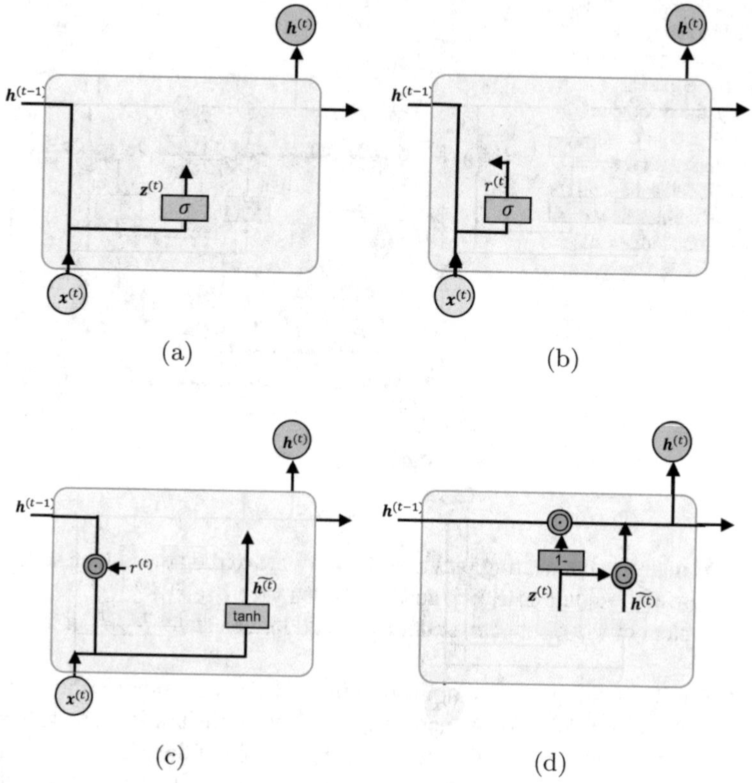

Fig. 7.8 (**a**) GRU update gate; (**b**) GRU reset gate; (**c**) New information added to the hidden state; and, (**d**) update GRU new hidden state

$$\boldsymbol{h}^{(t)} = (1 - z^{(t)}) \odot \boldsymbol{h}^{(t-1)} + z^{(t)} \odot \tilde{\boldsymbol{h}}^{(t)}. \tag{7.15}$$

The final hidden state of GRU is illustrated in Fig. 7.8d.

Key Insight Note that the output of any of the gates in LSTM or GRU are actually vectors so that different elements in those vectors will decide whether to keep or remove or add information. In that sense, the gates control information flow via multiple dimensions. For example, one element in the output vector of a gate (output of a sigmoid) can correspond to the age information. Another element may correspond to the history of heart disease. LSTM or GRU may decide to update the element corresponding to the age information with the updated age while keeping the element about heart disease history. Because the output is represented as vectors, LSTM or GRU can have the necessary flexibility to keep or update information selectively.

7.3.3 Bidirectional RNN

RNNs process input sequences in a specific order. For example, if the sequence is a list of clinical visits from a patient over time, the RNN model can follow the temporal order to process the earliest visits first, then go to the recent visits. In particular, when RNNs calculate the output or hidden state at time t, it will not be able to utilize any information from time $t+1, t+2, \ldots$. However, sometimes one may want to leverage the events before and after the current time. For example, when generating a representation of clinical notes, a word x embedding should consider the context before and after x. A bidirectional RNN allows the output of RNN to depend on both previous and future events. This is a common scenario, especially in modeling clinical notes. Thus the bidirectional RNNs are proposed. They are simply two RNNs: one processes input sequences in a forward direction, and one processes in a backward direction, as illustrated in Fig. 7.9. The output is computed based on the concatenation of the hidden states from both RNNs. The idea of bidirectional RNN can be extended to all RNN variants and yield bidirectional LSTM and bidirectional GRU models.

The computation of bidirectional RNN is given by

$$\overrightarrow{\boldsymbol{h}}^{(t)} = f(\boldsymbol{U}\boldsymbol{x}^{(t)} + \boldsymbol{W}\boldsymbol{h}^{(t-1)} + \boldsymbol{b}_1) \tag{7.16}$$

$$\overleftarrow{\boldsymbol{h}}^{(t)} = f(\boldsymbol{U}\boldsymbol{x}^{(t)} + \boldsymbol{W}\boldsymbol{h}^{(t+1)} + \boldsymbol{b}_1) \tag{7.17}$$

$$y^{(t)} = g(\boldsymbol{V}[\overrightarrow{\boldsymbol{h}}^{(t)}; \overleftarrow{\boldsymbol{h}}^{(t)}] + \boldsymbol{b}_2) \tag{7.18}$$

where $\overrightarrow{\boldsymbol{h}}^{(t)}$ indicates the hidden state from RNN processing in the forward direction, $\overleftarrow{\boldsymbol{h}}^{(t)}$ is the one in the backward direction, and $[\overrightarrow{\boldsymbol{h}}^{(t)}; \overleftarrow{\boldsymbol{h}}^{(t)}]$ corresponds to the concatenation of the hidden states from both directions.

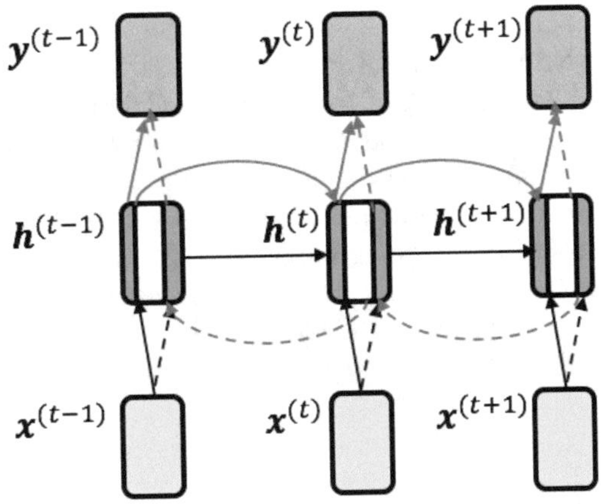

Fig. 7.9 Bidirectional RNN

7.3.4 Encoder-Decoder Sequence-to-Sequence Models

The sequence-to-sequence (in short "Seq2Seq") models [19, 145] are trained to map an input sequence to an output sequence via two RNN models. The first RNN (encoder) will process the input sequence $\mathcal{X}$ to obtain a fixed size vector $\boldsymbol{c}$ that represents the input sequence. The second RNN (decoder) will generate the output sequence $\mathcal{Y}$. Seq2Seq models have received great success in various tasks such as machine translation, speech recognition, and text summarization. In healthcare applications, researchers have used such a model to generate a list of medications based on a list of diagnoses [174]. Let us define input sequence $\mathcal{X}$ and output sequence $\mathcal{Y}$:

$$\mathcal{X} = (\boldsymbol{x}_1, \cdots, \boldsymbol{x}_I) = (\boldsymbol{x}_i)_{i=1}^I \tag{7.19}$$

$$\mathcal{Y} = (\boldsymbol{y}_1, \cdots, \boldsymbol{y}_J) = (\boldsymbol{y}_J)_{j=1}^J \tag{7.20}$$

where $\boldsymbol{x}_i \in \mathbb{R}^{N_x}$ is the i-th element in input sequence $\mathcal{X}$ and $\boldsymbol{y}_j \in \mathbb{R}^{N_y}$ the j-th element in input sequence $\mathcal{Y}$. Note that the length of input sequence I and that of the output sequence J can be different.

From a probabilistic perspective, a seq2seq model is to learn the conditional distribution of an output sequence $\mathcal{Y}$ conditioned on the input sequence $\mathcal{X}$, or formally $P(\mathcal{Y}|\mathcal{X})$. The seq2seq does not model $P(\boldsymbol{y}_1, \cdots, \boldsymbol{y}_J|\boldsymbol{x}_1, \cdots, \boldsymbol{x}_I)$ directly, instead it models the probability of $P(\boldsymbol{y}_j|\boldsymbol{y}_{j-1}, \cdots, \boldsymbol{y}_1, \mathcal{X})$, which is the probability of jth element of output sequence given elements of output sequence before jth element and the entire input sequence $\mathcal{X}$. Thus the conditional distribution $P_\theta(\mathcal{Y}|\mathcal{X})$ parameterized by θ can be expressed as the following product.

$$P_\theta(\mathcal{Y}|\mathcal{X}) = \prod_{j=1}^{J+1} P_\theta(\boldsymbol{y}_j|\boldsymbol{y}_{j-1}, \cdots, \boldsymbol{y}_1, \mathcal{X}) \tag{7.21}$$

where in practice $\mathcal{X}$ is represented as the output of the first RNN $\boldsymbol{c}$.

The learning of the seq2seq model mainly consists of the following two parts: (1) the generation of the fixed size hidden vector $\boldsymbol{c}$ from the input sequence $\mathcal{X}$, and (2) the generation of output sequence $\mathcal{Y}$ from the hidden vector $\boldsymbol{c}$. As illustrated in Fig. 7.10, the encoder is an RNN that processes input data points sequentially. During the process, the hidden state of the RNN changes according to $\boldsymbol{h}_t = f(\boldsymbol{h}_{t-1}, \boldsymbol{x}_t)$ where f is an activation function such as **tanh**. After reaching the end of the input sequence, the hidden state of the RNN becomes the context vector $\boldsymbol{c}$ for generating the output sequence.

$$\boldsymbol{c} = \boldsymbol{h}_T = f(\boldsymbol{h}_{T-1}, \boldsymbol{x}_T)$$

The decoder RNN generates the output sequence by predicting the next output $\boldsymbol{y}_t$ given the hidden state $\boldsymbol{h}_t$ and the context vector $\boldsymbol{c}$. In this case, both $\boldsymbol{y}_t$ and $\boldsymbol{h}_t$ are

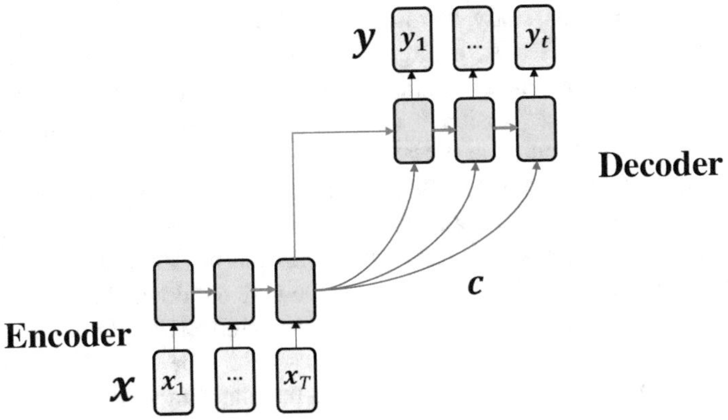

Fig. 7.10 Example of a sequence-to-sequence RNN architecture. An encoder RNN reads the input sequence $\mathcal{X}$ and learns the context, which is parameterized by weight $\boldsymbol{c}$. A decoder RNN generates the output sequence $\mathcal{Y}$ based on the context learned from the input. Here the blue arrows refer to the sequence of context vector. In contrast, the black arrow refers to conditional decoding using the encoding context

also conditioned on $\boldsymbol{y}_{t-1}$ and on the context $\boldsymbol{c}$. Hence, the hidden state of the decoder at time t is computed by $\boldsymbol{h}_t = g(\boldsymbol{h}_{t-1}, \boldsymbol{y}_{t-1}, \boldsymbol{c})$. Or similarly, the conditional distribution of the next output item becomes

$$P(\boldsymbol{y}_t|\boldsymbol{y}_{t-1}, \cdots, \boldsymbol{y}_1, \boldsymbol{c}) = g(\boldsymbol{h}_t, \boldsymbol{y}_{t-1}, \boldsymbol{c}).$$

where g is the decoding RNN with the final activation function that produces probabilities for multiclass problems, such as softmax.

A critical disadvantage of the seq2seq model is unable to remember long sentences due to a single fixed context vector. This disadvantage will be addressed by attention models described in Chap. 9.

7.4 Case Study: Early Detection of Heart Failure

Problem Choi et al. [30] studied an important prediction task for heart failure. The goal is to predict whether the patient will develop heart failure based on the recent history documented in their EHR data. Heart failure is a deadly condition with 50% mortality within 5 years of diagnosis [125]. Earlier detection of heart failure could lead to better outcomes through inexpensive treatment and lifestyle improvement. RNN can be a valuable tool for modeling such event sequences because it overcomes irregular lengths across patients. In practice, the number of visits per patient varies significantly as many patients may have just a single visit, but some patients may have over 100 visits. Traditionally it will be quite difficult to apply a single model to all the patients of different lengths. Thanks to the recurrent structure, RNN naturally applies to variable lengths of event sequences.

Data The data for this study were derived from outpatient EHR records over 10 years from Sutter Health, a large provider network in northern California. The dataset includes patient demographics, diagnosis information as International Classification of Disease version 9 (ICD-9) codes, medications, and procedure codes. The particular study is a case-control study, where 4178 HF cases are identified and matched with 29,139 control patients. More specifically, each HF case is identified with the corresponding HF diagnosis date. Then multiple control patients are matched to this HF case, where the controls are active patients in the same clinic with the same age and gender as the case but do not have HF. After the patient cohort is identified, 18 months of the structured EHR data before the index date are extracted for this study. For an HF case, the index date is the actual HF diagnosis date, but the index date for control is the matching case's diagnosis date.

Method The average number of clinical codes assigned to each patient was about 72, and 18,181 unique clinical codes are present in this dataset (6910 diagnosis codes, 6897 medication codes, and 4374 procedure codes) (Fig. 7.11).

Each raw event, such as ICD9 code 250.00 is represented as a one-hot vector of 18,181 dimensions, which is sequentially fed through a Gated Recurrent Unit (GRU) model. They also consider two other feature representations: One is based on clinical code hierarchy, which group diagnosis codes into 283 groups, medication codes into 96 groups, and procedure codes into 244 groups; The other is based on pre-trained word2vec embedding [111] of 100 dimensions over all the clinical events. Since

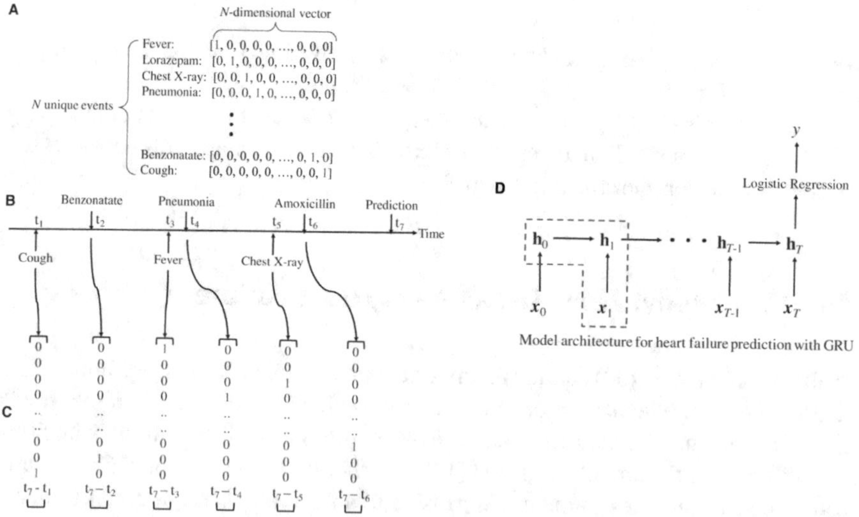

Fig. 7.11 (**a**) One-hot vector encoding of clinical events. (**b**) indicates the time at which the event occurs, assuming we make the prediction at time *t*7. The time duration between current and previous visits are appended as a feature at the end of all input vectors, as shown in (**c**). All the events are passed through a RNN model with binary classification at the end for HF shown in (**d**)

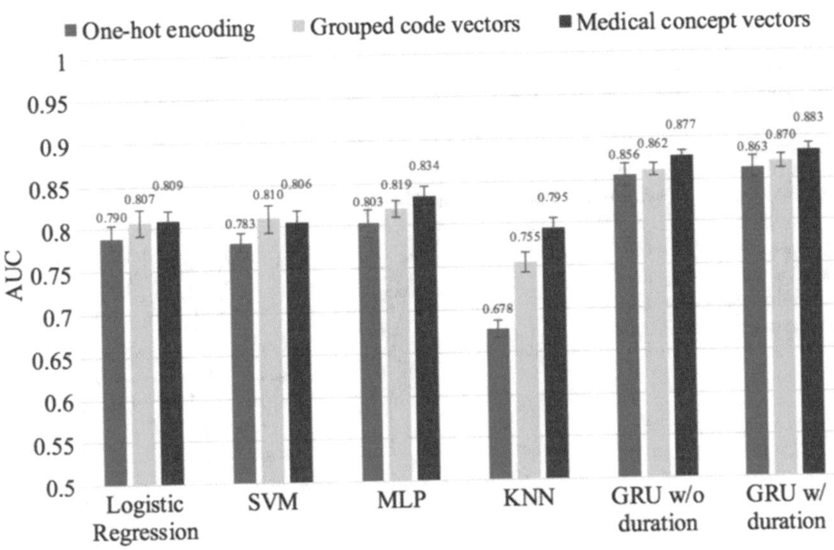

Fig. 7.12 GRU outperform all the methods for HF onset prediction. Medical concept vectors pretrained with Word2Vec outperforms knowledge driven features (aggregation using grouper such as CCS codes)

there is no temporal order of events recorded within a clinical visit, this work picks an arbitrary order of RNN and word2vec training events.

Results The GRU model consistently outperformed all the other methods, including logistic regression, support vector machine (SVM), multi-layer perceptron (MLP, i.e., DNN with 1 hidden layer), and k-nearest neighbor (KNN), with 0.883 AUC. Models trained using the word2vec embedding significantly outperformed models trained by one-hot vectors and outperformed models trained by grouped code vectors. The study shows that data-driven feature representation can be more effective than traditional knowledge-driven feature engineering (Fig. 7.12).

7.5 Case Study: Sequential Clinical Event Prediction

Problem Beyond predicting a specific disease such as HF, RNN has been used to predict all diagnoses and medications at every clinical visit. Choi et al. [23] studied whether the EHR history of patients can provide sufficient information to predict the future diagnoses and medication orders in the next visit. The specific goal is to predict 1183 diagnosis categories, 595 medication groups, and the duration to the next visit based on the patient's historical visits (Fig. 7.13).

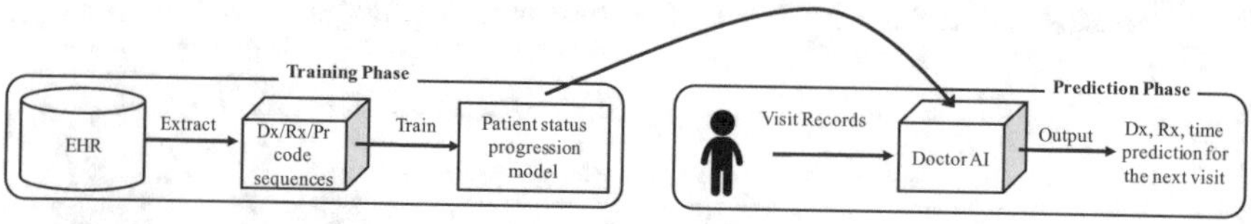

Fig. 7.13 Doctor AI system try to predict future clinical events using RNN

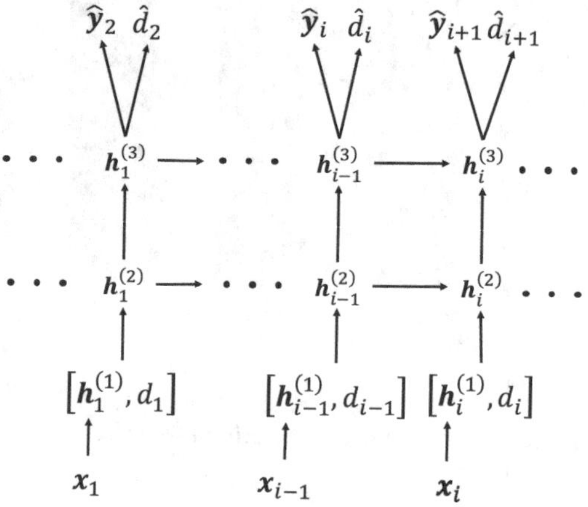

Fig. 7.14 2-layer RNN is applied to predict diagnosis- and medication groups and the time duration to the next visit

Data The dataset is the de-identified structured outpatient EHR data from 265K patients over 8 years from Sutter health, including diagnoses, medications, and procedure information at each visit. On average, each patient has about 55 visits in this dataset.

Method The input is a sequence of clinical visit $(t_i, \boldsymbol{x}_i)$ for $i = 1, \ldots, n$. Each visit pair represents the visit time t_i and visit vector $\boldsymbol{x}_i$ including ICD-9 diagnosis codes, procedure codes, or medication codes documented at t_i. Note that $\boldsymbol{x}_i$ is a multi-hot vector where all the corresponding dimensions of the medical codes documented at t_i will be 1, and other dimensions will be 0. For example, each patient has type-2 diabetes and takes metformin. The dimensions corresponding to type-2 diabetes and metformin will be 1, and others will be 0. Besides multi-hot vector $\boldsymbol{x}_i$, the time duration to the previous visit $d_i = t_i - t_{i-1}$ is also included as part of the input.

An initial embedding is introduced $\boldsymbol{h}_i^{(1)} = [\boldsymbol{x}_i{}^\top \boldsymbol{W}_{emb},\ d_i]$. Then a 2-layer GRU model is applied to process $[\boldsymbol{h}_i^{(1)}, d_i]$. The final output is the prediction of diagnosis and medication groups $\hat{y}_i$ and the duration to the next visit $\hat{d}_{i+1}$ as shown in Fig. 7.14.

Result The performance metrics for predicting diagnoses and medication groups was the top k recall defined as:

$$\text{top-}k \text{ recall} = \frac{\#\text{ of true positives in the top } k \text{ predictions}}{\#\text{ of true positives}}$$

Table 7.2 Accuracy of algorithms in forecasting future medical activities

	Dx,Rx,Time Recall @k			
Algorithms	$k = 10$	$k = 20$	$k = 30$	R^2
Most frequent codes	48.11	60.23	66.00	–
Logistic regression	36.04	46.32	52.53	0.0726
MLP	38.82	49.09	55.74	0.1221
2-layer RNN	**54.96**	**66.31**	**72.48**	**0.2534**

The bold values indicate the best performance numbers across all methods

Top-k recall mimics doctors' behavior conducting a differential diagnosis, where doctors list most probable diagnoses based on the patient's condition.

The performance metric for time duration prediction is the coefficient of determination R^2 as introduced in Eq. (3.12). It compares the accuracy of the prediction for the simple prediction by the mean of the target variable.

$$R^2 = 1 - \frac{\sum_i (y_i - \widehat{y_i})^2}{\sum_i (y_i - \overline{y_i})^2}$$

In addition, they measured the R^2 performance of $\log(d_i)$ instead of d_i directly.

Table 7.2 shows the RNN model outperforms standard classification methods such as logistic regression and simple multi-layer perceptron (MLP). It also demonstrates that simple heuristics such as predicting the most frequent codes in the patient history achieved much lower performance than RNN. Note that the prediction of future diagnosis and medication is much more accurate than the timing of the next visit.

Other important observations in this work include (1) RNN performs better when patients have a long history and (2) knowledge transfer across hospitals is possible with proper initialization of a pre-trained model from another hospital.

7.6 Case Study: De-identification of Clinical Notes

Problem Due to privacy, security, and legal challenges, sharing EHR data for research is hard. A common way to reduce the risk for sharing is to produce de-identified EHR records by removing sensitive protected health information (PHI) such as name, birth date, and address. The most challenging part of de-identification is on unstructured clinical notes as all the information is combined as a free text field. One has to identify the PHI in the notes and remove or replace them, which is time-consuming and extremely tedious and error-prone even for skilled human experts. Dernocourt et al. [36] developed a method to automatically de-identify the clinical notes by identifying then removing or replacing the protected health information (PHI) from the raw text.

Table 7.3 Statistics of the i2b2 and MIMIC-III datasets

Statitics	i2b2	MIMIC-III
Vocabulary size	46,803	69,525
Number of notes	1304	1635
Number of tokens	984,723	2,945,228
Number of PHI instances	28,867	60,725
Number of PHI tokens	41,355	78,633

Table 7.4 Performance comparison on de-identification tasks

	i2b2			MIMIC-III		
Model	Precision	Recall	F1	Precision	Recall	F1
Nottingham	99.000	96.400	97.680	–	–	–
MIST	91.445	92.745	92.090	95.867	98.346	97.091
CRF	98.560	96.528	97.533	99.060	98.987	99.023
RNN	98.320	97.380	97.848	99.208	99.251	99.229
CRF+RNN	97.920	97.835	97.877	98.820	99.398	99.108

Data Two datasets were used in this study: (1) i2b2 data from i2b2/UTHealth shared task Track 1 [140]; and (2) MIMIC-III data contains 61K ICU stays and 2 million clinical notes [82]. The detailed statistics are shown in Table 7.3.

Method The proposed model in [36] involves two bidirectional LSTMs: One for the character-level to extract features based on character combinations; The other one is based on the word-level plus the output embedding from the character-level bidirectional LSTM. The final PHI prediction is on each word.

Results Table 7.4 presents the performance on the test set in terms of precision, recall, and F1 score. Baselines include Nottingham (the winner of that i2b2 competition) [171], MITRE Identification Scrubber Toolkit (MIST)—the freely available program for de-identification and Conditional Random Field (CRF)—a popular method for sequential labeling. RNN is the neural network model. CRF+RNN concatenates the outputs of both CRF and RNN models. CRF+RNN provides the highest recall with a small sacrifice on precision because any token in the document will be marked as PHI if either CRF or RNN model considered that token as PHI.

7.7 Case Study: Learning to Prescribe Treatment Combination for Multimorbidity

Problem Managing patients with complex multimorbidity has long been recognized as a difficult problem due to complex disease and medication dependencies and the potential risk of adverse drug interactions. In this work [174], the authors studies the medication recommendation problem based on the list of diagnoses within a visit.

Data *MIMIC-3* The MIMIC-3 dataset [81] is a publicly available dataset consisting of medical records of 40K intensive care unit (ICU) patients over 11 years. It consists of 50,206 medical encounter records that associated with 6695 distinct diseases and 4127 drugs.

Sutter This dataset from Sutter Palo Alto Medical Foundation (PAMF) consists of 18-years longitudinal medical records of 258K patients between age 50 and 90. It contains 2,415,414 medical encounters associated with 8359 distinct diseases and 7516 drugs. Average number of diseases and drugs per record are 2.97 and 1.75 respectively.

Drugs in Sutter and MIMIC-3 are encoded using GPI[1] and NDC[2] codes, respectively. The GPI coding is inherently a multi-level ontology that identifies drugs from their primary therapeutic use down to unique interchangeable product regardless of manufacturer or package size. To conduct experiments at different granularity, we use the first and third level of GPI codes, resulting 93 and 982 distinct drug groups, respectively. We convert drugs in MIMIC-3 to GPI code using an open-source software from OHDSI.[3] The diagnoses in both datasets are represented using ICD-9 code.[4] In order to learn robust and nontrivial mapping between diseases and medications, We extract the records from each dataset with more than two diagnosis codes and filtered the records to include only top 2000 most common diagnosis codes, which covers 95.3% of all records (Fig. 7.15).

Method The authors in [174] use a seq2seq model from the diagnosis list to predict the medication list at each clinical visit. They further leverage reinforcement learning to fine tune the model parameters to ensure accuracy and completeness. They also incorporate external clinical knowledge into the design of the reinforcement reward to effectively prevent generating unfavorable drug combinations.

Let $\mathcal{X}$ denote the diagnosis space and $\mathcal{Y}$ denote the medication space. $\mathbf{R} = \{(X_1, Y_1), (X_2, Y_2), ...\}$ is a set of medical records where $X_k \subseteq \mathcal{X}$ is a diagnosis set $X_k = \{x_1^k, x_2^k, ..., x_{|X_k|}^k\}$ and $Y_k \subseteq \mathcal{Y}$ is a medication set $Y_k = \{y_1^k, y_2^k, ..., y_{|Y_k|}^k\}$, where $|X_k|$ and $|Y_k|$ are the cardinalities of X_k and Y_k, respectively. To avoid clutter, we omit k in the notation if there is no ambiguity. The objective of treatment recommendation is to select an optimal set of medications Y from all medications $\mathcal{Y}$ based on a diagnosis set X. Thus, we want to model the conditional probability $p(Y|X)$ and find the maximum likelihood solution Y^* (Fig. 7.15).

[1] http://www.wolterskluwercdi.com/drug-data/medi-span-electronic-drug-file/.

[2] http://www.fda.gov/Drugs/InformationOnDrugs/ucm142438.htm.

[3] http://www.ohdsi.org/.

[4] http://www.icd9data.com/2015/Volume1/default.htm.

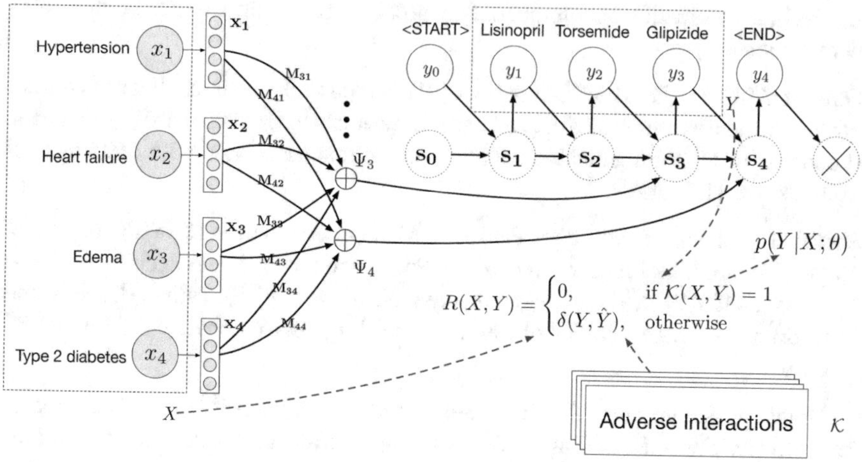

Fig. 7.15 An overview of our solution for treatment recommendation. Gray nodes indicate input diagnoses, white nodes denote output treatments, dashed nodes are state variables

Formally, the conditional probability of Y given X is decomposed as

$$p(Y|X) = \prod_{t=1}^{|Y|} p(y_t|X, y_1, y_2, ..., y_{t-1})$$

$$= \prod_{t=1}^{|Y|} p(y_t|\{x_1, x_2, ..., x_{|X|}\}, y_1, y_2, ..., y_{t-1}),$$

where x_i is the i-th diagnosis code in X and y_t is the t-th medication being selected, $\{...\}$ indicates a set of discrete instances. Each diagnosis x_i in X is $|\mathcal{X}|$-dimensional one hot vector and each medication y_t in Y is a $|\mathcal{Y}|$-dimensional one hot vector. We use distributed representation to encode both diagnosis and medications, that is, we leverage embedding matrix $\mathbf{W}_\mathcal{X}$ and $\mathbf{W}_\mathcal{Y}$ to project diagnosis x_i and medication y_j into a unified d-dimensional space. We use vector $\mathbf{x}_i, \mathbf{y_j} \in \mathbb{R}^d$ to denote the embedding of x_i and y_j respectively, where

$$\mathbf{x}_i = \mathbf{W}_\mathcal{X} x_i, \quad \mathbf{y_j} = \mathbf{W}_\mathcal{Y} y_i.$$

To model different degrees of contribution of each $x_i \in X$ to medication y_t at step t we leverage the attention mechanism. Let $\mathbf{s}_t \in \mathbb{R}^d$ be a variable summarizing the state at step t.

$$\mathbf{s}_t = g(\mathbf{s}_{t-1}, y_{t-1}, \Psi_t(X))$$

where $\Psi_t(\cdot)$ is an attention function that encode the compatibility between each $\mathbf{x}_i$ and the current state variable.

$$\Psi_t(X) = \sum_{i=1}^{|X|} \mathbf{M}_{ti}\mathbf{x}_i,$$

where $\mathbf{M} \in \mathbb{R}^{|X|\times|Y|}$ is an mapping matrix, in which each element $\mathbf{M}_{ti}$ indicates the contribution of the i-th diagnosis code x_i to generating the t-th medication y_t. We formulate mapping matrix $\mathbf{M}$ as

$$\mathbf{M}_{ti} = \frac{\exp(\alpha(\mathbf{x}_i, \mathbf{s}_{t-1}))}{\sum_{k=1}^{|X|} \exp(\alpha(\mathbf{x}_k, \mathbf{s}_{t-1}))}$$

where $\alpha(\mathbf{x}_i, \mathbf{s}_{t-1})$ is a function determines the weight for the i-th diagnosis code. $\alpha(\mathbf{x}, \mathbf{y})$ is implemented as a MLP that takes the concatenation of $\mathbf{x}$ and $\mathbf{y}$ as input. Now we can rewrite $\mathbf{s}_t$ as

$$\mathbf{s}_t = g([\Psi_t(X); \mathbf{y}_{t-1}], \mathbf{s}_{t-1})$$

where $[\cdot;\cdot]$ denotes the concatenation of two vectors, g can be defined as a RNN unit (e.g. we used GRU in our implementation). The prediction at step t is given by

$$y_t = \arg\max_{y\in\mathcal{Y}} \text{softmax}(\mathbf{s}_t).$$

Result LEAP were compared with the following baselines:

- *Rule-based:* This method recommends drugs based on an existing drug to disease mapping from the MEDI database [165]. For each disease, one of the drugs mentioned in the mapping is assigned.
- *K-Most frequent:* This is a simple baseline that retrieves the top K medications that most frequently co-occur with each disease as their treatment. We set $K = 1$ on Sutter dataset and $K = 3$ on MIMIC-3 dataset according to the performance on validate set.[5]
- *Softmax MLP:* We learn a multi-label classifier using a multi-layer perceptron with softmax output layer. Our implementation uses a 3-layer MLP. A global threshold is used to select positive medications. The value of the threshold and hyper parameters are tuned on a validation set using grid search.
- *Classifier Chains:* Classifier Chains [122] is a popular multi-label learning method that models the correlation between labels by a feeding both input and previous classification results into the latter classifiers. We use a multi-hot vector to encode input diagnosis set X and leverage SVM as binary classifiers for each label.

[5] It makes intuitive sense because patients in MIMIC-3 are sicker and usually require more medications as they visited the intensive care unit.

Table 7.5 Treatment recommendation performance on Sutter and MIMIC3 dataset. We evaluate the experimental results in terms of Jaccard Coefficient. Granularity indicates the level of GPI medication code we are using

	Sutter		MIMIC-3	
Granularity	1	3	1	3
Rule-based	0.3207	0.2770	0.2753	0.2354
K-most frequent	0.4283	0.3181	0.2609	0.2616
Softmax MLP	0.4908	0.3739	0.4897	0.3342
Classifier chains	0.4839	0.3620	0.4621	0.3204
LEAP w/o RL	0.5270	0.3936	0.5107	0.3865
LEAP	**0.5341**	**0.4073**	**0.5582**	**0.4342**

The bold values indicate the best performance numbers across all methods

Evaluation Metric Assume Y_i is the treatment set generated by the algorithm, and $\hat{Y}^i$ is the doctor prescription in the data. The Jaccard coefficient is defined as the size of the intersection divided by the size of the union of ground truth label set and predicted label set.

$$\text{Jaccard} = \frac{1}{K}\sum_{i}^{K}\frac{|Y_i \cap \hat{Y}_i|}{|Y_i \cup \hat{Y}_i|},$$

where K is the number of samples in test set (Table 7.5).

Quantitative experiments are conducted on two real world electronic health record datasets to verify the effectiveness of our solution. On both datasets, LEAP significantly outperforms baselines by up to 10–30% in terms of mean Jaccard coefficient (Table 7.5).

7.8 Exercises

1. What is the main difference between RNN and bidirectional RNN?
2. What is the main difference between LSTM and GRU?
3. What data are suitable for RNN to model? [multiple correct choices]
   (a) Clinical notes
   (b) Medical images
   (c) Longitudinal medical records
   (d) Time series such as electrocardiogram
4. Which of the following architectures is best for sequential diagnosis prediction is(i.e., predicting the disease diagnosis of the current visit based on a patient's visit history) as illustrated in Fig. 7.2?
5. What are the potential issues of backpropagation through time (BPTT) algorithm?

6. In the GRU model, can we replace tanh activation function with sigmoid activation in Eq. (7.14)? Why?
7. What is NOT true about bidirectional RNNs?
   (a) Two RNN models are trained from the opposite directions?
   (b) Hidden states of two RNNs are concatenated before predicting the output
   (c) Bidirectional RNNs are suitable for modeling languages.
   (d) Two RNN models have to be trained separately.
8. What is NOT true about the Seq2seq model?
   (a) Seq2seq model requires training two RNNs: one for encoding and another for decoding.
   (b) Seq2seq models can be used for machine translation applications.
   (c) Encoder RNN produces a context vector c which will be used as part of the input in the decoder RNN.
   (d) Seq2seq model ensures input sequence and output sequence to be the same length.
9. Which of the following is NOT true about RNN applications to healthcare?
   (a) We need training data of the same length to train RNN models.
   (b) RNN model can be used to model longitudinal EHR data.
   (c) The output of RNN models can be binary or multi-class classification.
   (d) RNN can also be used to model clinical notes.

Chapter 8
Autoencoders (AE)

8.1 Overview

So far, we have presented various deep learning models for supervised learning where output labels (e.g., heart failure diagnosis) are available in the training data. However, unlabeled data are the norm in many real-world applications. Next, we introduce the autoencoder, which is a popular unsupervised deep learning model.

In general, the autoencoder (AE) is an unsupervised and nonlinear dimensionality reduction model, which is widely used in many healthcare applications [5, 13, 94, 104, 113, 143, 144, 173]. An autoencoder maps inputs to an internal representation via an encoder and then maps the internal representation back to the input space through a decoder. The composition of encoder and decoder is called the reconstruction function. The autoencoder's objective tries to minimize the reconstruction loss, thus allowing AEs to focus on essential properties of the data while reducing the dimensionality.

Sparse autoencoders (SAE) and denoising autoencoders (DAE) are two AE variants. For SAE, the reconstruction loss is regularized via a sparsity penalty on internal representation so that the model tries to learn sparse representation. SAE was often used for unsupervised EHR phenotyping [94] or sparse EEG feature representation [100, 170, 173]. DAE introduces randomly corrupted inputs, through which the model would gain robustness towards missing data or noises. DAE was used for learning robust representations of patient phenotypes from EHRs [5, 13, 113]. In the summary, we will introduce several AEs, including stacked autoencoders, sparse autoencoders, denoising autoencoders and their healthcare applications (Table 8.1).

C. Xiao, J. Sun, *Introduction to Deep Learning for Healthcare*,
https://doi.org/10.1007/978-3-030-82184-5_8

Table 8.1 Notations for autoencoders

Notation	Definition
$\boldsymbol{x} \in \mathbb{R}^d$; X	Input vector; random variable of input data distribution
$\boldsymbol{h} \in \mathbb{R}^k$	Hidden layer
s_t	Hidden state at time t
$\boldsymbol{r}$; R	Reconstructed data; reconstructed data distribution

8.2 Autoencoders

An autoencoder is a neural network that aims to reconstruct the input data via a nonlinear dimensionality reduction. Formally, an autoencoder includes an encoder and a decoder:

- *Encoder* $f_\theta()$ transforms an input vector $\boldsymbol{x} \in \mathbb{R}^d$ into a hidden layer $\boldsymbol{h} \in \mathbb{R}^k$ (usually $k < d$):

$$\boldsymbol{h} = f_\theta(\boldsymbol{x}) = \sigma_1(\boldsymbol{W}\boldsymbol{x} + \boldsymbol{b})$$

  where $\boldsymbol{W} \in \mathbb{R}^{k\times d}$ is weight matrix, $\boldsymbol{b} \in \mathbb{R}^k$ is a bias vector and σ_1 is the input activation function.
- *Decoder* $g_{\theta'}()$ maps the hidden representation $\boldsymbol{h} \in \mathbb{R}^k$ back to a reconstructed vector

$$\boldsymbol{r} = g_{\theta'}(\boldsymbol{h}) = \sigma_2(\boldsymbol{W}'\boldsymbol{h} + \boldsymbol{b}')$$

  where $\boldsymbol{W'} \in \mathbb{R}^{d\times k}$ is weight matrix, $\boldsymbol{b'} \in \mathbb{R}^d$ is a bias vector and σ_2 the output activation function.

The procedure of encoding and decoding is depicted in Fig. 8.1. The encoder and the decoder are parameterized by $\theta = \{\boldsymbol{W}, \boldsymbol{b}\}$ and $\theta' = \{\boldsymbol{W}', \boldsymbol{b}'\}$, respectively. Note that without the nonlinear transformation σ_1, σ_2, the process becomes linear dimensionality reduction similar to Principal Component Analysis (PCA).

In general, the objective of AE is min $L(\boldsymbol{x}, \boldsymbol{r})$, where $L(\boldsymbol{x}, \boldsymbol{r}) \propto -\log p(\boldsymbol{x}|\boldsymbol{r})$. Here $L(\cdot)$ is a loss function such as squared error or cross-entropy loss. The choice of the loss function depends on the distribution of $\boldsymbol{x}$.

1. If $\boldsymbol{x} \in \mathbb{R}^d$ is a real-value vector following normal distribution, that is $\boldsymbol{x} \sim \mathcal{N}(\boldsymbol{r}, \sigma^2\boldsymbol{I})$, the squared loss $L(\boldsymbol{x}, \boldsymbol{r}) = ||\boldsymbol{x} - \boldsymbol{r}||^2$ is preferred.
2. If $\boldsymbol{x}$ is binary-valued, the decoder needs to produce a $\boldsymbol{r} \in \{0, 1\}^d$. Thus a sigmoid activation will typically be used in the decoder. This yields the choice of cross-entropy loss: $L(\boldsymbol{x}, \boldsymbol{r}) = -\sum_i [\boldsymbol{x}_i \log \boldsymbol{r}_i + (1 - \boldsymbol{x}_i) \log(1 - \boldsymbol{r}_i)]$.

In general, the formulation of autoencoders is an empirical risk optimization.

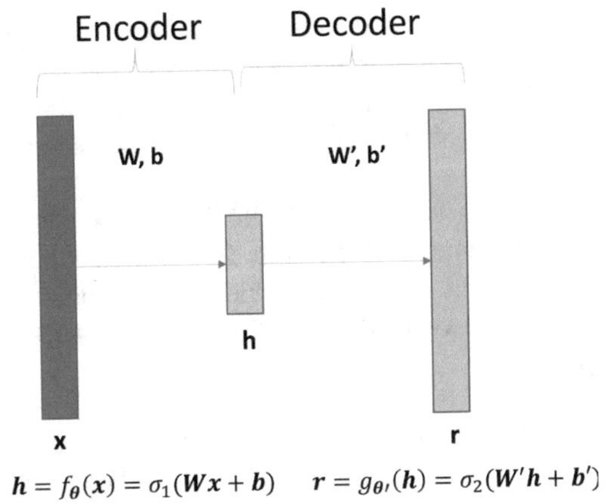

Fig. 8.1 Autoencoder model illustration

$$\hat{R}(f_\theta, g_{\theta'}, \boldsymbol{x}) = \sum_{i=1}^{n} L(\boldsymbol{x}_i, g_{\theta'}(f_\theta(\boldsymbol{x}_i)))$$

where $\boldsymbol{x}_i$ is the i-th input data point and $g_{\theta'}(f_\theta(\boldsymbol{x}_i))$ the reconstruction of $\boldsymbol{x}_i$.

To avoid overfitting or to enhance sparsity, we can add regularization on the model parameters θ or θ'.

$$\hat{R}_\lambda(f_\theta, g_{\theta'}, \boldsymbol{x}) = \sum_{i=1}^{n} L(\boldsymbol{x}_i, g_{\theta'}(f_\theta(\boldsymbol{x}_i))) + \lambda\Omega. \tag{8.1}$$

where Ω is the regularization function and $\lambda \geq 0$ is the regularization weight. For example, L1 regularization $\Omega = \sum |f_\theta(\boldsymbol{x}_i)|$ to impose sparsity constraint on the latent activations, or Kullback–Leibler divergence to penalize excessive activations which we will discuss below.

8.3 Sparse Autoencoders

Sparse autoencoders (SAE) [115] aim at imposing a sparsity constraint on the hidden layer of AEs. The idea is to have fewer neurons activated when applying to the input. The SAE constrains the neurons to be inactive most of the time (i.e., most neurons' output is 0). Specifically, we assume the activation function of hidden units is sigmoid, which means the output is between 0 and 1. We also denote $\hat{\rho}_j$ be the average activation of hidden unit j (averaged over all n data points) such that

$$\hat{\rho}_j = \frac{1}{n}\sum_{i=1}^{n} h_j[i]$$

where $h_j[i]$ represents the j-th hidden unit of the input data point i.

The SAE tries to enforce the constraint $\hat{\rho}_j = \rho$ where ρ is a sparsity parameter. For example, we can set the sparse parameter to be 0.05, which means each hidden unit is activated on 5% of the data points and is zero on 95% of the remaining data points.

To achieve this goal, the SAE adds a penalty term to the AE objective to penalize $\hat{\rho}_j$ that deviates significantly from ρ, and the penalty term that is mostly chosen is based on the Kullback–Leibler (KL) divergence $\mathcal{D}_{\mathrm{KL}}$ between $\hat{\rho}_j$ and ρ as given below. The total (KL) divergence $\mathcal{D}_{\mathrm{KL}}$ between $\hat{\rho}_j$ and ρ across all k hidden units is given by

$$\sum_{j=1}^{k} \mathcal{D}_{KL}(\rho||\hat{\rho}_j) = \sum_{j=1}^{k}(\rho \log \frac{\rho}{\hat{\rho}_j} + (1-\rho) \log \frac{1-\rho}{1-\hat{\rho}_j})$$

where k is the number of neurons in this hidden layer. Since the KL divergence reaches its minimum of 0 when $\hat{\rho}_j = p$ and grows to ∞ as $\hat{\rho}_j$ approaches 0 or 1, this penalty term based on KL can effectively enforce $\hat{\rho}_j$ to be close to ρ.

With the aforementioned penalty term, the new objective for SAE is given below.

$$\arg\min_{\theta,\theta'} \frac{1}{n} \sum_{i=1}^{n} L(\boldsymbol{x}_i, \boldsymbol{r}_i) + \gamma \sum_{j=1}^{k} \mathcal{D}_{KL}(\rho||\hat{\rho}_j) \tag{8.2}$$

where γ is the regularization weight and $\sum_{j=1}^{k} \mathcal{D}_{KL}(\rho||\hat{\rho}_j)$ is the sparsity regularization on the hidden units.

8.4 Stacked Autoencoders

When multiple autoencoders are stacked together such that outputs of each layer are used as inputs of the next layer, we have the stacked autoencoders. Formally, consider an autoencoder with K layers. Stacked autoencoders perform the encoding step by running each layer's encoding step in forward order and perform decoding by running each layer's decoding step in backward order. Given K layers of encoders and decoders each, we have the following formulation:

- *Encoder* of the first layer $f_\theta^{(1)}()$ transforms an input vector $\boldsymbol{x} \in \mathbb{R}^d$ into a hidden layer $\boldsymbol{h}^{(1)}$.

$$\boldsymbol{h}^{(1)} = f_\theta^{(1)}(\boldsymbol{x}) = \sigma_1(\mathbf{W}^{(1)}\boldsymbol{x} + \boldsymbol{b}^{(1)}).$$

Then the encoder of the k-th layer $f_\theta^{(k)}()$ transforms the output from the previous layer $\boldsymbol{h}^{(k-1)}$ into next hidden layer $\boldsymbol{h}^{(k)}$:

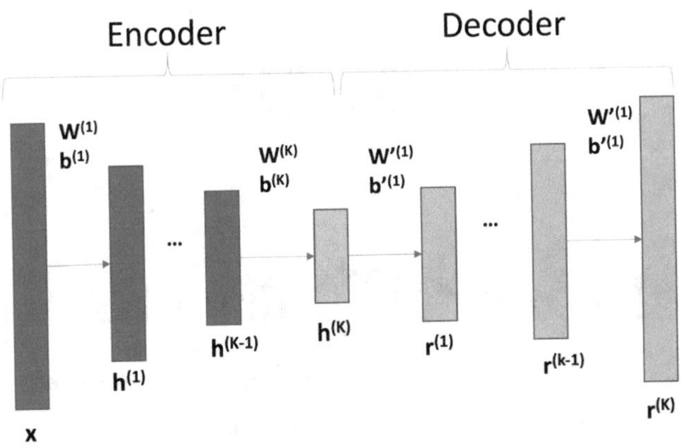

Fig. 8.2 Stacked autoencoder model of K layers

$$\boldsymbol{h}^{(k)} = f_\theta^{(k)}(\boldsymbol{x}) = \sigma_1(\boldsymbol{W}^{(k)}\boldsymbol{h}^{(k-1)} + \boldsymbol{b}^{(k)}).$$

- The initial input to the first layer decoder is the hidden representation from the K-th layer encoder, i.e., $\boldsymbol{r}^{(0)} = \boldsymbol{h}^{(K)}$. In general, the *decoder* of the k-th layer $g_{\theta'}^{(k)}()$ maps the hidden representation from the previous reconstruction layer $\boldsymbol{r}^{(k-1)}$ back to the next reconstruction vector:

$$\boldsymbol{r}^{(k)} = g_{\theta'}^{(k)}(\boldsymbol{r}^{(k-1)}) = \sigma_2(\boldsymbol{W'}^{(k)}\boldsymbol{r}^{(k-1)} + \boldsymbol{b'}^{(k)}).$$

8.5 Denoising Autoencoders

In [163], the authors proposed denoising autoencoders (DAE), which can learn more robust representation against noisy input. The idea is to add noises to the original input $\boldsymbol{x}$ to obtain corrupted version $\tilde{\boldsymbol{x}}$ and then try to reconstruct clean uncorrupted input $\boldsymbol{x}$ from noisy input $\tilde{\boldsymbol{x}}$ (Fig. 8.3).

- First, we corrupt the initial input $\boldsymbol{x}$ to obtain $\tilde{\boldsymbol{x}}$ by means of a stochastic mapping $\tilde{\boldsymbol{x}} \sim q_D(\tilde{\boldsymbol{x}}|\boldsymbol{x})$. Different types of noises can be created: (1) random Gaussian noises at all locations, (2) masking noises (a small number of locations are set to 0), (3) salt-and-pepper noises (a small number of locations are set to 0 or 1 at random).
- Then we pass the corrupted input $\tilde{\boldsymbol{x}}$ through a standard encoder:

$$\boldsymbol{h} = f_\theta(\tilde{\boldsymbol{x}}) = \sigma(\boldsymbol{W}\tilde{\boldsymbol{x}} + \boldsymbol{b})$$

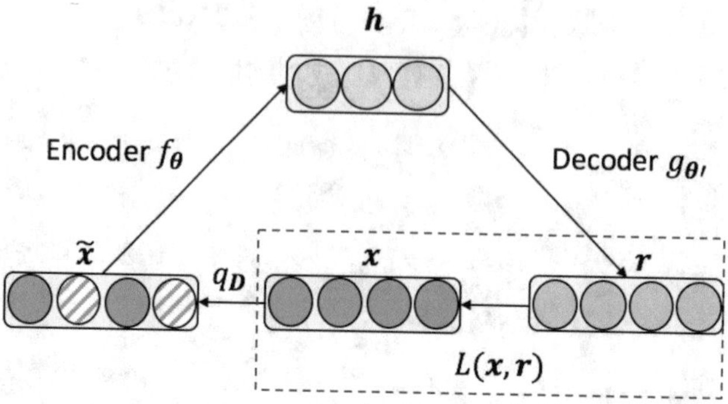

Fig. 8.3 A schematic representation of denoising autoencoders. The input data is stochastically corrupted via q_D to $\tilde{\boldsymbol{x}}$. It then be mapped to $\boldsymbol{h}$ via encoder f_θ and tries to reconstruct $\boldsymbol{x}$ via decoder $g_{\theta'}$ and produces reconstruction $\boldsymbol{r}$. The reconstruction error is measured by $L(\boldsymbol{x}, \boldsymbol{r})$

- Finally, the decoder will try to map $\boldsymbol{h}$ back to a reconstructed vector that is close to the original uncorrupted input $\boldsymbol{x}$:

$$\boldsymbol{r} = g_{\theta'}(\boldsymbol{h}) = \sigma(\boldsymbol{W}'\boldsymbol{h} + \boldsymbol{b}')$$

Note that denoising autoencoders try to minimize the reconstruction loss between the original $\boldsymbol{x}$ and the reconstruction $\boldsymbol{r}$ from the corrupted $\tilde{\boldsymbol{x}}$.

8.6 Case Study: "Deep Patient" via Stacked Denoising Autoencoders

Problem How to derive a general-purpose feature representation from EHR data? Authors of "Deep Patient" compared several unsupervised feature construction methods, including Stacked Denoising Autoencoders (SDA) for supporting predictive modeling tasks [113].

Data In "deep patient", patient representations were learned based on the EHR data from the Mount Sinai hospital and evaluated using disease classification and prediction tasks. In particular, the dataset includes over 700k patients with up to 12 years of patient history. The raw data include structured data such as diagnoses (ICD-9 codes), medications, procedures, lab tests, and unstructured clinical text. The clinical notes are processed with Open Biomedical Annotator [132]. They used the number of occurrences of all the events in their EHR data as the raw feature values. All the feature values were then normalized to lie between zero and one to reduce the data variance while preserving zero entries.

Table 8.2 Disease classification results in terms of area under the ROC curve (AUC-ROC), accuracy and F-score. The difference with the corresponding second best measurement is statistically significant

Patient representation	ROC-AUC	Accuracy	F-1
Raw feature	0.659	0.805	0.084
PCA	0.696	0.879	0.104
GMM	0.632	0.891	0.072
K-means	0.672	0.887	0.093
ICA	0.695	0.882	0.101
Deep patient	**0.773**	**0.929**	**0.181**

The bold values indicate the best performance numbers across all methods

Method A 3-layer stacked denoising autoencoders were used to process input feature vectors of patients in an unsupervised manner. In particular, 500 hidden units per layer are used for each layer. Then 5% random input locations were set to 0 for each layer. This can be viewed as simulating the presence of missed components in the EHRs (e.g., medications or diagnoses not recorded in the patient records), thus assuming that the input clinical data is a degraded or "noisy" version of the actual clinical situation. Sigmoid activations are used. Next, the learned encoding function is applied to the clean input, and the resulting hidden layer is the final patient representation. As a result, each patient was represented by a dense vector of 500 features.

Result The output of the stacked denoising autoencoder was compared with other well-known feature learning algorithms and demonstrated utility in various tasks. In particular, the following algorithms were used as baselines, including principal component analysis (PCA) with 100 principal components, k-means clustering with 500 clusters, Gaussian mixture model with 200 mixtures and full the covariance matrix, and independent component analysis with 100 principal components.

Then random forest classifiers were implemented to predict the probability that patients might develop a certain disease given their current clinical status using the learned features on a separate dataset of 200,000 patients. The training and evaluation follow a one-vs-all strategy. Prediction result performance was listed in Table 8.2. The main finding is that Deep Patient (i.e., DAE) significantly outperformed the unsupervised methods in the classification tasks. This result confirmed the DAE as an effective method for feature engineering from EHR data.

8.7 Case Study: Learning from Noisy, Sparse, and Irregular Clinical Data

Problem The study in [94] targeted unbiased deep phenotype discovery using large-scale EHR data. The paper argues that standard deep learning on its own cannot reliably learn compact longitudinal features from the noisy, sparse, and irregular observations typically existed in EHRs. To bridge the gap, this work first applied Gaussian process regression to transform the irregularly sampled lab results

(i.e., serum uric acid in this case) into a continuous longitudinal probability density over time and then learn phenotypes using sparse autoencoder (SAE) over the output of Gaussian process regression.

Data The data used in this work was extracted from Vanderbilt's Synthetic Derivative, a deidentified mirror of their production EHR. This mirror contains over 15 years of longitudinal clinical data on over 2 million individuals. The authors identified 4368 records of individuals with either gout or acute leukemia, but not both. We extracted the full sequence of uric acid values and measurement times from each record and associated it with the appropriate disease label. The disease label served as the reference standard for downstream evaluation but was not used in the feature learning. Roughly a third of the records were set aside as a final test set.

Method The paper proposed a framework consisting of the following two steps: the transformation step and the feature learning step. The transformation step assumed that there was an unobserved source function for each individual that represented the true uric acid concentration over time, and considered each uric acid sequence to be a set of possibly noisy samples taken from that source function. The authors use Gaussian process regression to learn the continuous uric acid function from limited samples of the lab results.

A sliding window of 30 days was applied on daily resampled data to construct patches in the feature learning step. A two-layer stacked sparse autoencoder was then trained on patches of 30-day long where the inputs are 30-dimensional vectors. The reason for using sparse autoencoder is to learn sparse features that will be used as new phenotypes.

To evaluate the effectiveness of the proposed method, three tasks were evaluated: (1) the face validity of the learned features as low-level, high-resolution phenotypes, (2) their ability to illuminate unknown disease population subtypes, and (3) their accuracy in distinguishing between disease phenotype signatures known to exist in the data but which were unknown to the feature learning algorithm.

Result To assess the quality of the learned features, they were evaluated using a supervised classification task unknown to the feature-learning algorithm. Since the features were not optimized for the evaluation task, the task serves as a generalized performance test. They were compared with expert features, which were optimized for the specific task. The selected learning task was to distinguish the known gout vs. leukemia phenotypes using only the uric acid sequences. The selected classification algorithm was logistic regression because a simple linear classifier is more likely to illuminate differences in feature quality than a more sophisticated algorithm.

Four supervised classifiers were trained for comparison: (1) a classifier using first-layer learned features, (2) a classifier using second-layer learned features, (3) a gold-standard classifier using expert-engineered features, (4) a baseline classifier using the sequence means as the only input feature. The first two classifiers evaluated the learned features. The gold-standard classifier was intended to estimate the upper-bound performance for the task. The baseline classifier was intended to

Table 8.3 Unsupervised features were as powerful as expert engineered features in distinguishing uric acid sequences from gout vs. leukemia

Classifier	AUC (training)	AUC [CI] (test)
First-layer learned features	0.969	0.972 [0.968, 0.979]
Second-layer learned features	0.965	0.972 [0.968, 0.979]
Expert engineered features	0.968	0.974 [0.966, 0.981]
Baseline (sequence mean only)	0.922	0.932 [0.922, 0.944]

establish how well a single basic feature can do on the task. Gout and leukemia disease labels were used as the class labels for all classifiers.

The performance was evaluated using the area under the Receiver Operating Characteristic curve (AUC) on a held-out test set. The experiment shows that features generated using Gaussian process regression followed by sparse autoencoders can achieve similar predictive performance as the expert features shown in Table 8.3.

8.8 Exercises

1. What are the main difference between autoencoder and principal component analysis?
2. What is the main difference between autoencoder and denoising autoencoder?
3. What is the most analogous method to Autoencoders?

   (a) K-means clustering
   (b) Principal component analysis
   (c) Support vector machine
   (d) Hierarchical clustering

4. Which of the following is NOT true about autoencoders?

   (a) It is an unsupervised method.
   (b) It is a lossless compression technique.
   (c) It is a dimensionality reduction method.
   (d) It is a feedforward neural network.

5. What is NOT true about sparse autoencoder?

   (a) It introduces sparsity in the latent code **h**.
   (b) Sigmoid activation function is used to produce latent code **h**.
   (c) The same loss function to the standard autoencoder is used for sparse autoencoder.
   (d) Sparsity level on each dimension of h needs to be specified.

6. What is NOT true about denoising autoencoder?
   (a) It adds random noise to the original input before applying the autoencoder model.
   (b) Its loss function is between reconstruction and the original input x without adding random noise.
   (c) It is more expensive to train because of random noise added to the original input.
   (d) It is more robust against noises thanks to the introduction of corrupted input.
7. What are the model parameters first learned in a stacked autoencoder as illustrated in Fig. 8.2?
8. What is NOT true about stacked autoencoder?
   (a) It applies multiple encoders first, then applies the corresponding decoders in reverse orders.
   (b) It is a deep neural network of 2K layers where K is the number of autoencoders.
   (c) It is trained in an end-to-end fashion as a single model using backpropagation.
   (d) It is trained sequentially as K separate autoencoders.
9. What other model is used before applying autoencoder in the phenotype discovery paper [94]?
10. Question 8 What is the variant of autoencoder model used in deep patient paper [113]?

Chapter 9
Attention Models

9.1 Overview

Accuracy and interpretability are two desirable properties of successful predictive models. Most of deep learning models try to achieve high accuracy without much consideration of interpretability. The attention mechanism is one rare occasion that allows neural network models to achieve both accuracy and interpretability [2]. Various attention mechanisms have been applied to EHR data [25, 28, 73, 174]. Furthermore, *attention mechanism* plays an essential role in many advanced neural network models such as memory networks and transformers, which will be discussed in Chap. 11.

9.2 Attention Mechanism

Beyond DNN, CNN, and RNN, the attention mechanism is another fundamental breakthrough in deep learning. It is a general strategy that can lead to many modeling variations. Next, we will introduce the key concepts of the attention mechanism and its healthcare applications.

Attention Based on Encoder-Decoder RNN Models The attention mechanism was originally proposed for improving sequence-to-sequence models with machine translation application. In particular, a sequence of words in a source language is mapped into a sequence of words in a target language, usually of different lengths [2]. For EHR modeling, attention mechanism can help explain the degree of relevancy between clinical events and target outcomes, e.g., [25, 28, 174].

The attention model extends the sequence-to-sequence (seq2seq) models using two RNNs as described in Sect. 7.3.4. In the original seq2seq model, the encoder RNN will map the input sequence into a fixed-length context variable $\boldsymbol{c}$. This "static"

C. Xiao, J. Sun, *Introduction to Deep Learning for Healthcare*,
https://doi.org/10.1007/978-3-030-82184-5_9

context variable $\boldsymbol{c}$ will be passed into each step of the decoder RNN to generate the output sequence. However, such seq2seq models have limited capacity in modeling long sequences as the information of the entire input has to be compressed into a single static context variable $\boldsymbol{c}$ [20].

Attention mechanism allows a "dynamic" context variable $\boldsymbol{c}$, which provides alignment and translation between source and target sequences. By optimizing alignment, the model aims to identify which parts of the source sequence are relevant to generate a given word in the target sequence. The translation optimization then combines the relevant information from the input sequence into a dynamic context variable for each output word.

The design of an attention model involves the following components:

1. **Annotation vectors** refer to the encoding of the input sequence;
2. **Alignment model** measures the relevance between pairs of input and output positions;
3. **Attention weight** is how much attention to the input words should be given when producing each output word;
4. **Context vector** is the dynamic summary of the input depending on the current output position.

Table 9.1 shows notations used in attention modeling.

Annotation Vector $\boldsymbol{h}$ To start with, we will first encode input sequence $\boldsymbol{x}$ into vectors $(\boldsymbol{h}_1, \cdots, \boldsymbol{h}_{T_x})$ for each input time step. In [2], the encoded inputs are referred to as "annotations" for each time step.

$$(\boldsymbol{h}_1, \cdots, \boldsymbol{h}_{T_x}) = \text{Encoder}(\boldsymbol{x}_1, \cdots, \boldsymbol{x}_{T_x})$$

The encoder can be an RNN (e.g., bidirectional LSTM [2]) or a CNN as in [53].

Table 9.1 Notations for attention mechanism

Notation	Definition
$\boldsymbol{x} = (x_1, \cdots, x_{T_x})$	Input sequence of length T_x
$\boldsymbol{h}, \boldsymbol{h}_i$	Annotation vector in general; ith annotation vector
$\boldsymbol{c}, \boldsymbol{c}_i$	Context vector in general; ith context vector
s_t	Hidden state at time t
$\boldsymbol{y} = (y_1, \cdots, y_{T_y})$	Output sequence of length T_y
$a()$	Alignment model (parameterized by a neural network)
a_{ij}	Attention weight of input word j for generating output word i
$I(\boldsymbol{x})$	Input feature map
$\boldsymbol{m}_i$	ith memory slot
$\boldsymbol{o}$	Output feature map
$\boldsymbol{r}$	Final response (decoded output)

Alignment Model $a(\cdot)$ To quantify the alignment between input and output, the alignment model e_{ij} measures how well the input around position j and the output at position i match. In particular, e_{ij} measures the relevance between the output hidden state $\boldsymbol{s}_{i-1}$ and the input annotation vector $\boldsymbol{h}_j$ at position j, which denotes as

$$e_{ij} = a(\boldsymbol{s}_{i-1}, \boldsymbol{h}_j).$$

Sometimes, we also refer to the output as the *query* and all the input as the *keys* and the final output embedding as the *value*. The reason is that the attention mechanism is analogous to similarity search, where the terminologies of a query, keys, and values is natural. These terms will be revisited later in Chap. 11 when we introduce memory networks.

The annotation function $a(\cdot)$ can be parameterized in several different ways:

- **Dot-product attention:** If $\boldsymbol{s}_{i-1}$ and $\boldsymbol{h}_j$ are of the same length, we can use simple inner product

$$a(\boldsymbol{s}_{i-1}, \boldsymbol{h}_j) = \boldsymbol{s}_{i-1}^\top \boldsymbol{h}_j;$$

- **General dot-product attention:** If $\boldsymbol{s}_{i-1}$ and $\boldsymbol{h}_j$ can be of the different lengths, we can introduce a weight matrix to align two vectors

$$a(\boldsymbol{s}_{i-1}, \boldsymbol{h}_j) = \boldsymbol{s}_{i-1}^\top \boldsymbol{W}_a \boldsymbol{h}_j;$$

- **Additive attention:** Or we can concatenate both vectors and pass them through a simple neural network such as

$$a(\boldsymbol{s}_{i-1}, \boldsymbol{h}_j) = \boldsymbol{v}_a^\top \tanh(\boldsymbol{W}_a[\boldsymbol{s}_{i-1}, \boldsymbol{h}_j] + \boldsymbol{b}_a).$$

Here $\boldsymbol{W}_a$ and $\boldsymbol{v}_a$ are model parameters to be learned.

Attention Weight a_{ij} is the normalized version of the output from the alignment model. In particular, a_{ij} assigns a probability of relevance of input position j to output position i. More precisely, the alignment model e_{ij} is normalized using a softmax function. Attention weight a_{ij} is computed by the softmax function

$$a_{ij} = \frac{\exp e_{ij}}{\sum_{k=1}^{T_x} \exp e_{ik}}$$

where e_{ij} is an alignment model above. The weight a_{ij} refers to the probability that the target word i is aligned to (or translated from) the source word j. Keep in mind that the first index of a_{ij} corresponds to the target, while the second index refers to the source. This particular index order is important for matrix multiplication as all a_{ij} will be represented as a matrix.

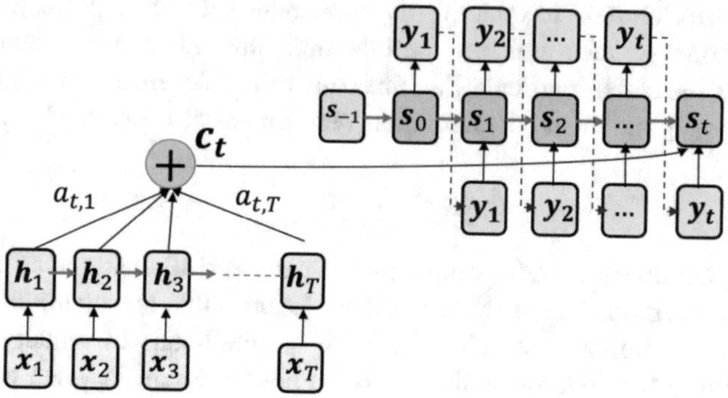

Fig. 9.1 Example of attention mechanism in neural machine translation. Here we can use any variant of RNN as encoder

Context Vector becomes dynamic for each position of the output, which denotes as $\boldsymbol{c}_i$. Mathematically, the context vector $\boldsymbol{c}_i$ is computed as the weighted sum of annotation vectors $\boldsymbol{h}_1, \ldots \boldsymbol{h}_{T_x}$:

$$\boldsymbol{c}_i = \sum_{j=1}^{T_x} a_{ij} \boldsymbol{h}_j$$

Decoder The decoding process will apply a function over the dynamic context vector $\boldsymbol{c}_i$ to generate the output hidden state $\boldsymbol{s}_i$ (e.g., another RNN). More specifically, the output hidden state $\boldsymbol{s}_i$ can be a function of previous hidden state $\boldsymbol{s}_{i-1}$, previous output y_{i-1} and current time context vector $\boldsymbol{c}_i$, represented as

$$\boldsymbol{s}_i = f(\boldsymbol{s}_{i-1}, y_{i-1}, \boldsymbol{c}_i)$$

as shown in Fig. 9.1. Finally, the output hidden state $\boldsymbol{s}_i$ can be fed into more layers to predict y_i for position i. Comparing to the seq2seq model, attention model has a distinct context vector $\boldsymbol{c}_i$ for each output hidden state. Then the output $\boldsymbol{y}_i$ will be generated from the output hidden state $\boldsymbol{s}_i$.

9.3 Case Study: Attention Model over Longitudinal EHR

Problem Longitudinal EHR data are represented as a sequence of visits over time. How to build an accurate and interpretable model over such temporal event sequences? Attention mechanism can be used to understand what part of historical information weighs more in making certain predictions. Authors in [25] proposed a two-level attention model to predict heart failure onset using longitudinal EHR data.

Data The dataset consists of electronic health records from Sutter Health. The EHR data include the encounter records, medication orders, procedure orders, and problem lists, visit records over multiple visits over time. The data are structured encoded with diagnosis, medication, and procedure codes. CCS medical grouper [34] is used to aggregate the codes into input variables (Table 9.2).

Method RETAIN [25] proposed an attention mechanism over time. Each visit $\boldsymbol{x}_i$ is represented by a multi-hot vector where each dimension corresponds to a medical code. Given a sequence of visits $\boldsymbol{x}_1, \ldots, \boldsymbol{x}_T$ from a patient, the goal [25] is to predict whether the patient will develop heart failure in future visits (Fig. 9.2).

First, RETAIN uses a linear projection to embed the visit information to preserve interpretability.

$$\boldsymbol{v}_i = \boldsymbol{W}_{emb}\boldsymbol{x}_i, \qquad \text{(Step 1)}$$

Table 9.2 Statistics of EHR dataset used in [25] (D:Diagnosis, R:Medication, P:Procedure)

Category	Statistics
# of patients	263,683
# of visits	14,366,030
# of medical code groups	615 (D:283, R:94, P:238)
Avg. # of visits per patient	54.48
Avg. # of codes in a visit	3.03
Max # of codes in a visit	62
Avg. # of Dx codes in a visit	1.83
Max # of Dx in a visit	42

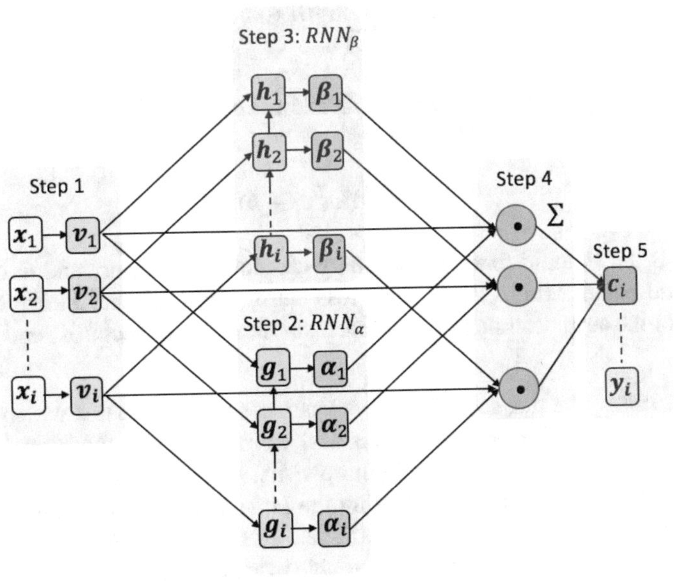

Fig. 9.2 Illustration of RETAIN's architecture

Second, RETAIN uses a two-level attention mechanism, which is the main methodology novelty of this work: one for the visit-level attention and variable-level attention with a visit. Instead of using dot product or additive attention like many previous works, the attention weights for RETAIN are modeled with two RNNs: RNN_α for visits and RNN_β for variables within visits. We assume that the query is the current visit (last visit for each patient). Hence the index of a query is ignored in the following description.

$$\begin{aligned} \boldsymbol{g}_i, \boldsymbol{g}_{i-1}, \ldots, \boldsymbol{g}_1 &= \text{RNN}_\alpha(\boldsymbol{v}_i, \boldsymbol{v}_{i-1}, \ldots, \boldsymbol{v}_1), \\ e_j &= \boldsymbol{w}_\alpha^\top \boldsymbol{g}_j + b_\alpha, \quad \text{for} \quad j = 1, \ldots, i \\ \alpha_1, \alpha_2, \ldots, \alpha_i &= \text{Softmax}(e_1, e_2, \ldots, e_i) \qquad \text{(Step 2: visit level)} \\ \boldsymbol{h}_i, \boldsymbol{h}_{i-1}, \ldots, \boldsymbol{h}_1 &= \text{RNN}_\beta(\boldsymbol{\beta}_i, \boldsymbol{\beta}_{i-1}, \ldots, \boldsymbol{\beta}_1) \\ \boldsymbol{\beta}_j &= \tanh\left(\boldsymbol{W}_\beta \boldsymbol{h}_j + \boldsymbol{b}_\beta\right) \quad \text{for} \quad j = 1, \ldots, i, \\ & \qquad \text{(Step 3: variable level)} \end{aligned}$$

where $\boldsymbol{g}_i \in \mathbb{R}^p$ is the hidden layer of RNN_α at time step i, $\boldsymbol{h}_i \in \mathbb{R}^q$ the hidden layer of RNN_β at time step i and $\boldsymbol{w}_\alpha \in \mathbb{R}^p$, $b_\alpha \in \mathbb{R}$, $\boldsymbol{W}_\beta \in \mathbb{R}^{m \times q}$ and $\boldsymbol{b}_\beta \in \mathbb{R}^m$ are the parameters to learn. Note that for prediction at each visit we compute a new set of attention weights α and $\boldsymbol{\beta}$ from RNN_α and RNN_β.

Next using the generated attentions, we obtain the context vector $\boldsymbol{c}_i$ for a patient up to the i-th visit as follows,

$$\boldsymbol{c}_i = \sum_{j=1}^{i} \alpha_j \boldsymbol{\beta}_j \odot \boldsymbol{v}_j, \qquad \text{(Step 4)}$$

where $\odot$ denotes element-wise multiplication. The context vector $\boldsymbol{c}_i \in \mathbb{R}^m$ is to predict the heart failure onset as follows,

$$\widehat{y}_i = \sigma(\boldsymbol{w}^\top \boldsymbol{c}_i + b). \qquad \text{(Step 5)}$$

where σ is the sigmoid function for binary classion of HF or not and $\boldsymbol{w} \in \mathbb{R}^m$ and $b \in \mathbb{R}$ are parameters to learn. The cross-entropy loss is used. Please check the spelling of the term “classion” in the sentence “The context vector...”, and correct if necessary.

Interpretation The risk score for a given patient can be computed with $\sigma(\boldsymbol{w}^\top \boldsymbol{c}_i + b)$ as shown above. To understand the risk, we need to find the most influential visits and influential variables within those visits. Finding the influential visits that contribute to prediction is derived using the largest α_i, which is straightforward. However, finding influential input variables (e.g., specific diagnosis codes) is slightly more involved. Given the k-th variable in visit j denoted as $x_{j,k}$, its influence score to the final prediction is

$$\omega(x_{j,k}) = \underbrace{\alpha_j \boldsymbol{w}^\top (\boldsymbol{\beta}_j \odot \boldsymbol{W}_{emb}[:, k])}_{\text{Contribution coefficient}} \cdot \underbrace{x_{j,k}}_{\text{Input}}$$

where $\boldsymbol{W}_{emb}[:, k]$ denotes the k-th column of embedding matrix $\boldsymbol{W}_{emb}$.

Result The interpretability of RETAIN is demonstrated in the HF prediction task. The patient suffered from skin problems, *skin disorder* (SD), *benign neoplasm* (BN), *excision of skin lesion* (ESL) for some time before showing symptoms of HF, *cardiac dysrhythmia* (CD), *heart valve disease* (HVD), and *coronary atherosclerosis* (CA), and then a diagnosis of HF (Fig. 9.3a). We can see that a high-risk score $\hat{y} = 0.2475$ and skin-related codes from the earlier visits made little contribution to HF prediction as expected. RETAIN properly puts much attention to the HF-related codes that occurred in recent visits.

To confirm RETAIN's ability to exploit the sequential information of the EHR data, we reverse the visit sequence of Fig. 9.3a and feed it to RETAIN. Figure 9.3b shows the contribution of the medical codes of the reversed visit record. HF-related codes in the past are still making positive contributions, but not as much as they did originally in Fig. 9.3a. The risk score, in this case, drops to 0.0905.

Figure 9.3c shows how the contributions of codes change when selected medication data are used in the model. We added two medications from day 219:

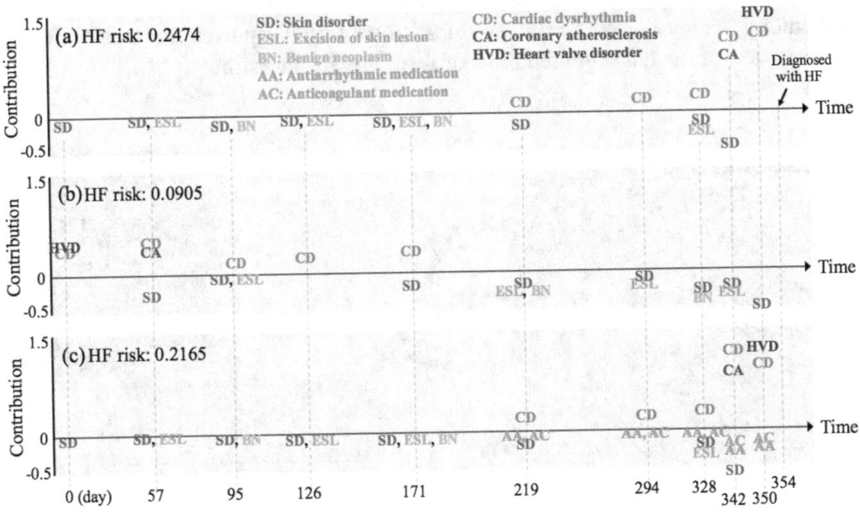

Fig. 9.3 (**a**) Temporal visualization of a patient's visit records where the contribution of variables for diagnosis of heart failure (HF) is summarized along the x-axis (i.e. time) with the y-axis indicating the magnitude of visit and code specific contributions to HF diagnosis. (**b**) Reverse the order of the visit sequence to see if RETAIN can properly take into account the modified sequence information. (**c**) Medication codes are added to the visit record to see how it changes the behavior of RETAIN. prediction (0.2165) in (**c**) is lower than that of (**a**) (0.2474). This suggests that taking proper medications can potentially help the patient in reducing their HF risk

antiarrhythmics (AA) and *anticoagulants* (AC), both of which are used to treat *cardiac dysrhythmia* (CD). The two medications have a negative weight and lowered the risk score from 0.2474 to 0.2165.

9.4 Case Study: Attention Model over a Medical Ontology

Problem Medical ontology represents a vast amount of medical knowledge, which are modeled as directed acyclic graphs (DAGs). Each node in the graph corresponds to a clinical concept such as heart failure. The edge represents the relation between concepts, e.g., heart failure is connected to heart disease. Those concepts are often organized hierarchically, as shown on the left side of Fig. 9.4. The question is how to construct a better patient representation that leverages both EHR data and knowledge DAGs.

Data In [28], the authors conduct heart failure (HF) prediction experiments on the same EHR data from Sutter health as described in Sect. 9.3. There are other tasks and datasets studied in [28], which are omitted for brevity.

Method GRAM [28] leverages the parent-child relationship of an ontology graph to learn robust representations from EHR data.

In the knowledge DAG, each node c_i such as a diagnosis code is assigned a basic embedding vector $\boldsymbol{e}_i$, We formulate a leaf node's final representation as a convex combination of the basic embeddings of itself and its ancestors:

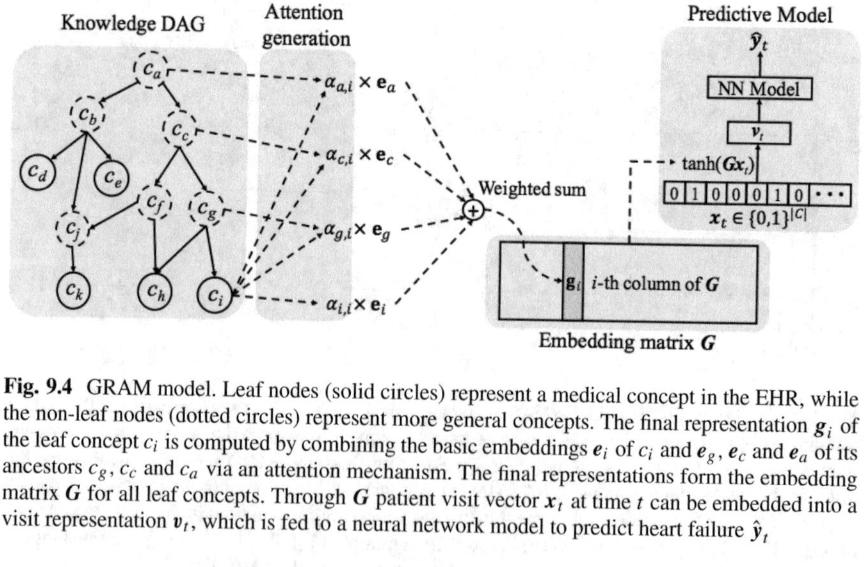

Fig. 9.4 GRAM model. Leaf nodes (solid circles) represent a medical concept in the EHR, while the non-leaf nodes (dotted circles) represent more general concepts. The final representation $\boldsymbol{g}_i$ of the leaf concept c_i is computed by combining the basic embeddings $\boldsymbol{e}_i$ of c_i and $\boldsymbol{e}_g$, $\boldsymbol{e}_c$ and $\boldsymbol{e}_a$ of its ancestors c_g, c_c and c_a via an attention mechanism. The final representations form the embedding matrix $\boldsymbol{G}$ for all leaf concepts. Through $\boldsymbol{G}$ patient visit vector $\boldsymbol{x}_t$ at time t can be embedded into a visit representation $\boldsymbol{v}_t$, which is fed to a neural network model to predict heart failure $\hat{\boldsymbol{y}}_t$

$$g_i = \sum_{j \in \mathcal{A}(i)} \alpha_{ij} \mathbf{e}_j, \qquad \sum_{j \in \mathcal{A}(i)} \alpha_{ij} = 1, \ \ \alpha_{ij} \geq 0 \text{ for } j \in \mathcal{A}(i),$$

where $\boldsymbol{g}_i$ denotes the final representation of the code c_i, $\mathcal{A}(i)$ the set of indices of the code c_i and c_i's ancestors, $\boldsymbol{e}_j$ the basic embedding of the code c_j and $\alpha_{ij} \in \mathbb{R}^+$ the attention weight on the embedding $\boldsymbol{e}_j$ when calculating $\boldsymbol{g}_i$. The attention weight α_{ij} is calculated by

$$\alpha_{ij} = \frac{\exp(f(\boldsymbol{e}_i, \boldsymbol{e}_j))}{\sum_{k \in \mathcal{A}(i)} \exp(f(\boldsymbol{e}_i, \boldsymbol{e}_k))}$$

where $f(\boldsymbol{e}_i, \boldsymbol{e}_j)$ is a scalar value representing the compatibility between the basic embeddings of $\boldsymbol{e}_i$ and $\boldsymbol{e}_k$. This function $f(\boldsymbol{e}_i, \boldsymbol{e}_j)$ is implemented with a multi-layer perceptron (MLP) with a single hidden layer or the additive attention,

$$f(\boldsymbol{e}_i, \boldsymbol{e}_j) = \boldsymbol{u}_a^\top \tanh(\boldsymbol{W}_a \begin{bmatrix} \boldsymbol{e}_i \\ \boldsymbol{e}_j \end{bmatrix} + \boldsymbol{b}_a)$$

where $\boldsymbol{W}_a$ is the weight matrix for the concatenation of $\boldsymbol{e}_i$ and $\boldsymbol{e}_j$, $\boldsymbol{b}$ the bias vector, and $\boldsymbol{u}_a$ the weight vector for generating the compatibility value. The constant l represents the dimension size of the hidden layer of $f(\cdot, \cdot)$.

Result GRAM and its variant achieved better results compared to RNN and its variants with the simple heuristics of generalizing medical codes to higher levels for the same heart failure onset prediction.

SimpleRollUp All input codes to the RNN are replaced with their direct parent codes in the CCS multi-level hierarchy.

RollUpRare The rare input codes to the RNN are replaced with their direct parents.

Table 9.3 shows the HF prediction performance on the Sutter HF cohort. GRAM consistently outperforms other baselines by 3–4% AUC.

Table 9.3 AUC of HF onset prediction when varying the training dataset size

Model	10%	20%	30%	40%	50%	60%	70%	80%	90%	100%
GRAM	**0.7981**	0.8217	**0.8340**	**0.8332**	0.8372	0.8377	0.8440	0.8431	0.8430	0.8447
RNN	0.7811	0.7942	0.8066	0.8111	0.8156	0.8207	0.8258	0.8278	0.8297	0.8314
SimpleRollUp	0.7799	0.8022	0.8108	0.8133	0.8177	0.8207	0.8223	0.8272	0.8269	0.8258
RollUpRare	0.7830	0.8067	0.8064	0.8119	0.8211	0.8202	0.8262	0.8296	0.8307	0.8291

The bold values indicate the best performance numbers across all methods

9.5 Case Study: ICD Classification from Clinical Notes

Problem Clinical notes are text documents created by clinicians for each patient encounter. They are typically accompanied by diagnosis codes and procedure codes, mainly used for reimbursement from insurance companies. Those diagnosis codes are manually assigned by human coders, which are labor-intensive and error-prone. Can a deep learning algorithm automate the medical code assignment based on clinical notes? Authors of [114] proposed an attention model to address this problem (Fig. 9.5).

Data In that study [114], discharge summaries from MIMIC-III data [81] are used. Each admission is tagged by human coders with a set of ICD-9 codes, describing both diagnoses and procedures during the patient's stay. There are 8921 unique ICD-9 codes present in our datasets, including 6918 diagnosis codes and 2003 procedure codes. The resulting dataset contains a set of 47,724 discharge summaries from 36,998 patients for training, with 1632 summaries and 3372 summaries for validation and testing, respectively.

Method Convolutional Attention for Multi-Label classification (CAML) [114] combines a convolutional architecture and an attention mechanism to model clinical text.

- *Input:* d_e-dimensional pre-trained embeddings for each word in the clinical document are horizontally concatenated into the input matrix $\boldsymbol{X} = [\boldsymbol{x}_1, \boldsymbol{x}_2, \ldots, \boldsymbol{x}_N]$, where N is the length of the document.
- *Convolution:* Adjacent word embeddings are combined using a convolutional filter $\boldsymbol{W}_c \in \mathbb{R}^{k \times d_e \times d_c}$, where k is the filter width, d_e the size of the input embedding, and d_c the size of the filter output. At each step n, they compute

$$\boldsymbol{h}_n = g(\boldsymbol{W}_c * \boldsymbol{x}_{n:n+k-1} + \boldsymbol{b}_c), \tag{9.1}$$

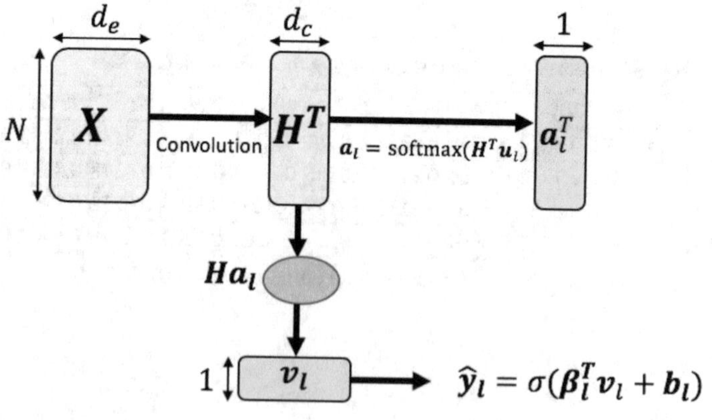

Fig. 9.5 CAML architecture

where $*$ denotes the convolution operator, g is an element-wise nonlinear transformation, and $\boldsymbol{b}_c \in \mathbb{R}^{d_c}$ is the bias.

- *Attention:* After convolution, the document is represented by the matrix $\boldsymbol{H} \in \mathbb{R}^{d_c \times N}$. For each label ℓ, they compute the matrix-vector product, $\boldsymbol{H}^\top \boldsymbol{u}_\ell$, where $\boldsymbol{u}_\ell \in \mathbb{R}^{d_c}$ is a vector parameter for label ℓ. They then pass the resulting vector through a softmax operator, obtaining a distribution over locations in the document,

$$\boldsymbol{\alpha}_\ell = \text{Softmax}(\boldsymbol{H}^\top \boldsymbol{u}_\ell),$$

The attention vector $\boldsymbol{\alpha}$ is then used to compute document representations for each label,

$$\boldsymbol{v}_\ell = \sum_{n=1}^{N} \alpha_{\ell,n} \boldsymbol{h}_n.$$

Input documents serve as the keys and each disease diagnosis label becomes a query in this case.

- *Classification:* Given the document representation $\vec{v}_\ell$, they compute a probability for label ℓ using another linear layer and a sigmoid transformation:

$$\hat{y}_\ell = \sigma(\boldsymbol{\beta}_\ell^\top \boldsymbol{v}_\ell + b_\ell),$$

where $\boldsymbol{\beta}_\ell \in \mathbb{R}^{d_c}$ is a vector of prediction weights, and b_ℓ is a scalar offset. The total cross-entropy loss across all labels is used $L = -\sum_\ell y_\ell \log(\hat{y}_\ell) + (1 - y_\ell)\log(1 - \hat{y}_\ell)$.

Result Our main quantitative evaluation involves predicting the full set of ICD-9 codes based on the MIMIC-III discharge summaries text. As shown in Table 9.4, the CAML model gives the strongest results on all metrics.

Table 9.4 Results on MIMIC-III full, 8922 labels. Here, "Diag" denotes Micro-F1 performance on diagnosis codes only, and "Proc" denotes Micro-F1 performance on procedure codes only

	AUC		F1				P@n	
Model	Macro	Micro	Macro	Micro	Diag	Proc	8	15
Logistic regression	0.561	0.937	0.011	0.272	0.242	0.398	0.542	0.411
CNN	0.806	0.969	0.042	0.419	0.402	0.491	0.581	0.443
Bi-GRU	0.822	0.971	0.038	0.417	0.393	0.514	0.585	0.445
CAML	**0.895***	**0.986***	**0.088**	**0.539***	**0.524***	**0.609***	**0.709***	**0.561***

The bold values indicate the best performance numbers across all methods

9.6 Case Study: Heart Disease Detection from Electrocardiography

Problem Electrocardiography (ECG) measures electrical activities of a heart and is a commonly used non-invasive diagnostic tool for heart diseases. The existing practice of ECG diagnosis is based on expert-defined patterns from ECG such as P-wave, QRS complex, and RR interval. However, deep learning provides a new set of powerful tools for analyzing ECG in a data-driven way. We have shown how CNN can be applied to ECG classification in Sect. 6.8. Authors of [73] proposed Multi-level knowledge-guide attention model (MINA) for classifying ECG signals.

Data The authors conducted all experiments using real-world ECG data from PhysioNet Challenge 2017 databases [32]. The dataset contains 8528 de-identified ECG recordings lasting from 9 s to just over the 60 s and sampled at 300 Hz by the AliveCor device, 738 from AF patients, and 7790 from controls predefined by the challenge. We first divided the data into a training set (75%), a validation set (10%), and a test set (15%) to train and evaluate in all tasks. Then, they process via a 10-second sliding window to produce segments of equal length of $n = 3000$. Thus ECG recording of a patient will become multiple 3000-dimensional segments. The objective is to differentiate segments of atrial fibrillation (AF) patients from those of controls.

Method An example of real-world ECG signals is shown in Fig. 9.6. ECG signals from AF patients and controls show different patterns at (1) *beat level*, (2) *rhythm level*, and (3) *frequency level*. Learning these patterns to support diagnoses has been an important research area in ECG analysis. For each level, MINA extracts level-specific domain knowledge features. It uses them to guide the attention models, including beat morphology knowledge that guides attentive CNN and rhythm knowledge that guides attentive RNN. MINA also performs attention fusion across time- and frequency domains.

MINA architecture is shown in Fig. 9.7. Given a single lead ECG signal $\boldsymbol{x} \in \mathbb{R}^n$, the goal is to predict the probability of AF based on $\boldsymbol{x}$. They firstly transform it into multi-channel signals with F channels across different frequency bands where ith signal is denoted as $\boldsymbol{x}^{(i)} \in \mathbb{R}^n$. They then split each $\boldsymbol{x}^{(i)}$ into M segments $\boldsymbol{s}^{(k)}$. Next they apply CNN and RNN consecutively on $\boldsymbol{s}^{(k)}$ to obtain beat level attention

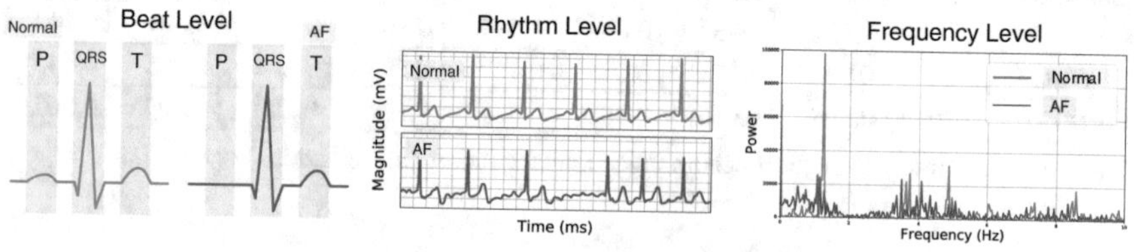

Fig. 9.6 Normal ECG signal and Abnormal ECG signal show different patterns across different levels

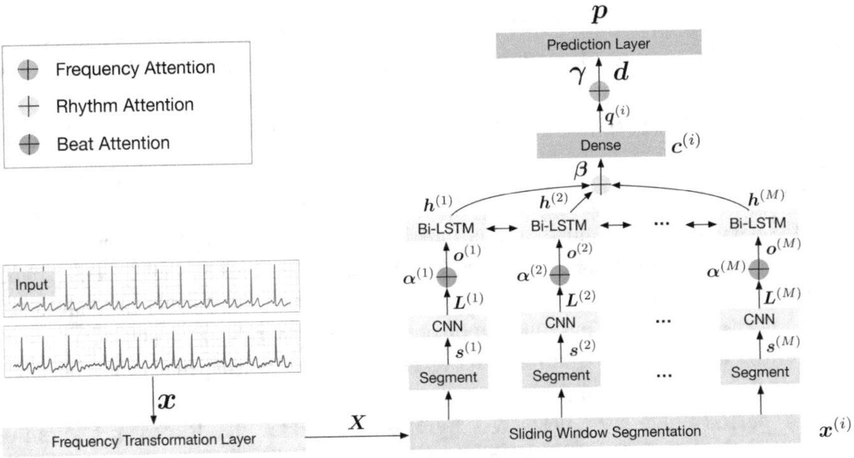

Fig. 9.7 Takes raw ECG signals as input and outputs probabilities of disease onset. used knowledge-guided attention to learn informative beat-, rhythm-, and frequency level patterns, and then performs attentive signal fusion for improved prediction

$\boldsymbol{o}^{(k)}, 1 \le k \le M$ and rhythm level attention $\boldsymbol{c}^{(i)}$. This follows by a fully connected layer that transforms $\boldsymbol{c}^{(i)}$ into $\boldsymbol{q}^{(i)}$. They then take weighted average to integrate $\boldsymbol{Q} = [\boldsymbol{q}^{(1)}, ..., \boldsymbol{q}^{(F)}]$ across all channels to output frequency attention $\boldsymbol{d}$, which will be used in prediction.

To compute multilevel attention weights $\boldsymbol{\alpha}, \boldsymbol{\beta}, \boldsymbol{\gamma}$, the attention mechanism can be regarded as a two-layer neural network: the 1st fully connected layer calculates the scores for computing weights; the 2nd fully connected layer computes the weights with via softmax activation.

In the first layer, the scores are computed based on the following features. (1) **Multilevel outputs** $\boldsymbol{L} \in \mathbb{R}^{K \times N}$, $\boldsymbol{H} \in \mathbb{R}^{J \times M}$, $\boldsymbol{Q} \in \mathbb{R}^{H \times F}$ extracted by this method. (2) **Domain knowledge features** including beat level $\boldsymbol{K}_\alpha \in \mathbb{R}^{E_\alpha \times N}$, rhythm level $\boldsymbol{K}_\beta \in \mathbb{R}^{E_\beta \times M}$, and frequency level $\boldsymbol{K}_\gamma \in \mathbb{R}^{E_\gamma \times F}$.

In the second layer, they concatenate model outputs and knowledge features to compute scores and attention weights.

$$\boldsymbol{\alpha} = softmax(\boldsymbol{V}_\alpha^T(\boldsymbol{W}_\alpha^T \begin{bmatrix} \boldsymbol{L} \\ \boldsymbol{K}_\alpha \end{bmatrix} \oplus \boldsymbol{b}_\alpha))$$

$$\boldsymbol{\beta} = softmax(\boldsymbol{V}_\beta^T(\boldsymbol{W}_\beta^T \begin{bmatrix} \boldsymbol{H} \\ \boldsymbol{K}_\beta \end{bmatrix} \oplus \boldsymbol{b}_\beta))$$

$$\boldsymbol{\gamma} = softmax(\boldsymbol{V}_\gamma^T(\boldsymbol{W}_\gamma^T \begin{bmatrix} \boldsymbol{Q} \\ \boldsymbol{K}_\gamma \end{bmatrix} \oplus \boldsymbol{b}_\gamma))$$

where, $\boldsymbol{W}_\alpha \in \mathbb{R}^{(K+E_\alpha)\times D_\alpha}$, $\boldsymbol{W}_\beta \in \mathbb{R}^{(J+E_\alpha)\times D_\beta}$, $\boldsymbol{W}_\gamma \in \mathbb{R}^{(H+E_\gamma)\times D_\gamma}$, $\boldsymbol{b}_\alpha \in \mathbb{R}^{D_\alpha}$, $\boldsymbol{b}_\beta \in \mathbb{R}^{D_\beta}$, $\boldsymbol{b}_\gamma \in \mathbb{R}^{D_\gamma}$ represent weights and biases in the first layer, $\boldsymbol{V}_\alpha \in \mathbb{R}^{D_\alpha \times 1}$, $\boldsymbol{V}_\beta \in \mathbb{R}^{D_\beta \times 1}$, $\boldsymbol{V}_\gamma \in \mathbb{R}^{D_\gamma \times 1}$ represent weights in the second layer. $\oplus$ is addition with broadcasting (i.e., to add the vector $\boldsymbol{b}_\alpha, \boldsymbol{b}_\beta, \boldsymbol{b}_\gamma$ to every column of the matrix).

Result The authors compare MINA with (1) **Expert**: A combination of extracted features used in AF diagnosis, including rhythm features, morphological features, and frequency features. Then, they build both logistic regression (**ExpertLR**) and random forest (**ExpertRF**) on above extracted features. (2) **CNN**: Convolutional neural networks with the same hyper-parameters in CNN, FC, and softmax as MINA. (3) **CRNN**: Convolutional recurrent neural networks; (4) **ACRNN**: Convolutional recurrent neural networks with attention.

The performance was measured by the area under the Receiver Operating Characteristic (ROC-AUC), Area under the Precision-Recall Curve (PR-AUC), and the F1 score. Table 9.5 shows MINA outperforms all baselines and shows 5.51% higher PR-AUC than the second-best models. Figure 9.8 shows interpretable results extracted from MINA.

Table 9.5 Performance comparison on AF prediction

	ROC-AUC	PR-AUC	F1
ExpertLR	0.9350 ± 0.0000	0.8730 ± 0.0000	0.8023 ± 0.0000
ExpertRF	0.9394 ± 0.0000	0.8816 ± 0.0000	0.8180 ± 0.0000
CNN	0.8711 ± 0.0036	0.8669 ± 0.0068	0.7914 ± 0.0090
CRNN	0.9040 ± 0.0115	0.8943 ± 0.0111	0.8262 ± 0.0215
ACRNN	0.9072 ± 0.0047	0.8935 ± 0.0087	0.8248 ± 0.0229
MINA	**0.9488** ± 0.0081	**0.9436** ± 0.0082	**0.8342** ± 0.0352

The bold values indicate the best performance numbers across all methods

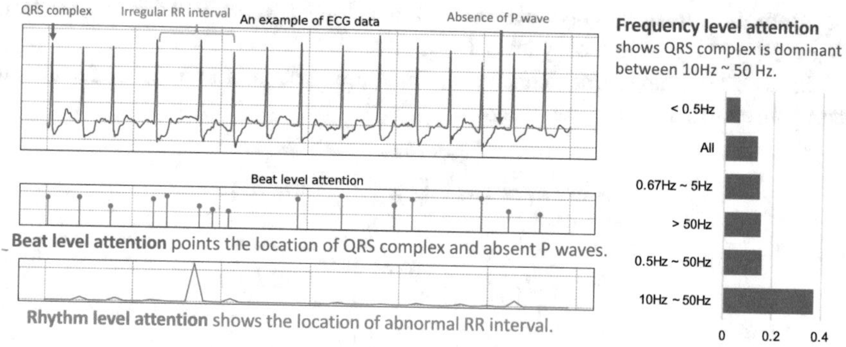

Fig. 9.8 From ECG signal of AF patient (left top), MINA learns beat level attention which points to the position of significant QRS complexes and abnormal P waves. Rhythm level attention shows the abnormal RR interval. The frequency channel that receives highest attention correspond to the frequency bands where QRS complex is dominant

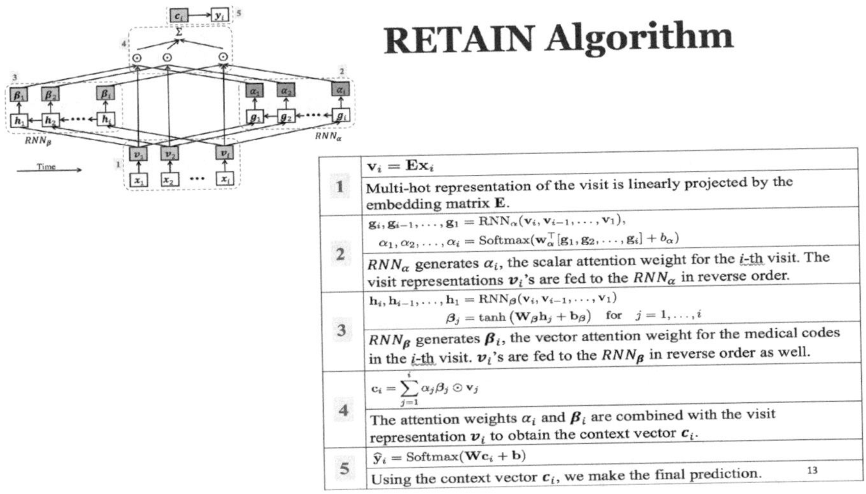

Fig. 9.9 RETAIN algorithm [25]

9.7 Exercises

1. What is the difference between sequence-to-sequence model with RNN and that with attention?
   For question 2–4, please refer to Fig. 9.1
2. What is the direct input to compute attention weight α_{ij}?
3. How to compute dynamic context vector c_i?
4. What are the direct input to decoder s_i?
5. Which steps compute attention weights in RETAIN method as shown in Fig. 9.9
6. In the CAML method[114], what other neural network architecture is used besides attention mechanism? And what is the clinical application of CAML?
7. What is the input data to MINA method [73]?

Chapter 10
Graph Neural Networks

10.1 Overview

Graphs are universal representations of pairwise relations with many real-world applications. In the healthcare domain, graphs are widely observed as relations of biomedical entities, including the graph structures of molecules [80, 103, 107], drug-drug interaction networks [108], protein-protein interaction networks [64, 178], and gene expression networks [99] and biomedical knowledge graphs and medical ontologies [28, 134]. Compared with other representations such as vectors or sequences, graphs are expressive models that can capture more complex interactions between heterogeneous biomedical concepts. Therefore, directly modeling graphs can be of great value to many biomedical applications.

Despite its success, deep learning methods are difficult to directly apply to graphs due to several challenges [175]: (1) *Irregular structure*: Graphs are flexibly represented by nodes and edges, which are more difficult to process than fixed-size input vectors and matrices. (2) *Heterogeneity of graphs*: In the biomedical domain, there are many different graphs, e.g., medical ontology graph, protein interaction graph, drug interaction graph. It is difficult to jointly model heterogeneous graphs. Even within a single graph, there can be different types of nodes and edges. For example, a medical ontology such as SNOMED contains many different types of relations. (3) *Large graphs*: Some graphs are small such as molecule graphs of tens of atoms and bonds, but some graphs are huge with hundreds of thousands of nodes and millions of edges, such as medical ontology graph like SNOMED. It is computationally expensive to process such large graphs.

Different neural network architectures have been proposed, including graph recurrent neural networks (graph RNN), graph convolutional neural networks (GCN), graph attention network (GAT), and graph autoencoders (GAEs). Among them, GCN receives most of the attention, which is the focus of this chapter [88]. GCNs extend feedforward neural networks to handle graphs (e.g., a biomedical network) by generalizing the concept of convolution operations from standard con-

C. Xiao, J. Sun, *Introduction to Deep Learning for Healthcare*,
https://doi.org/10.1007/978-3-030-82184-5_10

volutional neural networks. GCN and its variants have been applied to biomedical graphs [108, 134, 178]. In this chapter, we first overview the notation and tasks on graphs, then describe a few popular graph neural networks (GNNs) and finally present their applications on healthcare tasks such as drug discovery.

10.2 Notations and Tasks on Graphs

10.2.1 Notations and Operations

Graph is often denoted by $G =< V, E >$ where $V = \{v_1, v_2, \ldots, v_N\}$ is the set of N nodes and $E \subseteq V \times V$ the set of M edges connecting those nodes. Adjacency matrix of graph G is $\boldsymbol{A} \in \mathbb{R}^{N \times N}$, where $\boldsymbol{A}(i, :)$, $\boldsymbol{A}(:, j)$, $\boldsymbol{A}(i, j)$ denote the i-th row, the j-th column and the ij element, respectively. Often $\boldsymbol{A}$ is a binary matrix where ij element of value 1 indicates an edge from node i to node j and element of value 0 means no edge. We use $\boldsymbol{X} \in \mathbb{R}^{N \times D}$ to denote the feature matrix of nodes. Likewise, $\boldsymbol{Y} \in \mathbb{R}^{N \times M}$ denotes the label matrix of nodes, which is represented by N one-hot vectors. In particular, $\boldsymbol{X}(i, :)$ and $\boldsymbol{Y}(i, :)$ correspond to the feature vector and the label vector (e.g., a one-hot vector) for node v_i, respectively.

Normalization Instead of directly using the adjacency matrix, we often use a normalized adjacency matrix as input to graph neural networks. The common idea is to normalize the adjacency matrix $\boldsymbol{A}$ by the inverse degree matrix $\boldsymbol{D}$. Here the degree matrix $\boldsymbol{D} \in \mathbb{R}^{N \times N}$ is a diagonal matrix where its diagonal element $\boldsymbol{D}(i, i) = \sum_j \boldsymbol{A}(i, j)$ (the sum of the i-th row of $\boldsymbol{A}$). The different normalization options can computed: for example, (1) $\boldsymbol{P} = \boldsymbol{D}^{-1}\boldsymbol{A}$ where $\boldsymbol{P}(i, j)$ intuitively corresponds to the probability of jumping from node i to node j; and (2) $\boldsymbol{P} = \boldsymbol{D}^{-1/2}\boldsymbol{A}\boldsymbol{D}^{-1/2}$ which leads to a symmetric matrix.

Spectral Analysis Besides the adjacency matrix, another related matrix to a graph is the Laplacian matrix $\boldsymbol{L} = \boldsymbol{D} - \boldsymbol{A}$, which is often used for representing undirected graphs. Note that for undirected graphs $\boldsymbol{L}$ and $\boldsymbol{A}$ are symmetric, i.e., $\boldsymbol{L}(i, j) = \boldsymbol{L}(j, i)$ and $\boldsymbol{A}(i, j) = \boldsymbol{A}(j, i)$. Then a powerful linear algebra operation called eigen-decomposition can be applied on $\boldsymbol{L}$, denoted as $\boldsymbol{L} = \boldsymbol{Q}\boldsymbol{\Lambda}\boldsymbol{Q}^\top$ where $\boldsymbol{\Lambda}$ is a diagonal matrix with eigenvalues on the diagonal and $\boldsymbol{Q}$ are the corresponding eigenvectors. The eigen-decomposition on a Laplacian matrix is often referred to as spectral analysis. One popular application of spectral analysis is called *spectral clustering*, which performs a clustering operation on $\boldsymbol{Q}$ (e.g., k-means clustering on the rows of $\boldsymbol{Q}$). Spectral clustering is a simple and effective way to find node clusters on graphs. Spectral analysis is used in the initial graph convolutional network development [9], but later on, it is replaced with simpler and computationally more efficient neighborhood aggregation.

10.2.2 Tasks on Graphs

There are different tasks on graphs. At the most granular level, we have *node classification* and *link prediction*, whose targets are nodes and edges on a graph. On the intermediate level, we have *community detection* on graphs. Then on the entire graph level, we have *graph property classification* and *graph generation*. The common step to solve all these tasks is to convert input graph into vector representations. This process is called *graph embedding*. Mathematically, the objective of graph neural networks is to produce node embeddings $\{\boldsymbol{h}_1, \boldsymbol{h}_2, \ldots, \boldsymbol{h}_N\}$. These embeddings are also done with multiple layers of graph neural networks. Hence, we denote those embedding vectors of layer l as $\{\boldsymbol{h}_1^{(l)}, \boldsymbol{h}_2^{(l)}, \ldots, \boldsymbol{h}_N^{(l)}\}$. More precisely, $\boldsymbol{h}_i^{(l)} \in \mathbb{R}^F$ is the node embedding of v_i at layer l. Once node embeddings are obtained, we can solve all those tasks via standard machine learning approaches.

- **Node classification** is to classify each node in the graph into a set of predefined labels. For example, in epidemiology applications, we want to predict what diseases a patient is likely to have given a patient contact network. Given the embedding vectors of patient nodes and their corresponding labels, we can easily train a classifier to perform node classification. More formally, node classification aims at learning a function $f(\boldsymbol{h}_i)$ to estimate the target label y_i. For example, $f()$ can be a softmax function [88].
- **Link prediction** is to estimate the missing edges on a graph. For example, given a graph of known drug-protein interactions, we want to estimate the unknown drug-protein interactions. Formally, link prediction tries to learn a binary classification function $f(\boldsymbol{h}_i, \boldsymbol{h}_j)$ with two input node embedding $\boldsymbol{h}_i$ and $\boldsymbol{h}_j$. The goal is to estimate whether there should be a link between node v_i and v_j. For example, we can define the probability of the link between v_i and v_j as $\sigma(\boldsymbol{h}_i^\top \boldsymbol{h}_j)$ where $\sigma()$ is the sigmoid function [89].
- **Community detection** is to partition the graph into tight subgraphs (i.e., communities). For example, we want to find patient/disease clusters given a bipartite graph connecting two types of nodes (patients and diseases). This can be achieved by clustering the node embedding vectors. Spectral clustering can be one algorithm for this task.
- **Graph property prediction** is about predicting certain properties for the entire graph. For example, given existing molecular graphs (i.e., nodes are atoms and edges are bonds) and their associated drug properties, we want to estimate those drug properties on other unknown molecules. This task needs an embedding vector for the entire graph denoted by $\boldsymbol{h}_G$ which is a function over all the node embedding $\boldsymbol{h}_G = f(\boldsymbol{h}_1, \ldots, \boldsymbol{h}_N)$. For example, we can configure the readout operation as $\boldsymbol{h}_G = \text{Softmax}(\sum_i \boldsymbol{h}_i)$ [40]. Note that the *readout operation* is about creating an embedding for the entire graph from node embeddings.
- **Graph generation** is to produce new graphs based on existing graphs. One application in drug discovery is called *molecule generation* which is about

creating new molecules with desirable properties based on existing molecules. We will present a case study for this task in this chapter.

10.3 Graph Neural Networks

The main idea of a graph neural network is to pass messages across edges and aggregate those messages on nodes to compute node embedding vectors. For a graph $\boldsymbol{G}$ with N nodes, graph convolution with a kernel $\boldsymbol{g}$ is defined as

$$\boldsymbol{g} \star \boldsymbol{x} = \boldsymbol{U} g(\boldsymbol{\Lambda}) \boldsymbol{U}^\top \boldsymbol{x} \tag{10.1}$$

where $\boldsymbol{U}$ is the matrix of eigenvectors and $\boldsymbol{\Lambda}$ is the diagonal matrix that contains the eigenvalues of the normalized graph Laplacian matrix $\boldsymbol{L}_{norm} = \boldsymbol{I} - \boldsymbol{D}^{-1/2}\boldsymbol{A}\boldsymbol{D}^{-1/2}$, with $\boldsymbol{D}$ and $\boldsymbol{A}$ being the degree matrix and the adjacency matrix of the graph, and $g()$ is applied elementwise on $\boldsymbol{\Lambda}$. Since computing $\boldsymbol{U}$ and $\boldsymbol{\Lambda}$ can be very expensive (e.g., $O(N^3)$), most GNNs approximate the graph convolution operator instead. Next, we will describe different GNN methods for producing the node embedding vectors, including graph convolutional networks (GCN), message passing neural network (MPNN), and graph attention network (GAT).

10.4 Graph Convolutional Networks

Graph Convolutional Networks (GCN) is an approximation of the original GNN [88]. GCN produces node representations based on the input graph structure (e.g., adjacency matrix $\boldsymbol{A}$) and input node features $\boldsymbol{X}$. GCN models encode node information based on its neighbors on the graph. Intuitively GCN represents a node as a function of its neighbors like convolution operations in CNN. Iteratively GCN aggregates information from a node's local neighborhood to produce better features (or embedding) for that node. More formally,

$$\boldsymbol{h}_i^{(l+1)} = \sigma(\boldsymbol{h}_i^{(l)} \boldsymbol{W}^l + \frac{1}{d_i} \sum_{j \in \mathcal{N}_i} \boldsymbol{h}_j^{(l)} \boldsymbol{W}^l) \tag{10.2}$$

where $\boldsymbol{h}_i^{(l+1)}$ and $\boldsymbol{h}_i^{(l)}$ are the node embedding of v_i at layer $l+1$ and l, d_i is the degree of node i, $\mathcal{N}_i$ are the neighbors of v_i, $\boldsymbol{W}^{(l)}$ is the weight matrix at layer l and $\sigma()$ is the activation function such as ReLU.

In matrix form, the update equation becomes

$$\boldsymbol{H}^{(l+1)} = \sigma\left((\boldsymbol{I} + \boldsymbol{D}^{-1/2}\boldsymbol{A}\boldsymbol{D}^{-1/2})\boldsymbol{H}^{(l)}\boldsymbol{W}^{(l)}\right), \tag{10.3}$$

where $\boldsymbol{H}^{(l+1)}$ and $\boldsymbol{H}^{(l)}$ are the node embedding matrices at layer $l+1$ and l, $\boldsymbol{W}^{(l)}$ is the weight matrix at layer l, and $\boldsymbol{A}$ the adjacency matrix, $\boldsymbol{I}$ the identity matrix and $\boldsymbol{D}$ the degree matrix. Equation (10.3) can be rewritten as

$$\boldsymbol{H}^{(l+1)} = \sigma\left(\tilde{\boldsymbol{D}}^{-1/2}\tilde{\boldsymbol{A}}\tilde{\boldsymbol{D}}^{-1/2}\boldsymbol{H}^{(l)}\boldsymbol{W}^{(l)}\right),$$

where $\tilde{\boldsymbol{A}} = \boldsymbol{A} + \boldsymbol{I}$, $\tilde{\boldsymbol{D}}$ is a diagonal matrix with $\tilde{\boldsymbol{D}}(i,i) = \sum_j \tilde{\boldsymbol{A}}(i,j)$ and $\boldsymbol{W}^{(l)}$ is the weight matrix at layer l and $\sigma()$ is the activation function.

Loss Function for GCN depends on the tasks. The simplest setting is a supervised task like node classification. In that case, the loss function is

$$\mathcal{L} = \sum_i y_i \log(\sigma(\boldsymbol{h}_i^\top \boldsymbol{\theta})) + (1 - y_i)\log(1 - \sigma(\boldsymbol{h}_i^\top \boldsymbol{\theta}))$$

where y_i is the class label on v_i (e.g., healthy or sick if node is a patient) and $\boldsymbol{h}_i$ is the embedding of node v_i and $\boldsymbol{\theta}$ is the classification weight vector.

Remarks The advantages of GCN are (1) the weight matrix $\boldsymbol{W}^{(l)}$ is shared over all nodes; (2) the resulting embeddings are invariant to the node permutation; (3) Computationally more efficient $O(|E|)$. The limitations are (1) edge features are not supported, and (2) GCN can still be computationally expensive for very large graphs.

Speedup Graph Convolutional Networks

The computational bottleneck of GCN on large graphs is the neighborhood aggregation step, as shown in Eq. (10.2). In particular, many real-world graphs follow a power-law distribution where a small number of nodes can have many neighbors. Those "super-connected" nodes will cause expensive operations.

To alleviate this computational challenge, different sampling strategies have been proposed. GraphSAGE [63] uniformly samples a fixed number of neighbors for each node during training. FastGCN performs importance sampling over nodes by considering the nodes as independent and identically distributed random samples [17]. More specifically, FastGCN samples nodes layer by layer based on their normalized degrees, which achieves lower variance, faster speed, and higher accuracy.

10.5 Message Passing Neural Network (MPNN)

To extend GCN to a more general framework, a message passing neural network (MPNN) has been introduced [54], where node and edge features are supported, and many existing methods are covered under this MPNN framework [40, 84, 98, 131]. MPNN framework has two stages: the message passing stage and the readout stage.

- **Message passing stage** iteratively computes the message function $\boldsymbol{m}_v^{t+1}$ and then updates the node embedding $\boldsymbol{h}_v^{t+1}$.

$$\boldsymbol{m}_v^{(t+1)} = \sum_{w \in \mathcal{N}_v} M_t(\boldsymbol{h}_v^{(t)}, \boldsymbol{h}_w^{(t)}, \boldsymbol{e}_{vw})$$

$$\boldsymbol{h}_v^{(t+1)} = U_t(\boldsymbol{h}_v^{(t)}, \boldsymbol{m}_v^{(t+1)})$$

where $\boldsymbol{e}_{vw}$ is the edge features from node v to w, and $M_t()$ and $U_t()$ are message function and update functions, respectively. The message function $\boldsymbol{m}_v^{(t+1)}$ aggregates all the messages from node v's neighbors based on their node embedding $\boldsymbol{h}_w^{(t)}$ and edge features $\boldsymbol{e}_{vw}$. After that, the node embedding $\boldsymbol{h}_v^{(t+1)}$ is updated with the current node embedding $\boldsymbol{h}_v^{(t)}$ and newly aggregated message function $\boldsymbol{m}_v^{(t+1)}$.

- **Readout stage** produces an embedding vector for the entire graph $\boldsymbol{h}_G$ from the node embedding vectors

$$\boldsymbol{h}_G = R(\{\boldsymbol{h}_v^{(T)} | v \in G\})$$

where T is the total number of message passing iterations and $R()$ is the readout function.

Many different architectures (e.g., DNN, RNN) are introduced to specify those functions $M_t()$, $U_t()$ and $R()$.

Remarks The general MPNN can support edge features but require storing edge-based activations and can be much more expensive than GCN. MPNN is only applicable to small graphs such as molecule graphs.

10.6 Graph Attention Networks

The graph attention networks (GAT)[1] utilizes attention mechanism on graphs, which allows different weights to different nodes in the neighborhood. The input are a set of node embedding $\{\boldsymbol{h}_1^{(l)}, \boldsymbol{h}_2^{(l)}, \ldots, \boldsymbol{h}_N^{(l)}\}$ at layer l. And the output are the corresponding set of node embedding $\{\boldsymbol{h}_1^{(l+1)}, \boldsymbol{h}_2^{(l+1)}, \ldots, \boldsymbol{h}_N^{(l+1)}\}$ at layer $l + 1$. Here we assume the embedding vectors $\boldsymbol{h}_i^{(l)}, \boldsymbol{h}_i^{(l+1)} \in \mathbb{R}^F$ of size F. We ignore the subscript l when they are not ambiguous for simplicity.

The alignment model between node v_i and v_j is defined as

[1] The acronym GAN is associated with a more famous model called generative adversarial networks, which will be covered in a later chapter. Therefore, GAT was used instead.

$$e_{ij} = a(\boldsymbol{W}\boldsymbol{h}_i, \boldsymbol{W}\boldsymbol{h}_j)$$

where $\boldsymbol{W}$ is the weight matrix and $a()$ is $\texttt{LeakyReLU}(\boldsymbol{a}^\top[\boldsymbol{W}\boldsymbol{h}_i||\boldsymbol{W}\boldsymbol{h}_j])$ and $||$ indicates the vector concatenation. Here we only compute e_{ij} for nodes directly connected to v_i, i.e., $v_j \in \mathcal{N}_i$.

Hence, the graph attention weight between v_i and v_j is

$$\alpha_{ij} = \text{Softmax}(e_{ij}) = \frac{\exp(e_{ij})}{\sum_{v_j \in \mathcal{N}_i} \exp(e_{ij})}$$

The context vector is also constrained to the ones directly connected to v_i:

$$\boldsymbol{c}_i = \sum_{v_j \in \mathcal{N}_i} \alpha_{ij} \boldsymbol{W}\boldsymbol{h}_j.$$

Finally, the output node embedding is $\boldsymbol{h}_i^{(l+1)} = \sigma(\boldsymbol{c}_i)$ where $\sigma()$ is sigmoid or softmax function. To further improve the model stability, K independent attention models are computed and concatenated or averaged as the output node embedding, i.e., $\boldsymbol{h}_i^{(l+1)} = \sigma(\frac{1}{K}\sum_{k=1}^{K} \boldsymbol{c}_i^k)$.

Remarks Computationally, GAT is more efficient than MPNN with edge features due to the ease of parallel computation. Compared to GCN, GAT allows different importance to the neighboring nodes, making the model more flexible.

10.7 Case Study: Neural Fingerprint in Drug Molecule Embedding with GCN

Problem A chemical molecule compound is a graph structure characterized by atoms as nodes and chemical bonds as edges that connect atoms. A core computational problem is to extract a meaningful vector representation from a molecule graph. Such representation can then predict chemical properties associated with the molecule which is important for drug discovery.

Existing Approach Fingerprinting methods such as circular fingerprints are designed to encode the presence or absence of substructures in a molecule. The general idea is to apply a hash function on substructures of the molecule graphs and then index the results on a bit vector. The **hashing step** is to repeatedly extract subgraphs of variable sizes by expanding neighborhoods from each node in a molecule graph. Then it hashes those subgraphs into integers. Then in the **indexing** step, each resulting integer sets a specific bit to 1 in a long bit vector. This way, each molecule will be represented by a long bit vector (e.g., 1024 bits) where each bit corresponds to a particular substructure. One of the most commonly used fingerprint algorithms is the extended-connectivity circular fingerprints (ECFP) [124].

Table 10.1 Prediction accuracy of neural fingerprints compared to standard circular fingerprints

Dataset units	Solubility log Mol/L	Drug efficacy EC_{50} in nM	Photovoltaic efficiency percent
Predict mean	4.29 ± 0.40	1.47 ± 0.07	6.40 ± 0.09
Circular FPs + linear layer	1.84 ± 0.08	1.13 ± 0.03	2.62 ± 0.07
Circular FPs + neural net	1.40 ± 0.15	1.24 ± 0.03	2.04 ± 0.07
Neural FPs + linear layer	0.74 ± 0.09	1.16 ± 0.03	2.71 ± 0.13
Neural FPs + neural net	0.53 ± 0.07	1.17 ± 0.03	1.44 ± 0.11

Method Authors in [41] propose a differentiable fingerprint of molecules using GCNs. A GCN-like function was applied on the molecule data to output a real-valued vector for representing a molecule, analogous to circular fingerprint algorithms. The hash function in the circular fingerprint becomes the summation over node embeddings in a substructure. The indexing step becomes the accumulation of the softmax function over the summation result. In this case, the final representation of a molecule was obtained by aggregating representations of the neighborhoods of all atoms. The encoding procedure was graph convolutional in the sense that the neighborhood of each atom was aggregated to update the center atom, and the same local filter was applied for atoms with the same neighborhood size (e.g., ranged from 1 to 5) and their neighboring atoms.

Results Neural fingerprints were compared against circular fingerprints on a variety of domains: (1) Solubility: The aqueous solubility of 1144 molecules; (2) Drug efficacy: The half-maximal effective concentration (EC50) in vitro of 10,000 molecules against a sulfide-resistant strain of *P. falciparum*, the parasite that causes malaria; and (3) Organic photovoltaic efficiency: DFT simulation is used to estimate the photovoltaic efficiency of organic molecules [62]. A subset of 20,000 molecules from this dataset was used in the experiment.

The authors evaluated the generated fingerprints for several drug properties, including solubility, drug efficacy, and organic photovoltaic efficiency, with neural fingerprints outperformed traditional circular fingerprints as shown in Table 10.1.

10.8 Case Study: *Decagon* Modeling Polypharmacy Side Effects with GCN

Problem Polypharmacy, the use of multiple drugs together, is common in treating patients with multiple conditions. However, this combined use of drugs can cause a higher risk of adverse side effects. Among them, the adverse drug-drug interaction (DDI), in which one drug activity may change, favorably or unfavorably, if taken with another drug, is common among patients who have complex disease conditions. It is important to develop a complete profile of potential DDIs. However, the knowledge of drug interactions is often limited because these complex relationships are rare and are usually not observed in relatively small clinical testing. With the availability of massive health data, it is promising to infer unseen DDIs from multimodal health data by modeling it as a multi-typed link prediction task. Authors in [178] aim to solve this task via GCN models on heterogeneous graphs connecting drugs and target proteins.

Data To identify the side effects, the data used in this work are networks connecting drugs and proteins with three kinds of relations: drug to drug interactions (prediction targets), drug-protein interactions, and protein-protein interactions.

- To construct the **protein-protein interaction graph**, human protein-protein interaction (PPI) network is used [149]. The resulting network is an unweighted and undirected graph with 19,085 proteins and 719,402 physical interactions.
- To construct the **drug-protein interaction graph**, 8,083,600 interactions between 8934 proteins and 519,022 small chemicals are selected from the STITCH (Search Tool for InTeractions of CHemicals) database [148] to form an unweighted and undirected network.
- To form the **drug-drug interaction graph**, multiple sources are used, including SIDER (Side Effect Resource) database [91], OFFSIDES database, and TWOSIDES database [153]. In the end, the 964 commonly-occurring types of polypharmacy side effects that each occurred in at least 500 drug combinations are included in our dataset.

The **final dataset** has 645 drug and 19,085 protein nodes connected by 715,612 protein-protein, 4,651,131 drug-drug, and 18,596 drug-protein edges.

Method The polypharmacy side effect prediction is cast as a multi-relational link prediction problem on a graph connecting drugs and proteins. Formally, given a graph $G = (\mathcal{V}, \mathcal{R})$, a relation/edge between node v_i and v_j is represented as (v_i, r, v_j) where r is the relation type. Depending on the node types, the relations can be (1) physical bind between two proteins, (2) a target relationship between a drug and a protein, or (3) a side effect type between two drugs.

The encoder is a graph convolutional network with different parameters for different relation types. The encoding for a single layer this modified GCN is

$$\boldsymbol{h}_i^{(l+1)} = ReLU(\sum_r(\sum_{j\in\mathcal{N}_r^i} c_r^{ij}\mathbf{W}_r^{(l)}\boldsymbol{h}_j^{(l)} + c_r^i\boldsymbol{h}_i^{(l)}))$$

where $\boldsymbol{h}_i^{(l)}$ is the node embedding of v_i at layer l, r is the relation type, $\mathcal{N}_r^i$ is neighborhood of v_i of relation r, and $\mathbf{W}_r^{(l)}$ is the weight matrix of relation r at layer l, $c_r^{ij} = 1/\sqrt{|\mathcal{N}_r^i||\mathcal{N}_r^j|}$ and $c_r^i = 1/|\mathcal{N}_r^i|$.[2]

[2] $|\mathcal{N}_r^i|$ is the size of neighborhood $\mathcal{N}_r^i$.

The decoder is to predict the probability of links between nodes given the node embedding $\boldsymbol{h}_1, \boldsymbol{h}_2, \ldots, \boldsymbol{h}_N$. The decoder score (v_i, r, v_j) is

$$g(v_i, r, v_j) = \begin{cases} \boldsymbol{h}_i^\top \boldsymbol{D}_r \boldsymbol{R} \boldsymbol{D}_r \boldsymbol{h}_j^\top, & \text{if } v_i \text{ and } v_j \text{ are drugs} \\ \boldsymbol{h}_i^\top \boldsymbol{M}_r \boldsymbol{h}_j, & \text{if } v_i, v_j \text{ are both proteins or one drug and one protein.} \end{cases}$$

When v_i and v_j are both drugs, the model parameters include diagonal matrices $\boldsymbol{D}_r$ for each relation type r, and global weight matrix $\boldsymbol{R}$. Here $\boldsymbol{D}_r$ is a diagonal matrix providing relation specific weights by giving different weights for different latent dimensions in $\boldsymbol{h}_i$. And $\boldsymbol{R}$ is the global weight matrix across all relations. When at least one of v_i and v_j is protein, the model parameters are relation specific matrices $\boldsymbol{M}_r$.

The probability of the edge v_i, r, v_j is

$$p_r^{ij} = \sigma(g(v_i, r, v_j)).$$

The loss function is cross-entropy loss with negative sampling, which is similar to Word2Vec:

$$J_r(i, j) = -\log p_r^{ij} - \mathbb{E}_{n \sim P_r} \log(1 - p_r^{in}),$$

where the negative edges are random edges connecting to v_i. The total loss is $J = \sum_{(v_i, r, v_j)} J_r(i, j)$ (Fig. 10.1).

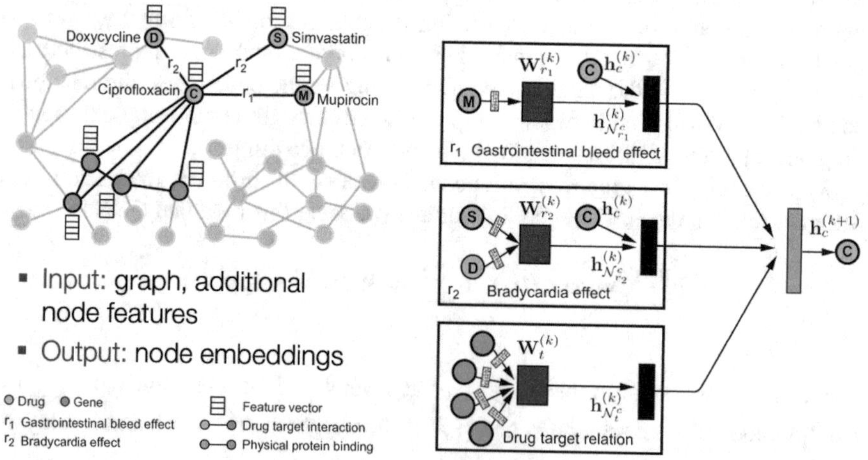

Fig. 10.1 Left: the illustration of the input graph containing edges between drug to protein, and protein to protein. The goal is to estimate the links between drugs which indicate different types of side effects. Right: the encoding process for a single node Ciprofloxacin involves three different relations: r1: Gastrointestinal bleed effect, r2: Bradycardia effect, r3: drug target relation

Table 10.2 The prediction results compared on Area under ROC curve (AUROC), area under precision-recall curve (AUPRC), and average precision at 50 (AP@50) for polypharmacy side effect prediction. Reported are average performance values for 964 side effect types

Approach	AUROC	AUPRC	AP@50
Decagon	0.872	0.832	0.803
RESCAL tensor factorization	0.693	0.613	0.476
DEDICOM tensor factorization	0.705	0.637	0.567
DeepWalk neural embeddings	0.761	0.737	0.658
Concatenated drug features	0.793	0.764	0.712

Table 10.3 The best and worst performing side effect types

Best performing side effects	AUPRCI	Worst performing side effects	AUPRC
Mumps	0.964	Bleeding	0.679
Carbuncle	0.949	Increased body temperature	0.680
Coccydynia	0.943	Emesis	0.693
Tympanic membrane perfor.	0.941	Renal disorder	0.694
Dyshidrosis	0.938	Leucopenia	0.695
Spondylosis	0.929	Diarrhea	0.705
Schizoaffective disorder	0.919	Icterus	0.707
Breast dysplasia	0.918	Nausea	0.711
Ganglion	0.909	Itch	0.712
Uterine polyp	0.908	Anaemia	0.712

Results The authors compared the performance of Decagon to other baseline approaches. Table 10.2 shows the GCN based method of different side effects allows Decagon to outperform other approaches. Across 964 side effect types, Decagon outperforms baselines approaches by 19.7% (AUROC), 22.0% (AUPRC), and 36.3% (AP@50).

To better understand Decagon's performance, the authors stratify performance by the side effect type. The best performing side effect types are presented in Table 10.3. Decagon models seem to perform particularly well on side effects with strong molecular underpinnings.

10.9 Case Study: Deep Learning Approach to Antibiotic Discovery

Problem Antibiotic drugs are essential for modern medicine. However, continued efficacy of existing antibiotics is uncertain due to the antibiotic resistance. Furthermore, due to the short course of use and the risk of antibiotic resistance, there is lack of economic incentive for new antibiotic development by pharmaceuticals. And the discovery of new antibiotics is becoming increasingly difficult.

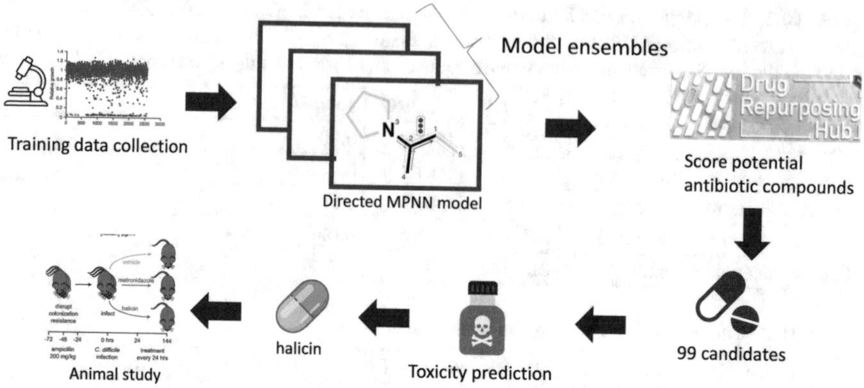

Fig. 10.2 The pipeline for developing a new antibiotic molecule

Approach and Results Authors in [139] performed predictions on multiple chemical libraries and discovered a molecule from drug repurposing hub that is structurally different from existing antibiotics with promising web lab experiment results. Figure 10.2 illustrates the analytic pipeline for identifying the new antibiotic molecule:

- The training dataset are collected by screening 1760 diverse drug molecules from FDA approved drug library, and 800 natural products using E. coli. The results are binarized as hit and non-hit. The authors use 80% growth inhibition as a hit cut-off. Among which 120 molecules are considered hits.
- Then a variant of MPNN algorithm (i.e., a directed MPNN model [172]) is used to convert molecule graphs into vector representation. In particular, each molecule is encoded as a graph with atoms as nodes and bond as edges. The node features include atom number, number of bonds, formal charge, chirality and number of bonded hydrogens, hybridization, aromaticity and atomic mass. The edge features include bond type (single, double, triple or aromatic), conjugation, ring membership, and stereochemistry. The details of those features are listed in Fig. 10.3. After directed MPNN, the resulting molecule will have an embedding representation. In addition, they also use RDKit (rdkit.org) to generate a list of domain features. Both MPNN embedding and domain features are concatenated as the final feature vector for a molecule.
- Using the final feature vectors, 20 classification models are computed and averaged to produce an ensemble classifier for predicting hit or non-hit. The model achieved AUC of 0.896. The 99 top ranked molecules are selected for further lab validation. Finally, the authors identified one molecule named Halicin as the new antibiotic candidate. They performed various animal experiments to show Halicin works much better than existing antibiotic Metronidazole. Furthermore, the structural diversity of Halicin is very different from other known molecules. In particular, they observe low Tanimoto similarity between Halicin and other known molecules in the training set.

Node features

feature	description	size
atom type	type of atom (ex. C, N, O), by atomic number	100
# bonds	number of bonds the atom is involved in	6
formal charge	integer electronic charge assigned to atom	5
chirality	unspecified, tetrahedral CW/CCW, or other	4
# Hs	number of bonded hydrogen atoms	5
hybridization	sp, sp2, sp3, sp3d, or sp3d2	5
aromaticity	whether this atom is part of an aromatic system	1
atomic mass	mass of the atom, divided by 100	1

Edge features

feature	description	size
bond type	single, double, triple, or aromatic	4
conjugated	whether the bond is conjugated	1
in ring	whether the bond is part of a ring	1
stereo	none, any, E/Z or cis/trans	6

Fig. 10.3 Node and edge features of a molecule graph and its dimensionalities

10.10 Case Study: *STAN* Spatio-Temporal Attention Network with GAT for Pandemic Prediction

Problem Pandemic diseases such as the novel coronavirus disease (COVID-19) has been spreading rapidly across the world and poses a severe threat to global public health. Up to the end of December 2020, COVID-19 has affected 19 million people and caused more than 332K deaths in the US, and caused significant disruption to people's daily life as well as substantial economic losses. Therefore, it is critical to predict the pandemic outbreak early and accurately to help design appropriate policies and reduce losses. In this work [51], we aim at developing a hybrid model for earlier and more accurate predictions for the number of infected cases in pandemics by (1) using patients' claims data from different counties and states that capture local disease status and medical resource utilization; (2) utilizing demographic similarity and geographical proximity between locations; and (3) integrating pandemic transmission dynamics into a deep learning model.

Data In this work, we used a US county-level dataset that consists of COVID-19 related data from two resources: Johns Hopkins University (JHU) Coronavirus Resource Center [20] and IQVIA's claims data [39]. The data from JHU Coronavirus Resource Center was collected from March 22, 2020 to June 10, 2020. It has the number of active cases, confirmed cases, and deaths related to COVID-19 for different US locations. We select states with more than 1000 confirmed cases by May 17 to ensure the data source accuracy, and finally we have 45 states and 193 counties in the dataset. For those counties, we set the number of cases before their respective first record dates as zero. The IQVIA's claims data is from the IQVIA US9 Database. We export patient claims data and prescription data from March

22, 2020 to June 10, 2020, from which we obtain the number of hospital and ICU visits and the term-frequency of each medical code per county per day. Detailed dataset descriptions are shown in Supplementary. The dataset has records for a total of 453,089 patients across the entire timespan of the JHU dataset. The 48 unique ICD-10 codes related to COVID-19 are listed in the Supplementary Material.

The input data to the STAN model includes dynamic data and static data. Dynamic data is a 3D tensor that includes location (e.g., states, counties, etc.), timestamp (e.g., days/weeks), and the dynamic features at each location (e.g., the number of active COVID-19 cases and the numbers of other related ICD codes). Static data is a 2D matrix that includes location and the static features for each location. We also form an attributed graph to capture the spatio-temporal epidemic/pandemic dynamics. In particular, we model the geographic proximity and demographic similarity between the different locations as edges in a location graph.

Method This work proposes a Spatio-Temporal Attention Network (STAN) for pandemic prediction using real-world evidence such as claims data and COVID-19 case surveillance data. We map locations (e.g., a county or a state) to nodes on a graph and construct the edges based on geographical proximity and demographic similarity between locations. Each node is associated with a set of static and dynamic features extracted from multiple real-world evidence in medical claims data that capture disease prevalence at different locations and medical resource utilization conditions.

- **Spatial correlation:** We utilize a graph attention network (GAT) to incorporate interactions of similar locations. In our setting, each location will receive information from its adjacent locations based on mobility to model spatio-temporal disease transmission patterns. This consideration is based on the real-world scenario that adjacent locations may have different impacts on the infectious status of the focused location. For example, if one city has a large population size and increasing infected cases, this city may have a more considerable impact on its adjacent counties.
- **Temporal correlation:** We input the graph embedding to Gated Recurrent Unit (GRU) network to learn temporal features using the location embeddings as input.
- **Transmission dynamics:** Then we predict the number of infected patients for a fixed period into the future while concurrently imposing physical constraints on predictions according to transmission dynamics of epidemiological models such as susceptible-infectious-removed (SIR) and susceptible-exposed-infectious-removed (SEIR). The idea is to use short-term prediction loss and long-term transmission dynamics constraint loss to regularize learned hidden representations of node embeddings (i.e., hidden state of the GRU)

Results We apply STAN to predict both state-level and county-level future number of infected cases, achieving up to 87% reduction in mean squared error compared to the best baseline model.

Table 10.4 Performance comparison for county-level predictions: Prediction window = 5 days

	MSE	MAE	CCC
SIR	93,512	151.33	0.40
SEIR	134,494	165.14	0.35
GRU	79,982	121.76	0.47
STAN	44,177	79.80	0.66

We compare STAN with the following baselines.

- SIR: the susceptible-infected-removed (SIR), a basic disease transmission model that uses differential equations to simulate an epidemic. S, I, and R represent the number of susceptible, infected, and recovered individuals.
- SEIR: the susceptible-exposed-infected-removed (SEIR) epidemiological model as another transmission dynamics constraint-based baselines. Compared to the SIR model, SEIR adds exposed population size to the equation.
- Gated Recurrent Unit (GRU): We input the latest number of infected cases into a naive GRU and predict future numbers.

We use the mean square error (MSE), mean absolute error (MAE) to evaluate our model. We also use the average concordance correlation coefficient (CCC) to evaluate the results. The CCC measures the agreement between two variables, and it is computed as:

$$CCC = \frac{2\rho\sigma_x\sigma_y}{\sigma_x^2 + \sigma_y^2 + (\mu_x - \mu_y)^2}$$

where μ_x and μ_y are the means of x and y, σ_x and σ_y are the standard deviations. Table 10.4 shows the prediction performance on the county level. STAN achieves much lower errors compared to all the baselines. More results are shown in [51].

10.11 Exercises

1. What is the main difference between graph convolutional network and graph attention network?
2. What applications for graph neural networks? (multiple correct choices).

    (a) Node classification
    (b) Link prediction
    (c) Graph generation
    (d) Anomaly detection
    (e) Graph property prediction
    (f) Community detection

3. What are the challenges of using neural networks on graphs? (multiple correct choices)
   (a) Arbitrary size
   (b) No fixed node ordering
   (c) Dynamic updates
   (d) Heterogeneous features
   (e) Small sample size
4. Which is not part of the input to graph neural networks?
   (a) Nodes
   (b) Edges
   (c) Node features
   (d) Importance weights of nodes
5. Which one is NOT a computational step in graph neural networks?
   (a) Define a neighborhood aggregation function
   (b) Define a loss function on the embeddings
   (c) Train a set of nodes based on local neighborhoods
   (d) Iteratively update the underlying graph structure
6. What is NOT true about GCN model?
   (a) It aims at learning node embeddings on graphs.
   (b) To achieve efficient training, various sampling strategies are introduced.
   (c) Aggregation over the neighborhoods is the bottleneck in training.
   (d) The number of parameters in GCN is proportional to the graph size.
7. In MPNN model illustrated in Fig. 10.4, what is the message passing update for node C?
   (a) $Mt(h_C, h_A, e_{CA}) + Mt(h_C, h_B, e_{CB})$
   (b) $Mt(h_C, h_A, e_{CA}) + Mt(h_C, h_B, e_{CB}) + Mt(h_C, h_E, e_{CE})$
   (c) $Mt(h_C, h_A, e_{CA}) + Mt(h_A, h_B, e_{AB}) + Mt(h_C, h_B, e_{CB})$
   (d) $Mt(h_C, h_B, e_{CB}) + Mt(h_C, h_E, e_{CE})$

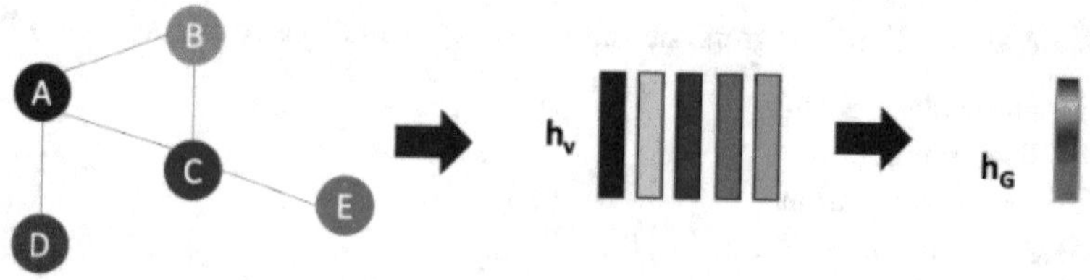

Fig. 10.4 MPNN exercise

8. What is NOT true about read-out operation in MPNN?
   (a) The read-out operation aims at generating an embedding for the entire graph.
   (b) Average or max pooling are common functions for read-out operation.
   (c) With RNN read-out, a random order over the nodes should be used.
   (d) Read-out operation is the most expensive step in training MPNN.
9. What is NOT true about GAT model?
   (a) Alignment weight e_{ij} is computed between node i and j.
   (b) GAT utilizes multi-head attention mechanism.
   (c) Attention weights are on all pairs of nodes in the graph.
   (d) GAT allows different importance to different neighbors via attention mechanism.
10. What are the different node types used in polypharmacy network described in Sect. 10.8? [multiple correct choices]
   (a) Drug molecules
   (b) Protein targets
   (c) Diseases
   (d) Side effects

Chapter 11
Memory Networks

Memory network is a powerful extension of attention models. The memory network models have shown initial successes in natural language processing such as question answering [60, 92, 112, 141, 166]. In particular, memory networks use external memory components to assist the deep neural networks in remembering and storing information. Various memory network based models have been proposed, such as [92, 112, 141]. In healthcare, memory networks can be valuable due to their capacities in utilizing medical knowledge and patient history, as shown in [134].

11.1 Original Memory Networks

Memory Networks [166] and Differentiable Neural Computers (DNC) [60] proposed to use external memory components to assist the deep neural networks in remembering and storing information. After that, various memory network models [92, 112, 141] have been proposed. The original memory networks are proposed for solving question answering in the natural language processing domain [92, 112, 141, 166].

At a high level, a memory network consists of memory $\boldsymbol{m}$ and the following four learning components.

1. **Input feature map** I converts the incoming input to the internal feature representation.
2. **Generalization** component G updates old memories given new input. We call this generalization as there is an opportunity for the network to compress and generalize its memories at this stage for some intended future use.
3. **Output feature map** O produces a new output in the feature representation space, given the new input and the current memory state.
4. **Response** component R converts the output embeddings into the response format desired. For example, a text description or a particular class label.

C. Xiao, J. Sun, *Introduction to Deep Learning for Healthcare*,
https://doi.org/10.1007/978-3-030-82184-5_11

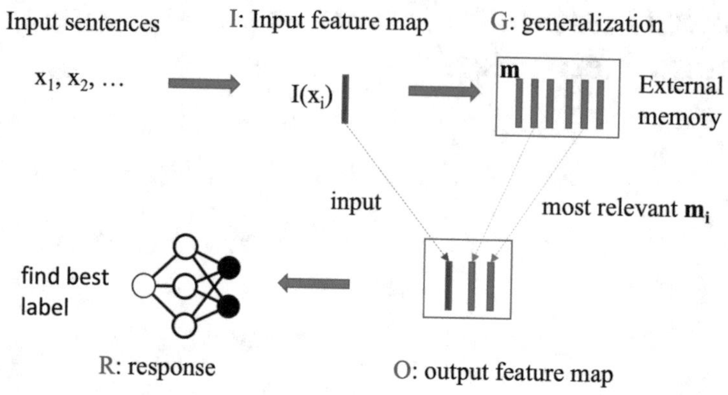

Fig. 11.1 Components of memory networks

Next, we illustrate the interaction between those components. Given an input $\boldsymbol{x}$ such as a sequence of words or sequence of clinical events, the flow of the memory network is given as follows.

1. First, we will convert $\boldsymbol{x}$ to an internal feature representation $I(\boldsymbol{x})$. Here the representation of inputs and memories can use all kinds of encodings such as a bag of words or multi-hot embeddings, RNN embedding.
2. Second, we store $I(\boldsymbol{x})$ into the memory, or update existing memory $\boldsymbol{m}_i$ with generalization and compression. Mathematically, it denotes as $\boldsymbol{m}_i = G(\boldsymbol{m}_i, I(\boldsymbol{x}), \boldsymbol{m})\forall i$. In the simplest form, G function just stores $I(\boldsymbol{x})$ into a memory slot $\boldsymbol{m}_i$ in memory bank $\boldsymbol{m}$.
3. Third, we compute the output feature o given the new input $I(\boldsymbol{x})$ and the current memory bank $\boldsymbol{m}$. This component tries to find the best matching memory slots based on some matching function $\boldsymbol{m}$: $o = O(I(\boldsymbol{x}), \boldsymbol{m})$. For example, Fig. 11.1 retrieves two most relevant memory slots to combine with input $I(\boldsymbol{x})$ as the output feature map.
4. Finally we map output o to give final response $r = R(o)$. We can choose any output decoders—for example, softmax for classification or RNN for sequence generation.

We need to specify the inference mechanism in O and R modules to implement the memory network with neural networks. One simple way is to use the input as a query to score all memory slots and retrieve the ones with highest scores: $o_1 = \arg\max_i S_O(x, \boldsymbol{m}_i)$ where S_O is the output scoring function that computes the similarity between input x and memory slot $\boldsymbol{m}_i$. This can be generalized to more than one memory slot. The response module will score the input and most relevant memory slots to generate the response. For example, if the response is a single word from a set W, the response will be $r = \arg\max_{w \in W} S_R([x, o_1], w)$ where S_R is the response scoring function between a word w and the combination of input x and most relevant memory o_1. In [166], the similarity function is

$S(x, y) = \Phi_x(x)^\top U^\top U \Phi_y(y)$ where $\Phi_x(x)$,$\Phi_y(y)$ are the input embeddings and U is the linear embedding matrix. Finally, the model is trained in a fully supervised fashion using the ranking loss of the output module and response module:

$$\underbrace{\sum_{\bar{f} \neq o_1} \max(0, \gamma - S_O(x, o_1) + s_O(x, \bar{f}))}_{\text{output module}} + \underbrace{\sum_{\bar{r} \neq r} \max(0, \gamma - S_R([x, o_1], r) + s_R([x, o_1], \bar{r}))}_{\text{response module}}$$

where $\bar{f}$ and $\bar{r}$ are the other choices than the correct label, and γ is the margin. In the paper [166], the top two output o_1 and o_2 are generated, which leads to a slightly more complicated expression. One major limitation of the original memory network is the lack of end-to-end training due to the arg max operations which break the gradient flows which is needed for backpropagation.

11.2 End-to-End Memory Networks

The original memory network [166] uses the arg max function to find the optimal memory slots and the best output. Later on, the authors [141] extended this "hard" attention with "soft" attention via softmax function, which leads to memory networks that can be trained in an end-to-end fashion.

This end-to-end memory network involves input $\boldsymbol{x}_1, \boldsymbol{x}_2, \ldots, \boldsymbol{x}_n$ stored in the memory bank and a query $\boldsymbol{q}$. And this network outputs an answer $\boldsymbol{a}$. For example, input $\boldsymbol{x}_i$ can be all the historical patient records in the EHR database. In contrast, query $\boldsymbol{q}$ is the record of the current patient, and the answer $\boldsymbol{a}$ can be the medication recommended for the current patient. Two different memory representations are constructed for the input: one input memory representation called the *keys*, and one output memory representation called the *values*. Figure 11.2 illustrates the architecture of the end-to-end memory network.

Input Memory (Keys) All the input $\boldsymbol{x}_1, \boldsymbol{x}_2, \ldots, \boldsymbol{x}_n$ are embedded via matrix $\boldsymbol{A}$ into a set of vectors $\boldsymbol{m}_1, \boldsymbol{m}_2, \ldots, \boldsymbol{m}_n$. For example, a simple linear embedding can be applied $\boldsymbol{m}_i = \boldsymbol{A}\boldsymbol{x}_i$. The query $\boldsymbol{q}$ is also embedded using a different matrix $\boldsymbol{B}$ to produce the embedded vector $\boldsymbol{u}$. For example, $\boldsymbol{u} = \boldsymbol{B}\boldsymbol{q}$. Then the similarity matching score between query embedding $\boldsymbol{u}$ and input embedding $\boldsymbol{m}_i$ can be computed as inner product followed by softmax:

$$p_i = \text{Softmax}(\boldsymbol{u}^\top \boldsymbol{m}_i).$$

Here p_i is the matching score between the query $\boldsymbol{u}$ and input $\boldsymbol{m}_i$. Once we calculated the matching scores from the query to all input embeddings, denoted by $p_1, p_2, \ldots, p_n$, we can retrieve the output embeddings with highest matching scores.

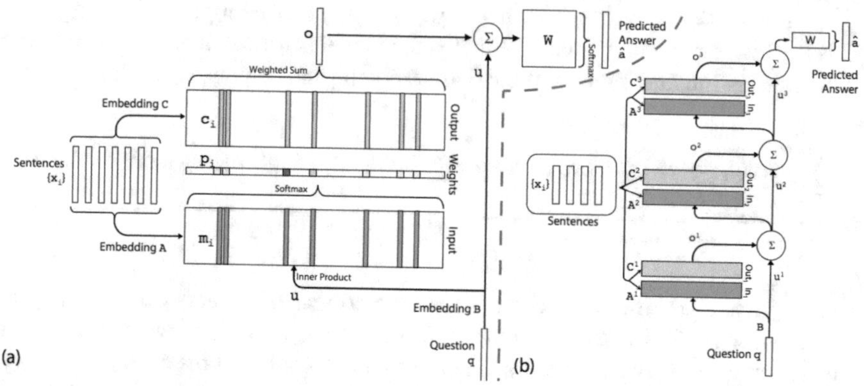

Fig. 11.2 End-to-end memory networks: (**a**) a single layer version, (**b**) multi-layer version

Output Memory (Value) Similar to input memory, the output memory are another set embedding vectors transformed from input $\boldsymbol{x}_1, \boldsymbol{x}_2, \ldots, \boldsymbol{x}_n$ via embedding matrix $\boldsymbol{C}$ via $\boldsymbol{c}_i = \boldsymbol{C}\boldsymbol{x}_i$. The response vector is the weighted sum of all output embedding $\boldsymbol{c}_1, \boldsymbol{c}_2, \ldots, \boldsymbol{c}_n$, namely

$$\boldsymbol{o} = \sum_i p_i \boldsymbol{c}_i.$$

Generating Final Prediction Both the response vector $\boldsymbol{o}$ and the query vector $\boldsymbol{u}$ are used to generate the final prediction:

$$\hat{\boldsymbol{a}} = \text{Softmax}(\boldsymbol{W}(\boldsymbol{o} + \boldsymbol{u})).$$

With this architecture, all the embedding matrix $\boldsymbol{A}, \boldsymbol{B}, \boldsymbol{C}$ and $\boldsymbol{W}$ are jointly trained using the cross-entropy loss between ground truth label $\boldsymbol{a}$ (a one-hot vector) and the prediction $\hat{\boldsymbol{a}}$.

Multiple Layers Multiple memory layers can be stacked:

- The input to layer $k + 1$ can be the sum between output $\boldsymbol{o}^k$ and the input $\boldsymbol{u}^k$ from layer k, namely, $\boldsymbol{u}^{k+1} = \boldsymbol{o}^k + \boldsymbol{u}^k$;
- Each layer will have its own embedding matrices $\boldsymbol{A}^k$, $\boldsymbol{B}^k$, $\boldsymbol{C}^k$;
- Finally the prediction per layer can be computed as $\hat{\boldsymbol{a}} = \text{Softmax}(\boldsymbol{W}\boldsymbol{u}^{k+1})$.

The authors proposed two ways to connect the parameters across layers.

- **Adjacent:** Output embedding matrix of layer k is the input embedding matrix for layer $k + 1$: $\boldsymbol{A}^{k+1} = \boldsymbol{C}^k$.
- **Layer-wise:** Tying input and output embeddings across all layers, i.e., $\boldsymbol{A}^1 = \boldsymbol{A}^2 = \ldots = \boldsymbol{A}^k$ and $\boldsymbol{C}^1 = \boldsymbol{C}^2 = \ldots = \boldsymbol{C}^k$. Then a linear mapping $\boldsymbol{H}$ is added between input layers: $\boldsymbol{u}^{k+1} = \boldsymbol{H}\boldsymbol{u}^k + \boldsymbol{o}^k$.

11.3 Self-Attention and Transformer

Self-attention is a more efficient strategy for computing attention scores among the original input without any dependency on RNN models. Standard attention models heavily rely on RNN as the annotation vectors $\boldsymbol{h}_i$ are the results of the encoder RNN and the hidden states $\boldsymbol{s}_i$ are also outputs of another RNN. Because of the sequential nature of RNN, the model training process leads to significant computational and optimization challenges. More specifically, attention models need all the hidden states $\boldsymbol{h}_1$ to $\boldsymbol{h}_T$ of the entire input sequence to compute the context vector $\boldsymbol{c}_i$. Such a training process is intrinsically sequential within an input example, limiting its ability to optimize training in parallel, which is computationally more efficient.

To address this parallel training challenge, *Transformer* model is proposed, which introduces a new type of attention without RNN [160]. The insight comes from a simple question "why don't we compute context vectors over $\boldsymbol{x}_i$ directly". We actually can, and the way to achieve this is through the *self-attention* mechanism. Conceptually, the self-attention model replaces the RNNs from the encoder and decoder completely with an attention mechanism with the input to itself.

The goal of transformer model is to "transform" an input embedding $\boldsymbol{x}_i$ into a better embedding $\boldsymbol{x}'_i$ that captures the contexts (or correlation) of $\boldsymbol{x}_i$ with all the other input. To achieve that, a query, keys, and values are introduced similar to an end-to-end memory network [142]. Here a query is a specific input $\boldsymbol{x}_i$, while keys and values are all input $\boldsymbol{x}_1, \boldsymbol{x}_2, \ldots, \boldsymbol{x}_n$. There are two steps involved:

- **Similarity search:** The idea is to compute similarity between query $\boldsymbol{x}_i$ and all input represented by $\boldsymbol{X} = [\boldsymbol{x}_1, \ldots, \boldsymbol{x}_n] \in \mathbb{R}^{d_x \times n}$. Instead of using original input $\boldsymbol{X}$, a linear embedding layer is introduced: $\boldsymbol{K} = \boldsymbol{W}^K \boldsymbol{X} \in \mathbb{R}^{d_K \times n}$ where $\boldsymbol{W}^K \in \mathbb{R}^{d_K \times d_x}$. Similarly, we linearly transform the query $\boldsymbol{q}_i = \boldsymbol{W}^Q \boldsymbol{x}_i \in \mathbb{R}^{d_K}$. A scaled dot product is computed as the similarity score vector $\boldsymbol{e}_i = \frac{\boldsymbol{K}^\top \boldsymbol{q}_i}{\sqrt{d_K}}$. The scaled dot product is very similar to a dot product $\boldsymbol{K}^\top \boldsymbol{q}_i$ but with additional $1/\sqrt{d_K}$ factor. The idea of $1/\sqrt{d_K}$ factor is to alleviate the concern that the softmax function of a high dimensional input may have an extremely small gradient. Like the standard attention mechanism, the attention weight is normalized by $\boldsymbol{a}_i = \text{softmax}(\boldsymbol{e}_i) \in \mathbb{R}^n$.
- **Value retrieval:** Based on the similarity score $\boldsymbol{a}_i$, we can retrieve or recombine the input to generate the output embedding $\boldsymbol{x}'_i = \boldsymbol{W}^V \boldsymbol{X} \boldsymbol{a}_i$.

Note that all weight matrices $\boldsymbol{W}^K, \boldsymbol{W}^V, \boldsymbol{W}^Q \in \mathbb{R}^{d_K \times d_x}$ are of the same size. The reason to have separate weight matrices is to avoid dependency and maximize potential parallelism in training. The self-attention mechanism eliminates any sequential dependency; hence the training can be done in parallel more easily.

Besides the self-attention mechanism, the Transformer model introduces a few other innovations, namely, **multi-head attention** and **positional embedding**.

- The idea of multi-head attention is to compute multiple $\boldsymbol{a}_i$ for the same input $\boldsymbol{x}_i$ with different sets of weight matrices, which is analogous to multiple filters in

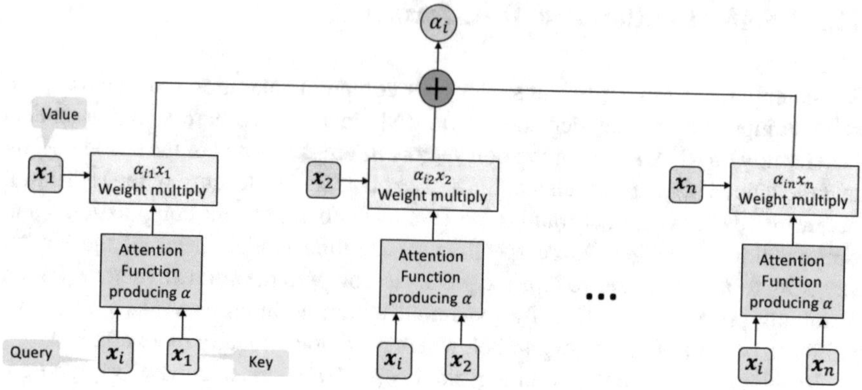

Fig. 11.3 Concept illustration of self-attention mechanism

CNN models. The benefit having multiple attention scores instead of one is to provide more robust estimate of the embedding.

- The positional embedding adds some features related to the position of $\boldsymbol{x}_i$ in the input sequence. This is important for natural language process application as a sequence corresponds to a sentence, and $\boldsymbol{x}_i$ is a word in the sequence. Therefore, where the word $\boldsymbol{x}_i$ appears in the sentence (at the beginning or the end) can be important (Fig. 11.3).

Now we understand the intuition and key components of the Transformer model. Next, we describe the overall algorithm, which follows an encoder and decoder architecture like a sequence-to-sequence model. Figure 11.4 illustrates the Transformer model.

Transformer Encoder The encoder can have multiple multi-head self-attention modules. The input embeddings (with optional positional embedding) are the input for the first layer. For subsequent layers, the output of the previous layer will be its input. The same input set will be used within each layer as keys, queries, and values to compute self-attention. The self-attention output will send through a feed-forward network layer with a skipped connection.

Transformer Decoder The decoder can also have multiple layers. Each layer is similar to the encoder but with different inputs. The input will be the output embedding of the decoder so far. Specifically, the input of the first layer will be the word embeddings generated so far. And subsequent layers will take the output of the previous layer as its input. Within each layer, a **masked multi-head self-attention** is computed with an appropriate mask so the attention will not be computed over the unseen words (i.e., those words to the right of the current word). For example, if the decoder output generates 5 tokens so far while the entire sequence has 20 tokens, the masked attention will not compute attention with the token 6–20 as they are not yet seen. The output is sent to another multi-head attention layer with the input embedding produced by the encoder. Finally, a feed-forward network layer

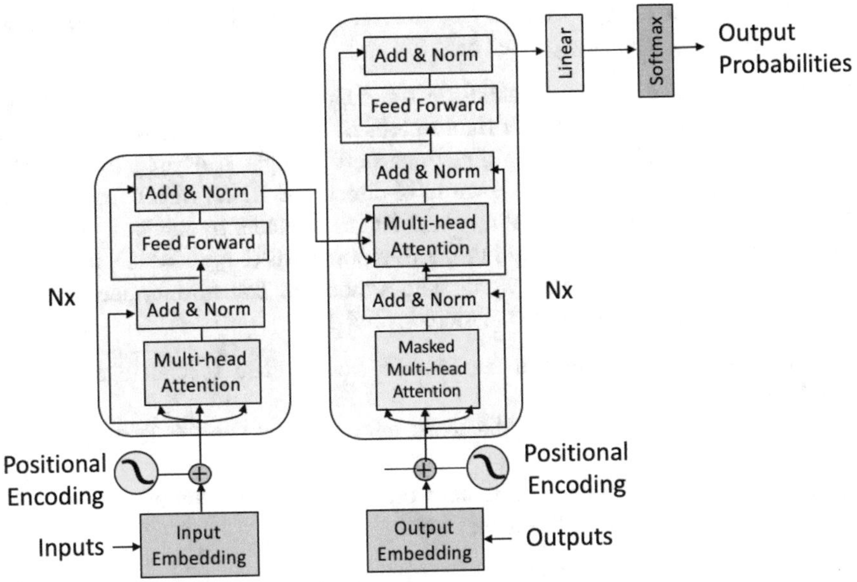

Fig. 11.4 The Transformer model architecture: The left side is the encoder and the right side is the decoder

like in encoder is applied at the end. The prediction task at position i is to predict next token at position $i + 1$ for all positions.

11.4 BERT: Pre-training of Deep Bidirectional Transformers

One important application of the Transformer is the BERT model for supporting natural language processing (NLP) tasks such as language understanding and question answering [37]. BERT stands for Bidirectional Encoder Representations from Transformers. The key ideas behind BERT are (1) context-specific pre-training and (2) masked language model.

Context Specific Pre-training Embedding vectors are the basis for deep learning models. In many tasks, people find it is useful to pre-train embedding from large datasets. For example, Word2Vec [110] and GloVe [117] are often used to generate pre-trained embeddings on large text corpus based on co-occurrence information between words. However, the same word will have the same embedding no matter what the contexts are. For example, although "bank account" and "river bank" have completely different meanings, the word "bank" will have the same embedding. BERT changed this assumption by introducing the context-specific embeddings, where the embedding of word x is dynamically computed based on the context of the sentence where x is in. BERT can be trained in an unsupervised fashion on a large corpus without any specific target label. If the labeled data exist, BERT also allows fine-tuning using the labeled data.

Masked Language Model Context-specific language models such as RNN are trained either from left to right or right to left. Bi-directional models are achieved by training 2 models from both directions (left to right and right to left) and concatenating the hidden states shown in bi-directional RNN. BERT introduces a new mechanism to achieve a bi-directional language model by randomly masking words. More specifically, by masking $k\%$ of input words (e.g., $k = 15$), the BERT model tries to predict the mask words with a modified Transformer decoder. The details of the masking procedure are more involved:

- 80% of the time we replace the masked word with a special token named [MASK];
- 10% of the time we replace the word with a random word from the entire vocabulary;
- 10% of the time we keep the original word unchanged. The purpose is to guide the BERT model towards this actual word.

The BERT model provides a power embedding method based on pre-training and masked language model, which have shown great performance on many real-world applications.

11.5 Case Study: Doctor2Vec—Doctor Recommendation for Clinical Trial Recruitment

Problem Massive electronic health records (EHRs) enable the success of learning accurate patient representations to support various predictive health applications. In contrast, doctor representation was not well studied, although doctors play pivotal roles in healthcare. How to construct the right doctor representations? How to use doctor representation to solve important health analytic problems? The authors of [8] study the doctor representation problem for the *clinical trial recruitment* application, which is about identifying the right doctors to help conduct the trials based on the trial description and patient EHR data of those doctors.

Method They propose Doctor2Vec, which simultaneously learns (1) doctor representations from EHR data and (2) trial representations from the description and categorical information about the trials. In particular, Doctor2Vec utilizes a *dynamic memory network* where the doctor's experience with patients is stored in the memory bank. The network will dynamically assign weights based on the trial representation via an attention mechanism. Figure 11.5 illustrates the overall framework of Doctor2Vec. Since each doctor sees a diverse set of patients, doctor representation should be dynamically constructed for a given trial instead of a static embedding vector staying the same for all trials. The authors achieved that by

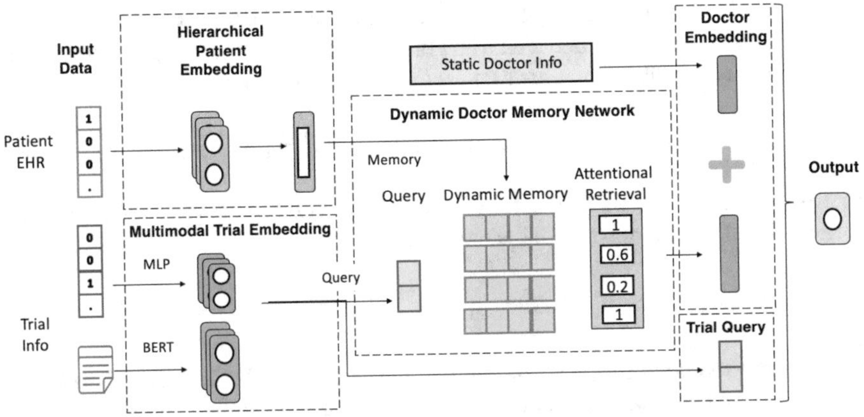

Fig. 11.5 Doctor2Vec Framework. (1) Hierarchical patient embedding: We obtain patient embeddings from patient visits using a Bi-LSTM with attention module. Unstructured text and categorical data are modeled using MLP and BERT, respectively. (2) Multimodal clinical trial information embedding: The obtained clinical trial embeddings from text and categorical data are concatenated together to form the query vector for the memory network. (3) Memory network module: This query vector is used to attend over the memory bank consisting of patient embeddings. The attention vector is used to obtain the final doctor embedding. The doctor embedding $\mathbf{Doc_{emb}}$ is combined with clinical trial embedding $\mathbf{Q_{emb}(I)}$ and static information about the doctors $\mathbf{Doc_{static}}$ to predict the enrollment rate of the clinical trial (output)

a dynamic memory network where patients are stored as memory vectors of the doctor. Using a trial embedding as a query, they fetch the relevant patient vectors from the memory bank and dynamically assemble a doctor representation for this trial.

Inspired by Weston et al. [166], four memory components **I**, **G**, **O**, **R** are proposed which mimics the architecture of modern computer in storing and processing information.

1. **Input Memory Representation**. This layer converts the patient representations to the input representation. They pass all the patient representations through a dense layer to obtain the input representations.

$$\mathbf{I_f(k)} = \mathbf{W_i I(k)} + \mathbf{b_i}$$

where $\mathbf{I(k)}$ and $\mathbf{I_f(k)}$ are input and final embedding of patient k.

2. **Generalization**. Typically generalization can be referred to as the process of updating memory representation for the memory bank. In our case, they use the patient representations to initialize the memory representation $\mathbf{M_d}$, which is the combination of all the patient representations. They then apply an LSTM layer to update the memory via multiple iterations.

$$\mathbf{M_d} = \mathrm{LSTM}(\mathbf{I_f(1)}, \cdots, \mathbf{I_f(k)}) \tag{11.1}$$

3. **Output**. In this step, the final output memory representation is generated. They calculate the relevance between trial embedding $\mathbf{Q_{emb}(l)}$ and doctor embedding $\mathbf{M_d}$ to obtain $\mathbf{A(k)}$ as the attention vector over patient representations.

$$\mathbf{A(k)} = \text{softmax}[\mathbf{Q_{emb}(l)^T M_d}] \tag{11.2}$$

4. **Response**. In this step, they obtain the final $\mathbf{Doc_{emb}}$ using the patient embeddings and attention weights over the patients.

$$\mathbf{Doc_{emb}} = \sum \mathbf{A(k) I_f(k)} \tag{11.3}$$

They use the doctor representation, composed of patients, and the clinical trial representation to obtain a final context vector. Besides dynamic doctor embedding $\mathbf{Doc_{emb}}$, they also include static information about doctors in the final embedding, such as their educational history, length of practice, length of practice into the feature vector. The resulting final embedding vectors are then fed into a fully connected layer and passed through a softmax to obtain class labels.

$$\mathbf{Y} = \text{Softmax}([\mathbf{Doc_{emb}}; \mathbf{Q_{emb}(l)}; \mathbf{Doc_{static}}])$$

where the input to Softmax are concatenation of dynamic doctor embedding $\mathbf{Doc_{emb}}$, trial query embedding $\mathbf{Q_{emb}(l)}$ and static doctor embedding $\mathbf{Doc_{static}}$.

The final prediction target is the trial enrollment rate for each doctor. The enrollment rate of a doctor is the number of patients enrolled by a doctor to the trial. And the enrollment rate is normalized by min and max values within each trial. Then the enrollment rate category is obtained by binning the continuous enrollment rate. They divide the continuous enrollment scores into five discrete classes ranging at 0–0.2, 0.2–0.4, 0.4–0.6, 0.6–0.8, 0.8–1.0. The five enrollment categories are used labels for classification.

Result Doctor2Vec is validated on large real-world trials and EHR data, including 2609 trials, 25K doctors and 430K patients.

They consider the following baselines.

1. Median Enrollment (Median). The current industry standard considers each therapeutic area's median enrollment rate as the estimated rate for all trials in that area.
2. Logistic Regression (LR). They combine the medication, diagnosis, procedure codes, and clinical trial information to create feature vectors and then apply LR to predict the enrollment rate category.
3. Random Forest (RF). They combine the medication, diagnosis, and procedure codes and clinical trial information to create feature vectors and then pass it to RF to predict the enrollment rate category.

Table 11.1 Doctor2Vec achieves the best performance on both metrics in predicting actual enrollment rate (regression task) and rate categories (classification task) compared to state-of-the-art baselines. Results of ten independent runs

	PR-AUC	R^2 Score
Median	0.571 ± 0.014	0.54 ± 0.072
LR	0.672 ± 0.041	0.314 ± 0.082
RF	0.731 ± 0.034	0.618 ± 0.034
AdaBoost	0.747 ± 0.002	0.684 ± 0.146
MLP	0.761 ± 0.019	0.762 ± 0.049
LSTM	0.792 ± 0.034	0.780 ± 0.621
DeepMatch	0.735 ± 0.068	0.821 ± 0.073
Doctor2Vec	$\mathbf{0.861 \pm 0.021}$	$\mathbf{0.841 \pm 0.072}$

The bold values indicate the best performance numbers across all methods

4. AdaBoost. They combine the medication, diagnosis, procedure codes, and clinical trial information to create feature vectors and then apply the AdaBoost classifier to predict the enrollment rate categories.
5. Multi-layer Perceptron (MLP). They use MLP to process doctor features. In this case, they obtain the doctor features by converting all the visit vectors associated with a doctor to a count vector of different diagnoses, medication, procedure codes. They convert categorical information of clinical trials to multi-hot vectors and obtain TF-IDF features from text information of clinical trials.
6. Long Short-Term Memory Networks (LSTM). They process all the temporally ordered visit vectors associated with a doctor using an LSTM. The embedding obtained from LSTM is concatenated with embedding obtained from categorical and text information of clinical trials to predict enrollment rate.
7. DeepMatch [56] In this model, the doctors' features are obtained by collecting the top 50 most frequent medical codes and passed through an MLP layer to obtain an embedding vector. This embedding is concatenated with embedding obtained from categorical and text information of clinical trials via MLP and TF-IDF to predict enrollment rate finally.

They conducted experiments for both classification (e.g., predict enrollment rate category) and regression (e.g., predict actual rate) tasks. Results are provided in Table 11.1. From the results, they observe that Doctor2Vec achieved the best performance in both settings.

In particular, Doctor2Vec demonstrated improved performance over the best baseline LSTM by up to 8.7% in PR-AUC. In the actual rate prediction task, Doctor2Vec gains 2.4% relative improvement in R^2 over the best baseline DeepMatch.

11.6 Case Study: Medication Recommendation

Problem How to select effective and safe medications? Can we perform medication recommendations based on medical history from EHR data and relevant

Table 11.2 Statistics of the data

# Patients	6350
# Clinical events	15,016
# Diagnosis	1958
# Procedure	1426
# Medication	145
Avg # of visits	2.36
Avg # of diagnosis	10.51
Avg # of procedure	3.84
Avg # of medication	8.80
Max # of diagnosis	128
Max # of procedure	50
Max # of medication	55
# Medication in DDI knowledge base	123
# DDI types in knowledge base	40

medical knowledge base such as drug-drug interactions (DDI) database? A good medication recommendation needs to perform recommendation based on longitudinal patient history and considers drug safety in their modeling, especially adverse drug-drug interactions (DDI). Authors [134] of proposed a memory network based approach called GAMENet for recommending medication.

Data The experiment is conducted using EHR data from MIMIC-III [81]. Here patients with more than one visit are included in the dataset. They used DDI knowledge from TWOSIDES dataset [152]. In this work, the Top-40 severity DDI types are transformed to ATC Third Level for integrating with MIMIC-III data. The dataset statistics are summarized in Table 11.2.

Method GAMENet model is a graph augmented memory network that embeds multiple knowledge graphs into the memory bank. GAMENet also enables attention-based memory search using query generated from longitudinal patient records. In particular, GAMENet not only stores the EHR graph and the drug-drug interaction graph as facts in Memory Bank (MB), but also inserts patient history to the Dynamic Memory (DM). Next, we present a high-level description of different modules in GAMENet, which is illustrated in Fig. 11.6.

- *Input medical embedding:* A visit $\boldsymbol{x}_t$ consists of $[\boldsymbol{c}_d^t, \boldsymbol{c}_p^t, \boldsymbol{c}_m^t]$ where each $\boldsymbol{c}_*^t$ is a multi-hot vector at the tth visit. The multi-hot vector $\boldsymbol{c}_*^t$ is binary encoded showing the existence of each medical codes recorded at the tth visit. A linear embedding is applied on the input vectors. We derive medical embeddings for $\boldsymbol{c}_d^t, \boldsymbol{c}_p^t$ for diagnosis codes and procedure codes separately at the tth visit as follows:

$$\boldsymbol{e}_*^t = \boldsymbol{W}_{*,e}\boldsymbol{c}_*^t$$

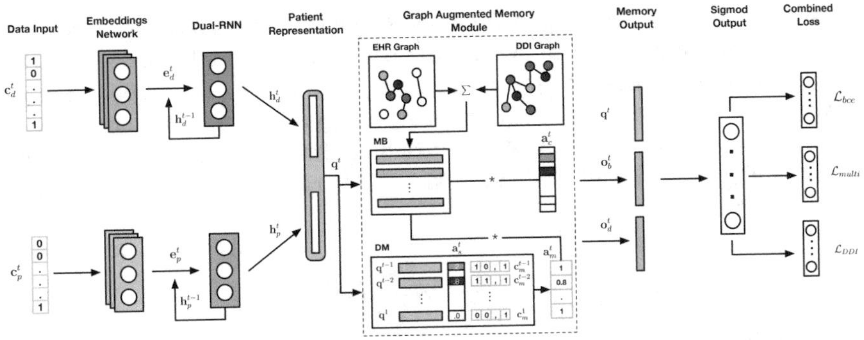

Fig. 11.6 GAMENet: At the tth visit, there are the multi-hot input vectors $\boldsymbol{c}^t_d$, $\boldsymbol{c}^t_p$ for diagnosis and procedure, respectively, which are mapped to embedding $\boldsymbol{e}^t_d$, $\boldsymbol{e}^t_p$ correspondingly. Then two separate RNN generates current hidden states on diagnosis $\boldsymbol{h}^t_d$ and procedure $\boldsymbol{h}^t_p$ based on embedding $\boldsymbol{e}^t_d$, $\boldsymbol{e}^t_p$. We use concatenated $\boldsymbol{h}^t_d$, $\boldsymbol{h}^t_p$ as query $\boldsymbol{q}^t$ (a.k.a. patient representation) to output $\boldsymbol{o}^t_b$ by reading from Memory Bank (MB) $\boldsymbol{M}_b$. Meantime, the Dynamic Memory (DM) stores key-value form history information along time and can be used to generate output $\boldsymbol{o}^t_d$. Finally, query and memory outputs are concatenated to make final medication recommendation. A combined loss is used to balance prediction performance and DDI

where $\boldsymbol{W}_{*,e} \in \mathbb{R}^{|C_*|\times d}$ is the embedding matrix to learn and $*$ can be either d for diagnosis or p for procedure. Thus a visit $\boldsymbol{x}_t$ is transformed to $\hat{\boldsymbol{x}}_t = [\boldsymbol{e}^t_d, \boldsymbol{e}^t_p, \boldsymbol{c}^t_m]$ where $\boldsymbol{e}^t_d$, $\boldsymbol{e}^t_p$ are diagnosis and procedure embeddings at time t, and $\boldsymbol{c}^t_m$ is the multi-hot vectors for medication at time t.

- *Patient representation:* The two RNNs are used for modeling diagnosis sequences and procedure sequences of patients, separately. Thus, the RNNs accept all patient history to produce hidden states to generate patient representation as a query $\boldsymbol{q}^t$. Formally, for each input vector in transformed clinical history $[\hat{\boldsymbol{x}}_1, \hat{\boldsymbol{x}}_2, \cdots, \hat{\boldsymbol{x}}_t]$, we retrieve $\boldsymbol{e}_d$, $\boldsymbol{e}_p$ and utilize RNN to encode visit-level diagnosis and procedure embeddings respectively as follows:

$$\boldsymbol{h}^t_d = RNN_d(\boldsymbol{e}^1_d, \boldsymbol{e}^2_d, \cdots, \boldsymbol{e}^t_d)$$
$$\boldsymbol{h}^t_p = RNN_p(\boldsymbol{e}^1_p, \boldsymbol{e}^2_p, \cdots, \boldsymbol{e}^t_p)$$

Finally, we can converts hidden states into a query vector as $\boldsymbol{q}^t = f([\boldsymbol{h}^t_d, \boldsymbol{h}^t_p])$ where we concatenate hidden diagnosis state $\boldsymbol{h}^t_d$ and procedure state $\boldsymbol{h}_p{}^t$ as the input patient health state. $f(\cdot)$ is a fully connected neural network with one hidden layer.

- *Static memory bank:* To leverage drug knowledge, we construct a graph augmented memory module that not only embeds and stores the EHR graph and the DDI graph as facts in Memory Bank (MB). Here graph convolution neural networks (GCN)[1] are used to construct the knowledge embedding vectors for medications to be stored in the memory bank. More formally, EHR graph and DDI graph are represented by two adjacency matrices $\boldsymbol{A}_e, \boldsymbol{A}_d$, respectively. $\boldsymbol{A}_e$ incorporates medication co-prescriptions (i.e., edges between drugs that are often co-prescribed together) while $\boldsymbol{A}_d$ encodes drug-drug interactions (i.e., two drugs with DDI are connected). Following the GCN procedure [88], each $\boldsymbol{A}_*$ is pre-processed as follows:

$$\tilde{\boldsymbol{A}}_* = \tilde{\boldsymbol{D}}^{-\frac{1}{2}}(\boldsymbol{A}_* + \boldsymbol{I})\tilde{\boldsymbol{D}}^{-\frac{1}{2}}$$

where $\tilde{\boldsymbol{D}}$ is a diagonal matrix such that $\tilde{\boldsymbol{D}}_{ii} = \sum_j \boldsymbol{A}_{ij}$ and $\boldsymbol{I}$ is an identity matrix. Then we applied a two-layer GCN on $\boldsymbol{A}_e$ and $\boldsymbol{A}_d$, respectively. The output $\boldsymbol{M}_b$ is generated as a weighted sum of the two graph embeddings.

$$\begin{aligned}
\boldsymbol{Z}_1 &= \tilde{\boldsymbol{A}}_e \tanh(\tilde{\boldsymbol{A}}_e \boldsymbol{W}_{e1})\boldsymbol{W}_1 \\
\boldsymbol{Z}_2 &= \tilde{\boldsymbol{A}}_d \tanh(\tilde{\boldsymbol{A}}_d \boldsymbol{W}_{e2})\boldsymbol{W}_2 \\
\boldsymbol{M}_b &= \boldsymbol{Z}_1 - \beta \boldsymbol{Z}_2
\end{aligned} \tag{11.4}$$

where $\boldsymbol{W}_{e1}, \boldsymbol{W}_{e2} \in \mathbb{R}^{|\mathcal{C}_m| \times d}$ are embedding matrices for EHR graph and DDI graph (each contains $|\mathcal{C}_m|$ number of d-dimensional vectors), $\boldsymbol{W}_1, \boldsymbol{W}_2 \in \mathbb{R}^{d \times d}$ are parameter matrices. All $\boldsymbol{W}_*$ are updated during the training phase. Then, medication/node embeddings $\boldsymbol{Z}_1, \boldsymbol{Z}_2 \in \mathbb{R}^{|\mathcal{C}_m| \times d}$ are computed using GCN. Finally we combine node embeddings $\boldsymbol{Z}_1$ and $\boldsymbol{Z}_2$ into $\boldsymbol{M}_b \in \mathbb{R}^{|\mathcal{C}_m| \times d}$ where β is a weighting variable to fuse both graphs. The combined embedding $\boldsymbol{M}_b$ for each medication will be stored into the memory bank.

- *Dynamic memory bank* stores patient history to Dynamic Memory (DM) as key-value pairs. The keys are the previous patient representation query $\boldsymbol{q}^{t'}, t' < t$, while the values are the corresponding multi-hot medication vectors $\boldsymbol{c}_m^{t'}, t' < t$ that are used in the past. Specifically, we can incrementally insert key-value pair after each visit step and treat $\boldsymbol{M}_d^t$ as a vectorized indexable dictionary as follows $\boldsymbol{M}_d^t = \{\boldsymbol{q}^{t'} : \boldsymbol{c}_m^{t'}\}_1^{t-1}$ where $\boldsymbol{M}_d^t$ is empty when $t = 1$. For clarity, we use $\boldsymbol{M}_{d,k}^t = [\boldsymbol{q}^1, \boldsymbol{q}^2, \cdots, \boldsymbol{q}^{t-1}] \in \mathbb{R}^{d \times |t-1|}$ to denote the key vectors and $\boldsymbol{M}_{d,v}^t = [\boldsymbol{c}_m^1; \boldsymbol{c}_m^2; \cdots; \boldsymbol{c}_m^{t-1}] \in \mathbb{R}^{|t-1| \times |\mathcal{C}_m|}$ to denote the value vectors at tth visit.
- *Medication recommendation:* We first query two memory banks MB and DM with current patient representation q^t to retrieve output $\boldsymbol{o}_b^t, \boldsymbol{o}_d^t$ as follows:

$$\boldsymbol{o}_b^t = \boldsymbol{M}_b^\top \overbrace{\text{Softmax}(\boldsymbol{M}_b \boldsymbol{q}^t)}^{\boldsymbol{a}_c^t}$$

[1] GCN will be covered in Chap. 10.

$$o_d^t = M_b^\top \overbrace{(M_{d,v}^t)^\top \underbrace{\text{Softmax}((M_{d,k}^t)^\top q^t)}_{a_s^t}}^{a_m^t}$$

Then we concatenate query q^t and their output from memory banks and perform the final classification

$$\hat{y}_t = \sigma([q^t, o_b^t, o_d^t])$$

Results

The performance of GAMENet is compared with the following baselines.

- **Nearest** will simply recommend the same combination medications at previous visit for current visit (i.e., $\hat{Y}_t = Y_{t-1}$)
- **Logistic Regression (LR)** is a logistic regression with L2 regularization. Here we represent the input data by sum of one-hot vector.
- **LEAP** [174] is an instance-based medication combination recommendation method.
- **RETAIN** [25] can provide a sequential prediction of medication combination based on a two-level neural attention model that detects influential past visits and significant clinical variables within those visits.
- **DMNC** [95] is a recent work of medication combination prediction via memory augmented neural network.

Table 11.3 compares the performance on accuracy and safety issues. Results show GAMENet has the highest score among all baselines for Jaccard, PR-AUC, and F1.

Table 11.3 Performance comparison of GAMENet and baseline methods

Methods	DDI rate	Δ DDI rate %	Jaccard	PR-AUC	F1	Avg # of med.
Nearest	0.0791	+1.80%	0.3911	0.3805	0.5465	14.77
LR	0.0786	+1.16%	0.4075	0.6716	0.5658	11.42
Leap	**0.0532**	**−31.53%**	0.3844	0.5501	0.5410	14.42
RETAIN	0.0797	+2.57%	0.4168	0.6620	0.5781	16.68
DMNC	0.0949	+22.14%	0.4343	0.6856	0.5934	20.00
GAMENet	0.0749	−3.60%	**0.4509**	**0.6904**	**0.6081**	14.02

The bold values indicate the best performance numbers across all methods

11.7 Case Study: Pre-training of Graph Augmented Transformers for Medication Recommendation

Problem G-BERT is another medication recommendation algorithm that extends the GAMENet model. Recall GAMENet utilizes memory networks for medication recommendation [134]. However, there are two limitations with GAMENet, which are addressed by G-BERT, a graph augmented Transformer model [133].

1. **Selection bias:** Data from patients who only have one hospital visit were discarded from training by GAMENet since it requires more than one visit to build a temporal prediction model like GAMENet. As a result, the training population is biased towards more severe patients with multiple inpatient visits.
2. **Lack of hierarchical knowledge:** Medical ontologies such as a diagnosis ontology follow hierarchical structures that were not utilized in GAMENet.

Method G-BERT is a model that first derives the initial embedding of medical codes from medical ontology using graph neural networks (**Ontology embedding**). Then, G-BERT constructs a variation of the BERT model on data from all patients of single or multiple visits (**Visit embedding**). Finally, we add a prediction layer to fine-tune the medication recommendation model (**Fine-tuning**). Figure 11.7 illustrates the model architecture of G-BERT.

Ontology Embedding

We constructed ontology embedding from diagnosis ontology $\mathcal{O}_d$ and medication ontology $\mathcal{O}_m$. Since the medical codes in raw EHR data can be considered leaf nodes in these ontology trees, we can enhance the medical code embedding using graph neural networks (GNNs) to integrate these codes' ancestors' information.

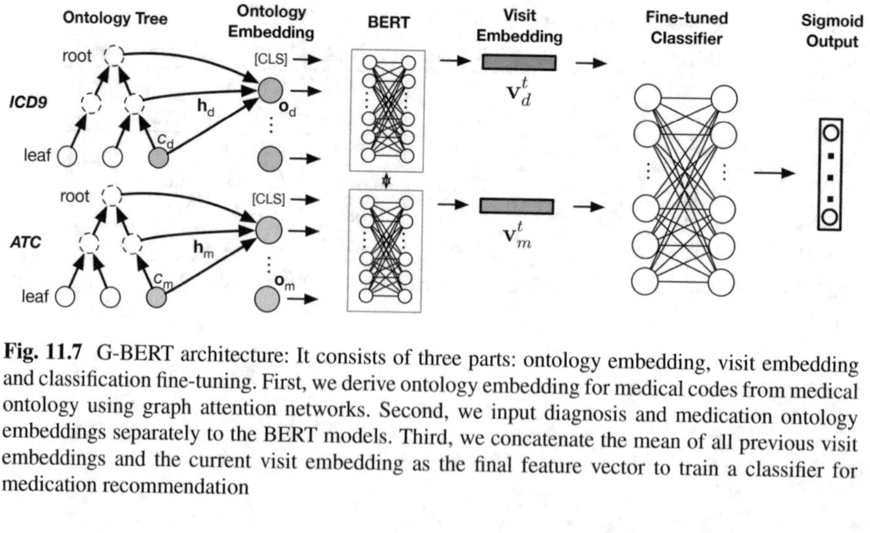

Fig. 11.7 G-BERT architecture: It consists of three parts: ontology embedding, visit embedding and classification fine-tuning. First, we derive ontology embedding for medical codes from medical ontology using graph attention networks. Second, we input diagnosis and medication ontology embeddings separately to the BERT models. Third, we concatenate the mean of all previous visit embeddings and the current visit embedding as the final feature vector to train a classifier for medication recommendation

Here we perform a two-stage procedure with a specially designed GNN for ontology embedding.

To start, we assign an initial embedding vector to every medical code $c_* \in \mathcal{O}_*$ with a learnable embedding matrix $\boldsymbol{W}_e \in \mathbb{R}^{|\mathcal{O}_*| \times d}$ where d is the embedding dimension. Here $\overline{\mathcal{C}_*}$ and $\mathcal{C}_*$ correspond to the set of non-leaf nodes and that of the leaf nodes, respectively.

Bottom-Up Stage For each non-leaf node $c_* \in \overline{\mathcal{C}_*}$, we obtain its enhanced medical embedding $\boldsymbol{h}_{c_*} \in \mathbb{R}^d$ as follows:

$$\boldsymbol{h}_{c_*} = g(c_*, ch(c_*), \boldsymbol{W}_e)$$

where $g(\cdot, \cdot, \cdot)$ is an aggregation function which accepts the target medical code c_*, its direct children $ch(c_*)$ and initial embedding matrix. Intuitively, the aggregation function can fuse information into the target node c_* from its direct children.

Top-Down Stage For the leaf nodes, we use the embedding matrix of non-leaf nodes $\boldsymbol{H}_e \in \mathbb{R}^{|\overline{\mathcal{O}}_*| \times d}$ in a top-down fashion to obtain their embeddings $c_* \in \mathcal{C}_*$.

$$\boldsymbol{o}_{c_*} = g(c_*, pa(c_*), \boldsymbol{H}_e)$$

where $g(\cdot, \cdot, \cdot)$ accepts the target medical code c_* and its parents $pa(c_*)$.

The option for the aggregation function $g(\cdot, \cdot, \cdot)$ is flexible, including *sum*, *mean*. Here we choose the one from graph attention networks (GAT) [161]. For example, for the top-down stage, the aggregation function is

$$g(c_*, p(c_*), \boldsymbol{H}_e) = \|_{k=1}^{K} \sigma \left(\sum_{j \in \mathcal{N}_{c_*}} \alpha_{c_*,j}^k \boldsymbol{W}^k \boldsymbol{h}_j \right)$$

where $\|$ represents concatenation of the K-dimensional output from the multi-head attention mechanism, σ is a nonlinear activation function, $\boldsymbol{W}^k \in \mathbb{R}^{m \times d}$ is the k-th weight matrix for input transformation, and $\alpha_{c_*,j}^k$ are the corresponding k-th normalized attention coefficients computed as follows:

$$\alpha_{c_*,j}^k = \frac{\exp\left(\text{LeakyReLU}(\boldsymbol{a}^\top[\boldsymbol{W}^k \boldsymbol{h}_{c_*} || \boldsymbol{W}^k \boldsymbol{h}_j])\right)}{\sum_{k \in \mathcal{N}_{c_*}} \exp\left(\text{LeakyReLU}(\boldsymbol{a}^\top[\boldsymbol{W}^k \boldsymbol{h}_{c_*} || \boldsymbol{W}^k \boldsymbol{h}_k])\right)} \tag{11.5}$$

where $\mathcal{N}_{c_*}$ is the neighbors of c_* which is $ch(c_*) \cup c_*$ in bottom-up stage and $pa(c_*) \cup c_*$ in top-down stage, respectively. $\boldsymbol{a} \in \mathbb{R}^{2d/K}$ is a learnable weight vector and LeakyReLU is a nonlinear activation function introduced in Sect. 4.1.1.

As shown in Fig. 11.7, ontology hierarchies for diagnosis and medications are constructed based on ICD and Anatomical Therapeutic Chemical (ATC) Classification, respectively.

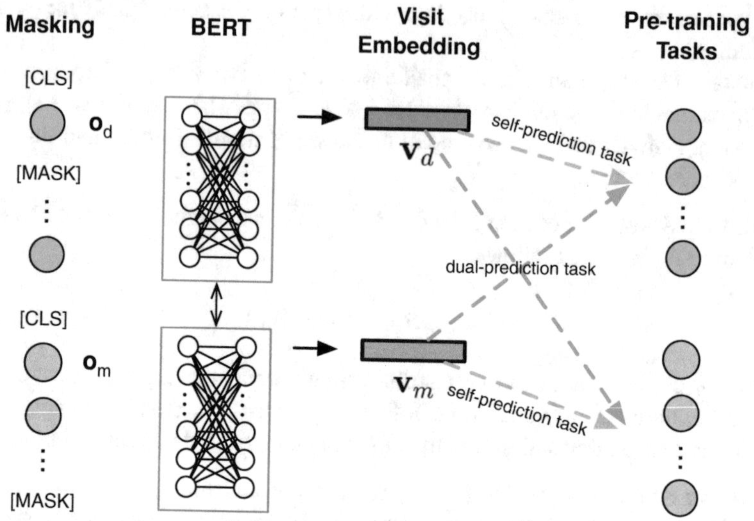

Fig. 11.8 Graphical illustration of pre-training procedure. We firstly randomly mask the input medical codes using a *[MASK]* symbol. **Orange arrow**: self-prediction task takes $\boldsymbol{v}_m$ or $\boldsymbol{v}_d$ as input to restore the original medical codes with the same type. **Green arrow**: dual-prediction task takes one type of visit embedding such as $\boldsymbol{v}_m$ or $\boldsymbol{v}_d$ and tries to predict the other type of medical codes

Visit Embedding
Similar to BERT, a multi-layer Transformer architecture is used to compute the visit embeddings. More specifically, the Transformer model maps a sequence of tokens (ontology embeddings of medical codes) to another sequence of embeddings (Fig. 11.8).

To generate a visit embedding summarizing all medical codes within the visit, a special token *[CLS]* is introduced to separate all the medical codes between visits. And the output embedding for *[CLS]* corresponds to the overall embedding for the entire visit. Formally, the visit embedding $\boldsymbol{v}_*^t \in \mathbb{R}^d$ for a patient at the t-th visit is the first element of the output from the Transformer model:

$$\boldsymbol{v}_*^t = \text{Transformer}(\{[CLS]\} \cup \{\boldsymbol{o}_{c_*}^t | c_* \in C_*^t\})[0] \tag{11.6}$$

where [0] means the first element of the output sequence, *[CLS]* is a special token as in BERT indicating the first position of each visit of a specific type, visit type $*$ can be diagnosis and medication. In fact, it is more reasonable to use Transformers as encoders (multi-head attention based architecture) than RNN for visit embedding since medical codes within one visit are unordered. Also, the positional embedding is not used in G-BERT as the unordered nature of medical codes within a visit.

Pre-training Before predicting medications, we need to learn better embeddings for medical codes using data from all visits. Many existing temporal models, such as RNN, require two or more visits per patient to train a model. However, there are many patients with only a single visit, which before G-BERT are mostly ignored in model training.

The pre-training strategy of G-BERT utilizes the data of those single visits. In particular, G-BERT modified the original pre-training tasks, i.e., Masked language model task and Next Sentence prediction task to **self-prediction task** and **dual-prediction task**. The idea to conduct these tasks is to visit embedding, absorb enough information about what it is made of, and predict.

Thus, for the **self-prediction task**, we want the visit embedding v_* to recover *what it is made of*, i.e., the input medical codes $\mathcal{C}_*$ limited by the same type for each visit as follows:

$$\begin{aligned}\mathcal{L}_{se}(\boldsymbol{v}_*, \mathcal{C}_*^{(n)}) &= -\log p(\mathcal{C}_*^{(n)} | \boldsymbol{v}_*) \\ &= -\sum_{c_* \in \mathcal{C}_*^{(n)}} \log p(c_* | \boldsymbol{v}_*) + \sum_{c_* \in \{\mathcal{C}_* \backslash \mathcal{C}_*^{(n)}\}} \log p(c_* | \boldsymbol{v}_*)\end{aligned}$$

where $\mathcal{C}_*^{(n)}$ is the medical codes set of the n-th patient, $* \in \{d, m\}$ indicating diagnosis and medication respectively. And we minimize the binary cross entropy loss $\mathcal{L}_{se}$. For instance, assume that the n-th patient takes 10 different medications out of total 100 medications which means $|\mathcal{C}_m^{(n)}| = 10$ and $|\mathcal{C}_m| = 100$. In such case, we instantiate and minimize $L_{se}(\boldsymbol{v}_m, \mathcal{C}_m^{(n)})$ to produce high probabilities among 10 taken medications captured by $-\sum_{c_* \in \mathcal{C}_m^{(n)}} \log p(c_* | \boldsymbol{v}_m)$ and lower the probabilities among 90 other medications captured by $\sum_{c_* \in \{\mathcal{C}_m \backslash \mathcal{C}_m^{(n)}\}} \log p(c_* | \boldsymbol{v}_m)$. In practice, Sigmoid$(f(\boldsymbol{v}_*))$ is applied after a fully connected neural network $f(\cdot)$ with one hidden layer. G-BERT also uses specific symbol [MASK] to randomly replace the 15% original medical codes $c_* \in \mathcal{C}_*$.

The **dual-prediction task** predicts different types of medical codes based on the other types of codes. For example, we want to predict multiple medications given only the diagnosis codes. Inversely, we can also predict unknown diagnosis given the medication codes. Formally, predicting diagnoses based on medication embedding $p(\mathcal{C}_d | \boldsymbol{v}_m)$ and predicting medications based on diagnosis embedding $p(\mathcal{C}_m | \boldsymbol{v}_d)$ lead the following loss:

$$\mathcal{L}_{du} = -\log p(\mathcal{C}_d | \boldsymbol{v}_m) - \log p(\mathcal{C}_m | \boldsymbol{v}_d)$$

The probability scores $p(\mathcal{C}_d | \boldsymbol{v}_m)$ and $p(\mathcal{C}_m | \boldsymbol{v}_d)$ are learned from two DNN models with a hidden layer Sigmoid$(f_1(\boldsymbol{v}_m))$, Sigmoid$(f_2(\boldsymbol{v}_d))$. This is a direct adaptation of the next sentence prediction task.

Thus, our final pre-training optimization objective can simply be combining the aforementioned losses, as shown in Eq. (11.7).

$$\mathcal{L}_{pr} = \mathcal{L}_{se}(\boldsymbol{v}_d, \mathcal{C}_d^{(n)}) + \mathcal{L}_{se}(\boldsymbol{v}_m, \mathcal{C}_m^{(n)}) + \mathcal{L}_{du} \tag{11.7}$$

Fine Tuning
After obtaining pre-trained visit representation for each visit, we aggregate all the visit embedding and add a prediction layer for the medication recommendation task. To be specific, from pre-training on all visits, we have a pre-trained Transformer encoder, which can then be used to get the visit embedding $\boldsymbol{v}_*^{\tau}$ at time τ. The known diagnosis codes C_d^t at the prediction time t is also represented using the same model as $\boldsymbol{v}_*^t$. Concatenating the mean of previous diagnoses visit embeddings and medication visit embeddings, also the last diagnoses visit embedding, we built a DNN based prediction layer to predict the recommended medication codes as:

$$\boldsymbol{y}_t = \text{Sigmoid}(\boldsymbol{W}_1[(\frac{1}{t}\sum_{\tau<t}\boldsymbol{v}_d^{\tau})||(\frac{1}{t}\sum_{\tau<t}\boldsymbol{v}_m^{\tau})||\boldsymbol{v}_d^t] + b)$$

where $\boldsymbol{W}_1 \in \mathbb{R}^{|\mathcal{C}_m|\times 3d}$ is a learnable transformation matrix.

Given the true labels $\hat{\boldsymbol{y}}_t$ at each time stamp t, the loss function for the whole EHR sequence (i.e. a patient) is

$$\mathcal{L} = -\frac{1}{T-1}\sum_{t=2}^{T}(\boldsymbol{y}_t^{\mathsf{T}}\log(\hat{\boldsymbol{y}}_t) + (1-\boldsymbol{y}_t^{\mathsf{T}})\log(1-\hat{\boldsymbol{y}}_t)) \tag{11.8}$$

Results We used EHR data from MIMIC-III [81]. We utilize data from patients with both single visits and multiple visits in the training dataset as the pre-training data source (multi-visit data are split into visit slices). In this work, we transform the drug coding from NDC to ATC Third Level. The statistics of the datasets are summarized in Table 11.4.

Different baseline methods include

1. **Logistic Regression (LR)** is logistic regression with L1/L2 regularization. Here we represent sequential multiple medical codes by the sum of the multi-hot vector of each visit.
2. **LEAP** [174] is an instance-based medication combination recommendation method that formalizes the task in a multi-instance and multi-label learning framework. It utilizes an encoder-decoder based model with an attention mechanism to build complex dependency among diseases and medications.

Table 11.4 Statistics of the data (dx for diagnosis, rx for medication)

Stats	Single-visit	Multi-visit
# of patients	30,745	6350
Avg # of visits	1.00	2.36
Avg # of dx	39	10.51
Avg # of rx	52	8.80
# of unique dx	1997	1958
# of unique rx	323	145

3. **RETAIN** [25] makes sequential prediction of medication combination and diseases prediction based on a two-level neural attention model that detects influential past visits and clinical variables within those visits.
4. **GRAM** [28] injects domain knowledge (ICD9 Dx code tree) to **tanh** via attention mechanism.
5. **GAMENet** [134] is the method to recommend accuracy and safe medication based on memory neural networks and graph convolutional networks by leveraging EHR data and Drug-Drug Interaction (DDI) data source. For a fair comparison, we use a variant of GAMENet without DDI knowledge and procedure codes as input renamed as GAMENet^{-}.
6. **G-BERT** is our proposed model which integrated the GNN representation into Transformer-based visit encoder with pre-training on single-visit EHR data.

To measure the prediction accuracy, we used the Jaccard Similarity Score (Jaccard), Average F1 (F1), and Precision-Recall AUC (PR-AUC). Jaccard is defined as the size of the intersection divided by the size of the union of ground truth set $Y_t^{(k)}$ and predicted set $\hat{Y}_t^{(k)}$.

$$\text{Jaccard} = \frac{1}{\sum_k^N \sum_t^{T_k} 1} \sum_k^N \sum_t^{T_k} \frac{|Y_t^{(k)} \cap \hat{Y}_t^{(k)}|}{|Y_t^{(k)} \cup \hat{Y}_t^{(k)}|}$$

where N is the number of patients in the test set and T_k is the number of visits of the kth patient.

Table 11.5 compares the performance on the medication recommendation task. Incorporating both hierarchical ontology information and pre-training procedure, the end-to-end model G-BERT has more capacity and achieve comparable results with others.

G-BERT performs better than all the baseline methods including the GAMENet model.

Table 11.5 Performance on medication recommendation task

Methods	Jaccard	PR-AUC	F1	# of parameters
LR	0.4075	0.6716	0.5658	–
GRAM	0.4176	0.6638	0.5788	3,763,668
LEAP	0.3921	0.5855	0.5508	1,488,148
RETAIN	0.4456	0.6838	0.6064	2,054,869
GAMENet^{-}	0.4401	0.6672	0.5996	5,518,646
GAMENet	0.4555	0.6854	0.6126	5,518,646
G-BERT	**0.4565**	**0.6960**	**0.6152**	3,034,045

The bold values indicate the best performance numbers across all methods

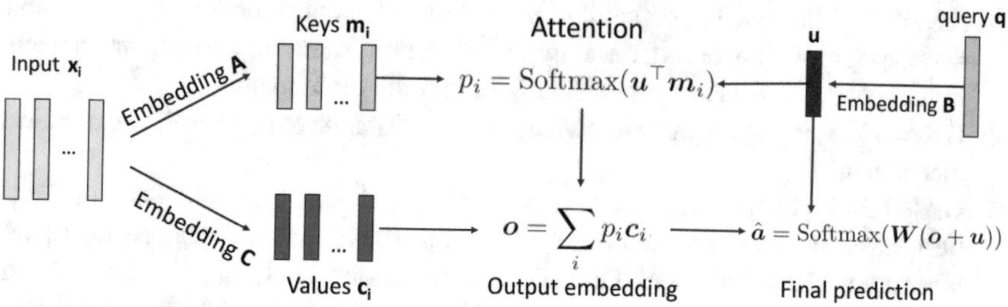

Fig. 11.9 End-to-end memory network exercise

11.8 Exercises

1. What is the main difference between the end-to-end memory network and the self-attention/transformer?
2. What is the most innovative step in the original memory network model and why?
3. What is NOT true about end-to-end memory networks as illustrated in Fig. 11.9?

   (a) It removes the arg max operation in the original memory networks so that gradient can be computed at all the steps.
   (b) The size of the embeddings in keys, values, and query are all the same.
   (c) Multi-layer end-to-end memory network can be created via multiple embedding matrices for keys and values
   (d) The model parameters are $\boldsymbol{A}$, $\boldsymbol{B}$, $\boldsymbol{C}$ and $\boldsymbol{W}$ matrices.

4. What is NOT true about self attention?

   (a) Three versions of embeddings of the input X are produced namely $\mathbf{Q}$, $\mathbf{K}$, $\mathbf{V}$.
   (b) The main reason to have multiple embedding matrices of $\mathbf{X}$ is to be able to apply and learn those embeddings independently in parallel.
   (c) The temporal dependency in the input sequences is essential in self-attention models.
   (d) Multiple versions of self-attention are concatenated together to produce more robust embedding, which is called multi-head self attention.

5. What are the method ideas used in Transformer encoder? [multiple correct choices]

   (a) Self attention
   (b) Positioning encoding
   (c) Multi-head attention
   (d) Residual connection

6. What are method ideas used in Transformer decoder? [multiple correct choices]
   (a) Masked attention
   (b) Self attention
   (c) Residual connection
   (d) Recurrent neural networks
7. What is NOT true about BERT model?
   (a) BERT provides a masked language model.
   (b) BERT masks x% of input words and try to predict them with other words.
   (c) BERT uses a transformer based model.
   (d) BERT provides static embeddings for all words.
8. What is the healthcare application in Doctor2Vec?
9. What is the healthcare application in GameNet?
10. What are the method ideas behind G-BERT? [multiple correct choices]
    (a) Medical ontology is used to embed medical concepts.
    (b) BERT model can be used to pre-train on large number of clinical visits.
    (c) Temporal dependencies across visits are important in prediction.
    (d) Multi-task learning is useful in clinical applications.

Chapter 12
Generative Models

Generative models are a broad area of machine learning models for producing realistic data samples based on training datasets. For instance, images are a popular kind of data for which we might create generative models. Each image is regarded as a data point of thousands or millions of dimensions (pixels). What the generative models can do is to learn the distribution that captures the dependencies between pixels and hence produce realistic image examples. Generative models have several advantages over discriminative models. For example, they are more effective in modeling high-dimensional probability distributions, which are often seen in many application domains, including healthcare. A key benefit of generative models is the ability to produce new data samples that resemble the real data. Thus we can achieve data augmentation: creating realistic synthetic examples like real examples in the dataset.

The Generative adversarial networks (GAN) [58] and the variational autoencoders (VAE) are two popular approaches for generative models [47, 74, 93, 123]. They have also been used in healthcare data augmentation: creating either more training data to avoid overfitting or more labeled data to reduce label acquisition costs. For example, GAN has been used in the healthcare domain to generate continuous medical time series [43] and discrete codes [16, 29, 169].

We will first introduce the GAN techniques and then focus on describing the variational autoencoders (VAEs). Then, we will present how GAN and VAE are applied to healthcare tasks.

12.1 Generative Adversarial Networks (GAN)

GAN is an approach for data generation via a game-theoretical process. The main idea behind GAN is to train two neural networks: a *generator* and a *discriminator*. The generator takes random noise as input and generates samples, while the

C. Xiao, J. Sun, *Introduction to Deep Learning for Healthcare*,
https://doi.org/10.1007/978-3-030-82184-5_12

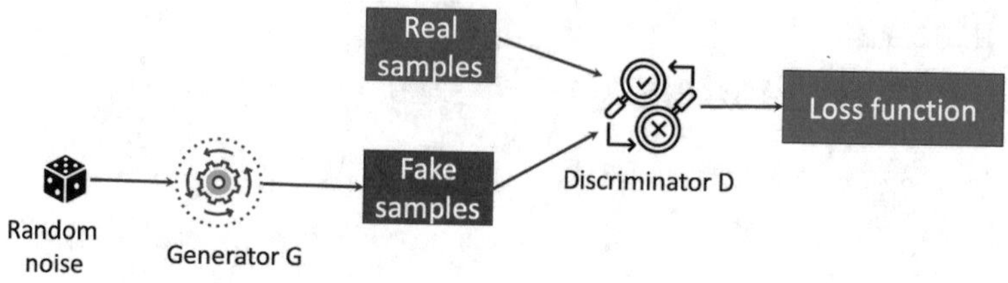

Fig. 12.1 The conceptual framework of Generative adversarial networks

discriminator takes both the real samples and the generated samples as input and tries to distinguish between the two. The two networks are trained alternatively after training each network for a few epochs, with the expectation that this competition will drive the generator to produce more and more realistic samples and the discriminator to have better distinguishing power. The iterative process is illustrated in Fig. 12.1.

12.1.1 The GAN Framework

Formally, GAN is a probabilistic model containing observed variables $\boldsymbol{x}$ and latent variables z. There are two players in the game: a *generator* and a *discriminator*, are represented by two functions, each of which is differentiable, both with respect to its inputs and to its parameters. The discriminator is a function D that takes $\boldsymbol{x}$ as input and is parameterized by θ_D. The generator is defined by a function G that takes z as input and is parameterized by θ_G. When z is sampled from some prior distribution P_d, $G(z)$ will yield a sample of $\boldsymbol{x}$ drawn from P_m. Here G is usually represented by a deep neural network.

Both players have cost functions that are defined in terms of their parameters. Each player's cost depends on the other player's parameters, but can only control its own parameters. This can be viewed as an optimization problem such that the discriminator tries to minimize $L_D(\theta_D, \theta_G)$ by controlling θ_D and the generator aims to minimize $L_G(\theta_D, \theta_G)$ by controlling θ_G. The solution to this optimization problem is a local minimum where all neighboring points have greater or equal cost. The solution to a game is a Nash equilibrium. In this setting a local minimum is (θ_G, θ_D) that minimize L_D with respect to θ_D, and also minimize L_G with respect to θ_G.

To train the GAN, on each step we sample one minibatch (e.g., 10 examples) from real data $\boldsymbol{x}$ and another minibatch of synthetic examples generated based on z drawn from model's prior. Then two gradient steps are calculated to minimize both L_D and L_G.

12.1.2 The Loss Function of Discriminator

The loss function is an important component in the GAN framework. As the cost function of the discriminator, most GAN models use the cross-entropy loss to minimize the discrepancy of two mini-batches of data; one from the real dataset with label 1, and the other synthetic one from the generator with label 0. The cross-entropy loss of the discriminator is given below.

$$L_D(\theta_D, \theta_G) = -\mathbb{E}_{\boldsymbol{x} \sim p_{data}(\boldsymbol{x})}[\log D(\boldsymbol{x})] - \mathbb{E}_{z \sim p_z(z)}[\log(1 - D(G(z)))] \quad (12.1)$$

Training the discriminator is to minimize the above cross-entropy loss. The first term of Eq. (12.1) corresponds to the negative log-likelihood of real samples being classified as real, while the second term corresponds to the negative log-likelihood of synthetic samples being classified as fake.

12.1.3 The Loss Function of Generator

Previously we introduced the loss function of the discriminator. We also need to define the generator's cost function. There are several strategies we can consider, for example, zero-sum game, maximum-likelihood game, etc. For the zero-sum game where we have $L_D = L_G$, the entire game can be summarized with a value function specifying the discriminator's payoff, as given by $V(\theta_D, \theta_G) = -L_D(\theta_D, \theta_G)$. The zero-sum game strategy will lead to the following objective:

$$\min_{\theta_G} \max_{\theta_D} V(\theta_D, \theta_G) = \mathbb{E}_{\boldsymbol{x} \sim p_{data}(\boldsymbol{x})}[\log D(\boldsymbol{x})] + \mathbb{E}_{z \sim p_z(z)}[\log(1 - D(G(z)))]$$

where $G(z)$ is a generated sample from distribution z, $D(x)$ is the estimated probability that x is a real data sample, when $D(x) = 1$ it means D regards x as a real sample with probability one, while $D(x) = 0$ it means D regards x as a synthetic sample with probability one. The discriminator's goal is to maximize V, while the overall goal is to minimize the max of V.

In practice, such minimax strategy can be difficult to optimize. This is due to the discriminator and the generator minimize the same cross-entropy loss. When the discriminator successfully rejects generator samples with high confidence, the generator's gradients will vanish, which leads to vanishing gradient problems. To solve this problem, we update the target used to construct the cross-entropy cost for the generator as the following.

$$L_G = -\mathbb{E}_z \log D(G(z)) \quad (12.2)$$

For this strategy, the generator maximizes the log probability of the discriminator being mistaken to ensure that each player has a strong gradient when that player is losing the game.

12.1.4 *Caveats of GAN*

Training GAN models is still an open problem for several reasons: There are no reliable metrics to indicate the model convergence. Also it has been observed that over-training can lead to performance degradation. As a result, we have to rely on alternative strategies to determine the quality of models. For example, users still heavily depend on visual inspection on the quality of image generation with GAN. Another known issue with GAN model is called model collapse, which means the generator keeps generating the same examples with limited variety. Mode collapse is a much bigger issue as the main use case of generative models is to create diverse examples, while mode collapse restricts the GAN model to produce diverse samples. Both topics are still being actively researched as of in year 2020. As practitioners of GAN, we need to be aware of these modeling limitations.

12.2 Variational Autoencoders (VAE)

Variational autoencoder (VAE) is another popular generative model for creating realistic data samples. VAE is in the intersection of deep learning and probabilistic graphical models. VAE has also been used in health applications such as molecule generation [57]. Next we will first introduce VAE models from deep learning perspective and then present the probabilistic model behind VAE.

12.2.1 *VAE from Deep Learning Perspective*

VAE is an extension of autoencoder model by providing more regularization on the structure of the latent embeddings.

Review of Autoencoder

Recall an autoencoder includes an encoder and an decoder:

- *Encoder* $f_\theta()$ transforms an input vector $\boldsymbol{x} \in \mathbb{R}^d$ into a hidden layer $\boldsymbol{h} \in \mathbb{R}^k$ (usually $k < d$):

$$h = f_\theta(x) = \sigma_1(Wx + b)$$

where $W \in \mathbb{R}^{k\times d}$ is weight matrix, $b \in \mathbb{R}^k$ is a bias vector and σ_1 is the input activation function.

- *Decoder* $g_{\theta'}()$ maps the hidden representation $h \in \mathbb{R}^k$ back to a reconstructed vector

$$r = g_{\theta'}(h) = \sigma_2(W'h + b')$$

where $W' \in \mathbb{R}^{d\times k}$ is weight matrix, $b' \in \mathbb{R}^d$ is a bias vector and σ_2 the output activation function.

The objective of autoencoder is to minimize the loss function $\min L(x, r)$, where $L(x, r) \propto -\log p(x|r)$. Here $L(\cdot)$ is a loss function such as squared error or cross-entropy loss.

The **main limitation** of this standard autoencoder formulation is the lack of structure constraints on the latent embedding h. As a result, a small perturbation on h can lead to large reconstruction errors. Variational autoencoder (VAE) tries to address this limitation by introducing a generative process in the latent embedding h.

VAE as Two Neural Networks

Like autoencoders, VAE model introduces two neural networks: one encoder called the *inference network*, and one decoder called the *generative network*.

The inference network (encoder) encodes the input x as a distribution by learning $q_\theta(z|x)$. Then we sample points from the encoding distribution $q_\theta(z|x)$ to obtain latent embedding z. Finally, the generative network (decoder) produces realistic data points x' by learning another distribution $p_\phi(x|z)$.

More specifically, the encoder assumes Gaussian distribution:

$$q_\theta(z|x) \sim \mathcal{N}(\mu_x, \Sigma(x)), \quad p_\phi(z) \sim \mathcal{N}(\mathbf{0}, I).$$

The loss function for a data point x is the regularized log-likelihood:

$$l_x = -\mathbb{E}_{x\sim D}\left[\log p(x|z) + \mathbb{D}_{\mathrm{KL}}(q_\theta(z|x)\|p_\phi(z))\right]$$

where $\log p(x|z)$ corresponds to the log-likelihood of x and $\mathbb{D}_{\mathrm{KL}}(q_\theta(z|x)\|p_\phi(z))$ is the regularization term.

Figure 12.2 shows the architecture of VAE. The encoder is a neural network. Its input is a data point x, its output is a hidden representation z, and has weights and biases θ. The encoder learn an efficient compression of the data into this lower-dimensional space note that the lower-dimensional space is stochastic: the encoder outputs parameters to $q_\theta(z|x)$, which is a Gaussian probability density. We

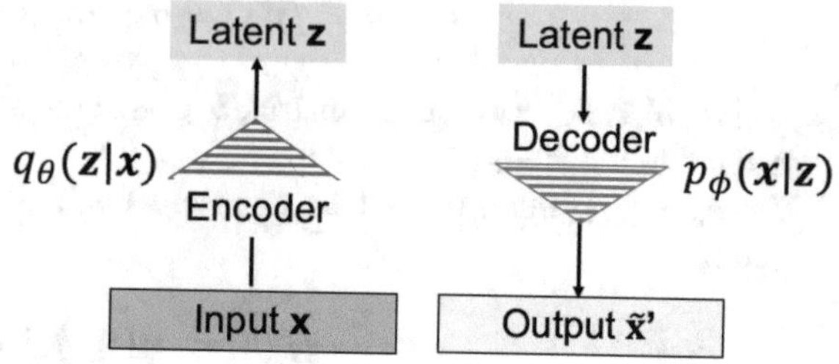

Fig. 12.2 The conceptual framework of variational autoencoders

can sample from this distribution to get noisy values of the representations z. The decoder is another neural net that captures $p_\phi(x|z)$. Its input is the representation z. It outputs the parameters to the probability distribution of the data, and has weights and biases ϕ. The decoder learns to reconstruct an input data given its latent representation.

Next we will explain the probabilistic view of VAE and the idea of reparametrization trick to bypass sampling to enable end-to-end model training.

12.2.2 *VAE from Probabilistic Model Perspective*

The VAE is one type of latent variable models. It assumes that a set of data $\boldsymbol{x}$ is generated by an underlying distribution $p(z)$, where z is a (potentially high-dimensional) latent vector which we could sample from according to some probability distribution $p(z)$. In another word, given a random variable $f_{\boldsymbol{\phi}}(z)$ which is parameterized by a vector $\boldsymbol{\phi}$, the goal of VAE is to optimize $\boldsymbol{\phi}$ such that when we sample z from $p(z)$, $f_{\boldsymbol{\phi}}(z)$ will have higher probability to be similar to data points in $\boldsymbol{x}$. Here to allow for $\boldsymbol{x}$ to depend on z more explicitly, we further replace $f_{\boldsymbol{\phi}}(z)$ with a distribution $p_{\boldsymbol{\phi}}(\boldsymbol{x}|z)$ and formally represent the data generation concept using an optimization problem:

$$p(\boldsymbol{x}) = \int p_{\boldsymbol{\phi}}(\boldsymbol{x}|z)p(z)dz. \tag{12.3}$$

Here we can have flexible choices for the distribution of $p_{\boldsymbol{\phi}}(\boldsymbol{x}|z)$. In VAE, we often choose Gaussian distribution such that $p_{\boldsymbol{\phi}}(\boldsymbol{x}|z) = \mathcal{N}(\boldsymbol{x}|f_{\boldsymbol{\phi}}(z), \sigma^2 * \boldsymbol{I})$.

Justification of the VAE Loss

The VAE model is formulated to approximately maximize the objective given by Eq. (12.3). The key questions are how to define the latent variables z to better capture the latent information, and how to solve the integral over z.

For the definition of the latent variable z, VAEs asserts that samples of z can be drawn from a Gaussian distribution $\mathcal{N}(0, \boldsymbol{I})$. The key is to notice that provided powerful function approximators (e.g., $f_{\boldsymbol{\phi}}(z)$ as a deep neural network), we can simply learn a function which maps our independent, normally-distributed z values to whatever latent variables might be needed for the model, and then map those latent variables to $\boldsymbol{x}$. However, this will result in a slow sampling process, since most $p(\boldsymbol{x}|z)$ will be nearly zero and have low contribution in estimating $p(\boldsymbol{x})$.

To speed up the sampling process, VAE attempts to sample values of z that are likely to have produced $\boldsymbol{x}$ and compute $p(\boldsymbol{x})$ from them. This key idea motivates us to define a new function $q_{\boldsymbol{\theta}}(z|\boldsymbol{x})$ parameterized by $\boldsymbol{\theta}$ to provide the distribution over z values that are likely to produce $\boldsymbol{x}$. The relationship between $\mathbb{E}_{z\sim q}\, p(\boldsymbol{x}|z)$ and $p(\boldsymbol{x})$ is considered the foundation of variational Bayesian methods.

The Kullback–Leibler divergence $\mathbb{D}_{\mathrm{KL}}$ between $p(z|\boldsymbol{x})$ and $q(z)$ is given below.

$$\begin{aligned} \mathbb{D}_{\mathrm{KL}}(q(z)\|p_{\boldsymbol{\phi}}(z|\boldsymbol{x})) &= \mathbb{E}_{z\sim q}[\log q(z) - \log p_{\boldsymbol{\phi}}(z|\boldsymbol{x}))] \\ &= \mathbb{E}_{z\sim q}[\log q(z) - \log p_{\boldsymbol{\phi}}(\boldsymbol{x}|z)) - \log p(z)] + \log p(\boldsymbol{x}) \end{aligned} \tag{12.4}$$

Rearranging Eq. (12.4), we can derive Eq. (12.5).

$$\log p(\boldsymbol{x}) - \mathbb{D}_{\mathrm{KL}}(q(z)\|p_{\boldsymbol{\phi}}(z|\boldsymbol{x})) = \mathbb{E}_{z\sim q}[\log p_{\boldsymbol{\phi}}(\boldsymbol{x}|z))] - \mathbb{D}_{\mathrm{KL}}(q(z)\|p_{\boldsymbol{\phi}}(z)) \tag{12.5}$$

Then we further define $q(z)$ as $q_{\boldsymbol{\theta}}(z|\boldsymbol{x})$ to create the dependency on $\boldsymbol{x}$. Thus we can re-write Eq. (12.5) as Eq. (12.6), the core function of VAE.

$$\begin{aligned} &\log p(\boldsymbol{x}) - \mathbb{D}_{\mathrm{KL}}(q_{\boldsymbol{\theta}}(z|\boldsymbol{x})\|p_{\boldsymbol{\phi}}(z|\boldsymbol{x})) \\ &= \mathbb{E}_{z\sim q}[\log p_{\boldsymbol{\phi}}(\boldsymbol{x}|z))] - \mathbb{D}_{\mathrm{KL}}(q_{\boldsymbol{\theta}}(z|\boldsymbol{x})\|p_{\boldsymbol{\phi}}(z)) \end{aligned} \tag{12.6}$$

For Eq. 12.6, its left hand side is the quantity we want to maximize: $\log p(\boldsymbol{x})$ while simultaneously minimizing the KL divergence $\mathbb{D}_{\mathrm{KL}}(q_{\boldsymbol{\theta}}(z|\boldsymbol{x})\|p_{\boldsymbol{\phi}}(z|\boldsymbol{x}))$.

VAE Based on Variational Approximation

To understand the posterior probability $p_{\boldsymbol{\phi}}(z|\boldsymbol{x})$, we leverage the Bayes theorem:

$$p_{\boldsymbol{\phi}}(z|\boldsymbol{x}) = \frac{p_{\boldsymbol{\phi}}(\boldsymbol{x}|z)p(z)}{p_{\boldsymbol{\phi}}(\boldsymbol{x})}.$$

The challenge is to compute $p_{\boldsymbol{\phi}}(\boldsymbol{x})$, which $p_{\boldsymbol{\phi}}(\boldsymbol{x}) = \int p_{\boldsymbol{\phi}}(\boldsymbol{x}, z)dz$ due to the integration over all z.

A common remedy in variational Bayes is to approximate the posterior $p_{\boldsymbol{\phi}}(z|\boldsymbol{x})$ with a tractable variational posterior $q_{\boldsymbol{\theta}}(z|\boldsymbol{x})$ defined by an inference network with parameters $\boldsymbol{\theta}$ to approximate the actual posterior $p_{\boldsymbol{\phi}}(z|\boldsymbol{x})$ (i.e., the generative network). Here we can measure the Kullback–Leibler (KL) divergence between

$p_{\phi}(z|\boldsymbol{x})$ and $q_{\theta}(z|\boldsymbol{x})$:

$$\mathbb{D}_{\mathrm{KL}}(q_{\theta}(z|\boldsymbol{x})\|p_{\phi}(z|\boldsymbol{x})) = \mathbb{E}_{q_{\theta}(z|\boldsymbol{x})}\left[\log\frac{q_{\theta}(z|\boldsymbol{x})}{p_{\phi}(\boldsymbol{x},z)}\right]$$

In this vein, the log-evidence $\log p_{\phi}(\boldsymbol{x})$ admits a lower bound called *Evidence Lower BOund*(ELBO) based on Jensen's inequality:

$$\begin{aligned}\log p_{\phi}(\boldsymbol{x}) = & \log\int q_{\theta}(z|\boldsymbol{x})\tfrac{p_{\phi}(\boldsymbol{x},z)}{q_{\theta}(z|\boldsymbol{x})}dz \\ \geq & \underbrace{\int q_{\theta}(z|\boldsymbol{x})\log\frac{p_{\phi}(\boldsymbol{x},z)}{q_{\theta}(z|\boldsymbol{x})}dz}_{\text{Evidence Lower Bound (ELBO)}}\end{aligned} \tag{12.7}$$

The loss of evidence lower bound, ELBO as given by Eq. (12.9), now is the new variational objective to optimize. Because of the following Eq. (12.8), minimizing the KL divergence is equivalent to maximizing the ELBO.

$$\log p_{\phi}(\boldsymbol{x}) = \underbrace{\mathbb{E}_{q_{\theta}(z|\boldsymbol{x})}\left[\log\frac{p_{\phi}(\boldsymbol{x},z)}{q_{\theta}(z|\boldsymbol{x})}\right]}_{\text{ELBO}} + \mathbb{D}_{\mathrm{KL}}(q_{\theta}(z|\boldsymbol{x})\|p_{\phi}(z|\boldsymbol{x})). \tag{12.8}$$

Then we can maximize ELBO with respect to θ and ϕ. Note that ELBO can be further represented as the following.

$$\mathrm{ELBO}(\boldsymbol{x};\boldsymbol{\phi},\boldsymbol{\theta}) = \mathbb{E}_{q_{\theta}(z|\boldsymbol{x})}[\log p_{\phi}(\boldsymbol{x}|z)] - \mathbb{D}_{\mathrm{KL}}(q_{\theta}(z|\boldsymbol{x})\|p_{\phi}(z)) \tag{12.9}$$

Such a variational treatment resembles an autoencoder, where the inference network $q_{\theta}(z|\boldsymbol{x})$ encodes a training example $\boldsymbol{x}$ into a latent representation z, and the generative network decodes the latent z and reconstructs the data from the probabilistic model $p(\boldsymbol{x})$, such that it is as close to $\boldsymbol{x}$ as possible. Between the two parts in ELBO, the expectation term is the negative reconstruction loss, whereas the KL divergence term serves as a regularization that encourages the variational posterior to stay close with the prior.

The loss function for data $\boldsymbol{x}$ is specified as

$$l_x = -\mathbb{E}_{x\sim D}\left[\log p(\boldsymbol{x}|z) + \mathbb{D}_{\mathrm{KL}}(q_{\theta}(z|\boldsymbol{x})\|p_{\phi}(z))\right]$$

where the first term corresponds to the reconstruction loss and the second term is the regularization term. Typically the encoder $q_{\theta}(z|\boldsymbol{x})$ is modeled with Gaussian distribution with mean $\mu(\boldsymbol{x})$ and variance $\Sigma(\boldsymbol{x})$, i.e., $q_{\theta}(z|\boldsymbol{x}) \sim \mathcal{N}(\mu(\boldsymbol{x}),\Sigma(\boldsymbol{x}))$ And the prior distribution $p(z) \sim \mathcal{N}(0,\boldsymbol{I})$.

12.2.3 Reparameterization Trick

The sampling process for z in VAE is problematic from a training perspective because it breaks the flow of gradient during backpropagation. The reparameterization trick is a method to bypass the need for sampling in the VAE model so that backpropagation can be done from end to end in VAE.

As illustrated in Fig. 12.3, the forward pass of this network works fine and, if the output is averaged over many samples of $\boldsymbol{x}$ and z, produces the correct expected value. However, we need to back-propagate the error through a layer that samples z from $q(z|\boldsymbol{x})$, which is a non-continuous operation and has no gradient. We use a strategy which we call the "reparameterization trick" to solve this problem. The reparameterization trick moves the sampling step to an input layer. Given the mean and covariance of $q(z|\boldsymbol{x})$, i.e., $\mu(\boldsymbol{x})$ and $\Sigma(\boldsymbol{x})$, we can sample from $\mathcal{N}(\mu(\boldsymbol{x}), \Sigma(\boldsymbol{x}))$ by firstly sampling $\epsilon \sim \mathcal{N}(0, \boldsymbol{I})$ as part of the input, then we compute the sample $z = \mu(\boldsymbol{x}) + \Sigma^{1/2}(\boldsymbol{x}) * \epsilon$.

Thus we compute the gradient of the following loss function.

$$l_x = \mathbb{E}_{x \sim D}\left[-\mathbb{E}_{\epsilon \sim \mathcal{N}(0,I)}[\log p(\boldsymbol{x}|z = \mu(\boldsymbol{x}) + \Sigma^{1/2}(\boldsymbol{x}) * \epsilon)] + \mathbb{D}_{\text{KL}}(q_\theta(z|\boldsymbol{x}) \| p_\phi(z))\right]$$

That is, given a fixed $\boldsymbol{x}$ and ϵ (i.e., the extra input from reparametrization), this function is deterministic and continuous in the parameters of $p_\phi()$ and $q_\theta()$. Hence, the backpropagation can work as the gradient can be computed. At test time, when we want to generate new samples, we simply input prior samples from $z \sim \mathcal{N}(0, \boldsymbol{I})$ into the decoder.

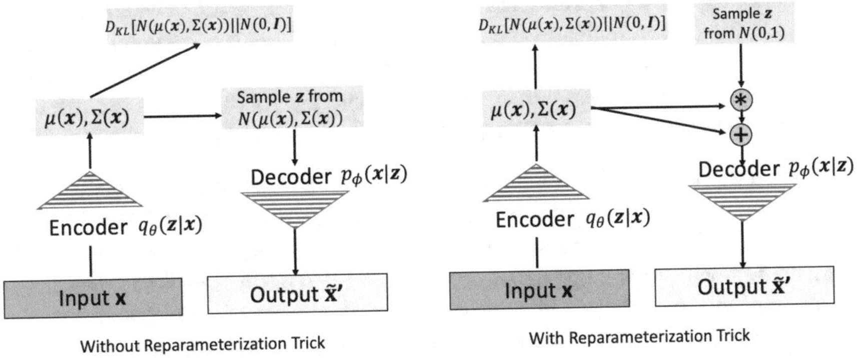

Fig. 12.3 A training-time VAE implemented as a feed-forward neural network, where $p(\boldsymbol{x}|z)$ is Gaussian. This left one does not have the "reparameterization trick", the right is with it. Red shows sampling operations that are non-differentiable. The feed-forward behavior of these networks is identical, but back-propagation can be applied only to the right network

12.3 Case Study: Generating Patient Records with GAN

Problem The adoption of EHR systems does not automatically lead to easy access to EHR data for researchers. One reasons behind limited access stems from the fact that EHR data are composed of personal identifiers, which in combination with potentially sensitive medical information, induces privacy concerns. As a result, access to such data for secondary purposes (e.g., research) is regulated, as well as controlled by the healthcare organizations that are at risk if data are misused or breached. The review process by legal departments and institutional review boards can take months, with no guarantee of access. This process limits timely opportunities to use data and may slow advances in biomedical knowledge and patient care. To address this limitation, the MedGAN [29] was introduced to generate realistic synthetic EHR data. MedGAN is a neural network model that generates high-dimensional, multi-label discrete variables that represent the events in EHRs (e.g., diagnosis of a certain disease or treatment of a certain medication).

Data The datasets in this study were from Sutter Palo Alto Medical Foundation (PAMF), which consists of 10-years of longitudinal medical records of 258K patients. From this dataset, they extracted diagnoses, medications and procedure codes, which were then respectively grouped by Clinical Classifications Software (CCS) for ICD codes, Generic Product Identifier Drug Group and for CPT.

Method MedGAN [29] tries to generate static patient vectors (e.g., binary or count vectors of diagnosis categories) using GAN. More specificialy, they assume there are $|\mathcal{C}|$ discrete variables (*e.g.*, diagnosis, medication or procedure codes) in the EHR data that can be expressed as a fixed-size vector $\boldsymbol{x} \in \mathbb{Z}_+^{|\mathcal{C}|}$, where the value of the i-th dimension indicates the number of occurrences (i.e., counts) of the i-th variable in the patient record. In addition to the count variables, a visit can also be represented as a binary vector $\boldsymbol{x} \in \{0, 1\}^{|\mathcal{C}|}$, where the ith dimension indicates the absence or occurrence of the i-th variable in the patient record.

Since the generator G is trained by the error signal from the discriminator D via backpropagation, the original GAN can only learn to approximate discrete patient records $\boldsymbol{x} \in \mathbb{Z}_+^{|\mathcal{C}|}$ with continuous values. In this work, an autoencoder is used to learn continuous embeddings of discrete variables that can be applied to decode the continuous output of G. This allows the gradient flow from D to the decoder Dec to enable the end-to-end fine-tuning. As depicted by Fig. 12.4, an autoencoder consists of an encoder $Enc(\boldsymbol{x}; \theta_{enc})$ that compresses the input $\boldsymbol{x} \in \mathbb{Z}_+^{|\mathcal{C}|}$ to $Enc(\boldsymbol{x}) \in \mathbb{R}^h$, and a decoder $Dec(Enc(\boldsymbol{x}); \theta_{dec})$ that decompresses $Enc(\boldsymbol{x})$ to $Dec(Enc(\boldsymbol{x}))$ as the reconstruction of the original input $\boldsymbol{x}$. The objective of the autoencoder is to minimize the reconstruction error:

$$\frac{1}{m}\sum_{i=0}^{m} ||\boldsymbol{x}_i - \boldsymbol{x}'_i||_2^2 \tag{12.10}$$

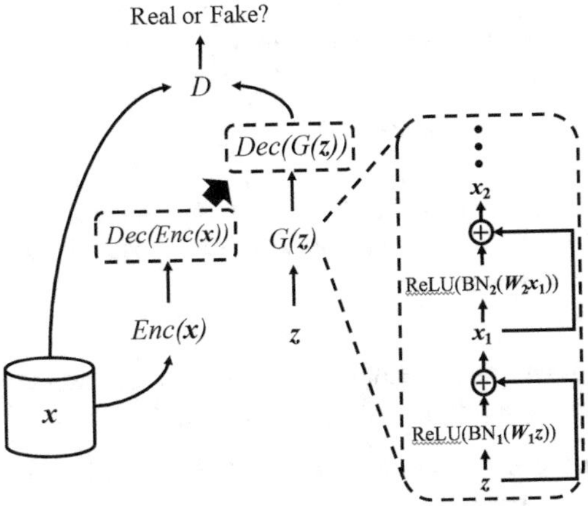

Fig. 12.4 Architecture of MedGAN: The binary or count input vector $\boldsymbol{x}$ are computed from EHR data, z is the random prior for the generator G; G is a feed-forward network with shortcut connections (right-hand side figure); An autoencoder (i.e, the encoder Enc and decoder Dec) is learned from $\boldsymbol{x}$; The same decoder Dec is used after the generator G to construct the discrete output. The discriminator D tries to differentiate real input $\boldsymbol{x}$ and discrete synthetic output $Dec(G(z))$

$$\frac{1}{m}\sum_{i=0}^{m} \boldsymbol{x}_i \log \boldsymbol{x}'_i + (1-\boldsymbol{x}_i)\log(1-\boldsymbol{x}'_i) \tag{12.11}$$

$$\text{where } \boldsymbol{x}'_i = Dec(Enc(\boldsymbol{x}_i))$$

where m is the size of the mini-batch. They use the mean squared loss (Eq.(12.10)) for count variables and cross entropy loss (Eq.(12.11)) for binary variables. For count variables, They use rectified linear units (ReLU) as the activation function in both Enc and Dec. For binary variables, They use tanh activation for Enc and the sigmoid activation for Dec.

With the pre-trained autoencoder, They can allow GAN to generate distributed representation of patient records (i.e., the output of the encoder Enc), rather than generating patient records directly. Then the pre-trained decoder Dec can pick up the right signals from $G(z)$ to convert it to the patient record $Dec(G(z))$. The discriminator D is trained to determine whether the given input is a synthetic sample $Dec(G(z))$ or a real sample $\boldsymbol{x}$. The architecture of MedGAN is depicted in Fig. 12.4. MedGAN is trained in a similar fashion as the original GAN as follows,

$$\theta_d \leftarrow \theta_d + \alpha \nabla_{\theta_d} \frac{1}{m}\sum_{i=1}^{m} \log D(\boldsymbol{x}_i) + \log(1 - D(\boldsymbol{x}_{z_i}))$$

$$\theta_{g,dec} \leftarrow \theta_{g,dec} + \alpha \nabla_{\theta_{g,dec}} \frac{1}{m} \sum_{i=1}^{m} \log D(\boldsymbol{x}_{z_i})$$

where $\boldsymbol{x}_{z_i} = Dec(G(z_i))$

Finally rounding operations are performed to the values of $Dec(G(z))$ to their nearest integers to ensure that the discriminator D is trained on discrete values instead of continuous values.

Results Various of baselines methods are compared. To assess the effectiveness of our methods, we tested multiple versions of MedGAN:

- **GAN:** We use the same architecture as MedGAN with the standard training strategy, but do not pre-train the autoencoder.
- **GAN**$_P$: We pre-train the autoencoder (in addition to the GAN).
- **GAN**$_{PD}$: We pre-train the autoencoder and use minibatch discrimination [129].
- **GAN**$_{PA}$: We pre-train the autoencoder and use minibatch averaging.
- **MedGAN:** We pre-train the autoencoder and use minibatch averaging. We also use batch normalization and a shortcut connection for the generator G.

They also compare the performance of MedGAN with several popular generative methods as below.

- **Random Noise (RN):** Given a real patient record $\boldsymbol{x}$, we invert the binary value of each code (i.e., dimension) with probability 0.1. This is not strictly a generative method, but rather it is a simple implementation of a privacy protection method based on randomization.
- **Independent Sampling (IS):** For the binary variable case, we calculate the Bernoulli success probability of each code in the real dataset, based on which we sample binary values to generate the synthetic dataset. For the count variable case, we use the kernel density estimator (KDE) for each code then sample from that distribution.
- **Stacked RBM (DBM):** We train a stacked Restricted Boltzmann Machines [68], then, using Gibbs sampling, we can generate synthetic binary samples. There are studies that extend RBMs beyond binary variables [52, 69, 157]. In this work, however, as our goal is to study MedGAN's performance in various aspects, we use the original RBM only.
- **Variational Autoencoder (VAE):** We train a variational autoencoder [87] where the encoder and the decoder are constructed with feed-forward neural networks.

The evaluation task is the **dimension-wise prediction**. It indirectly measures how well the model captures the inter-dimensional relationships of the real samples. After training the models with R to generate S, we choose one dimension k to be the label $\boldsymbol{y}_{R_k} \in \{0, 1\}^N$ and $\boldsymbol{y}_{S_k} \in \{0, 1\}^N$. The remaining $R_{\backslash k} \in \{0, 1\}^{N \times |C|-1}$ and $S_{\backslash k} \in \{0, 1\}^{N \times |C|-1}$ are used as features to train two logistic regression classifiers LR_{R_k} and LR_{S_k} to predict $\boldsymbol{y}_{R_k}$ and $\boldsymbol{y}_{S_k}$, respectively. Then, we use the model LR_{R_k}

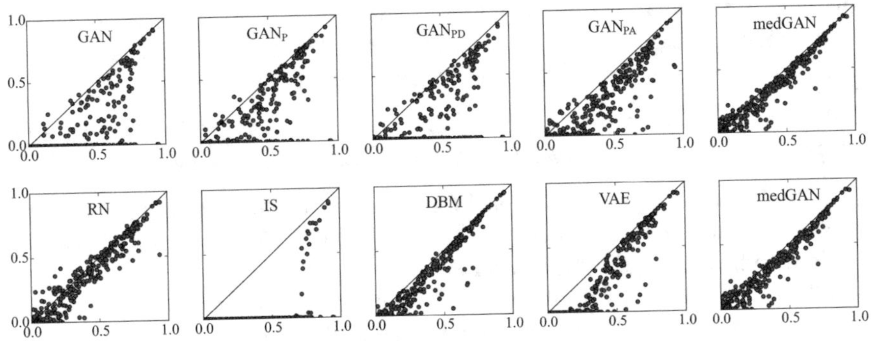

Fig. 12.5 Scatterplots of dimension-wise prediction results. Each dot represents one of 615 codes. The x-axis represents the F1-score of the logistic regression classifier trained on the real dataset A. The y-axis represents the F1-score of the classifier trained on the synthetic counterpart generated by each model. The diagonal line indicates the ideal performance where the real and synthetic data show identical quality. (**a**) Dimension-wise prediction performance of various versions of MedGAN. (**b**) Dimension-wise prediction performance of baseline models and MedGAN

and LR_{S_k} to predict label $\boldsymbol{y}_{T_k} \in \{0, 1\}^n$ of the test set T. We can assume that the closer the performance of LR_{S_k} to that of LR_{R_k}, the better the quality of the synthetic dataset S. We use F1-score to measure the prediction performance, with the threshold set to 0.5.

Figure 12.5a shows the dimension-wise prediction performance of various versions of MedGAN. The full MedGAN again shows the best performance as it did in the dimension-wise probability task. Although the advanced versions of MedGAN do not seem to dramatically increase the performance as they did for the previous task, this is due to the complex nature of inter-dimensional relationship compared to the independent dimension-wise probability. Figure 12.5b shows the dimension-wise prediction performance of baseline models compared to MedGAN. As expected, IS is incapable of capturing the inter-dimensional relationship, given its naive sampling method. VAE shows similar behavior as it did in the previous task, showing weakness at predicting codes with low occurrence probability. Again, DBM shows comparable, if not slightly better performance to MedGAN, which seems to come from its binary nature.

12.4 Case Study: Molecule Generation Using VAE

Problem Drug discovery is about designing novel molecules with desirable properties. Standard drug discovery approaches depend on high throughput screening over a large molecule library and some local search strategies such as genetic programming. Deep generative models especially GAN and VAE can provide new strategies to produce high quality and novel molecules for drug discovery. Here we present one simple application of VAE for tackling the molecule generation task.

The goal is to convert a discrete molecule representation in SMILES string into a continuous representation of embedding vectors with better chemical properties. The authors of [57] utilize VAE model to generate the embedding vectors.

Data Since VAE is an unsupervised method, it enjoys the benefit of leveraging a large number of molecules. Two datasets are utilized in the training:

- QM9 dataset is a dataset designed for testing machine learning prediction on chemical properties [55]. It consists of 133,885 molecules with up to nine heavy atoms from the range C, O, N and F.
- ZINC database is a free database of commercially-available compounds for virtual screening containing over 250,000 drug-like molecules [138].

Method The input molecules are represented by SIMILES strings which contains 22 distinct characters in QM9 and 35 distinct characters in ZINC. The encoder uses 1D convolution layerswith various filter sizes followed by a fully connected layer. The decoder includes 3 layers of gated recurrent units (GRUs). Besides the decoder, there is a separate prediction network of two fully connected layers from the latent embeddings to the output properties. The properties used in training include logP, QED, SAS for ZINC and HOMO energies, LUMO energies, and the electronic spatial extent (R^2).

Results One main objective is to test if the VAE can generate realistic molecules with similar properties to the input. As a baseline to compare against, genetic algorithm (GA) is used, which generate molecules with a list of hand-designed rules [164]. Table 12.1 illustrates describe the methods (the first column) whether it is the statistics directly from the data (Data), genetic algorithm (GA), or Variational Autoencoder (VAE). The training dataset (the second column) is either ZINC or QM9. Their corresponding number of molecules (real or generated) are presented in the third column (samples). The property columns on logP, SAS and QED show the average scores and their standard deviation. The last column indicates the percentage of those molecules already in ZINC database. We can observe that molecules generated by VAE are more similar to the ones in the real dataset (ZINC or QM9) compared to those generated by GA method. Moreover, those generated molecules by VAE are more novel as most of them are not already in the ZINC database.

Table 12.1 Comparison with different algorithms on ZINC and QM9 datasets

Method	Dataset	Samples	logP	SAS	QED	% in ZINC
Data	ZINC	249K	2.46 (1.43)	3.05 (0.83)	0.73 (0.14)	100
GA	ZINC	5303	2.84 (1.86)	3.80 (1.01)	0.57 (0.20)	6.5
VAE	ZINC	8728	2.67 (1.46)	3.18 (0.86)	0.70 (0.14)	5.8
Data	QM9	134k	0.30 (1.00)	4.25 (0.94)	0.48 (0.07)	0.0
GA	QM9	5470	0.96 (1.53)	4.47 (1.01)	0.53 (0.13)	0.018
VAE	QM9	2839	0.30 (0.97)	4.34 (0.98)	0.47 (0.08)	0.0

12.5 Case Study: *MolGAN* an Implicit Generative Model for Small Molecular Graphs

Problem Finding new chemical compounds with desired properties is an important task for drug discovery. However, the task is challenging since the space of synthesizable molecules is vast and search in this space proves to be very difficult. To side-step the expensive search procedures, recent advances in deep generative models for graph-structured data offer a new angle to directly generate molecular graphs. Among others, the MolGAN [10] is such a work that GANs to operate directly on graph-structured data for molecule generation. It also further leverages reinforcement learning objective to encourage the generation of molecules with specific desired chemical properties.

Data The experiments of MolGAN is conducted on QM9 data [121], which is a subset of the massive 166.4 billion molecules GDB-17 chemical database [126]. QM9 contains 133,885 organic compounds up to 9 heavy atoms: carbon (C), oxygen (O), nitrogen (N) and fluorine (F).

Method The MolGAN model takes molecule graph data as input, and generates new molecules that resemble the input molecules. It consists of three main components: a generator, a discriminator and a reward network. The generator takes a sample from a prior distribution and generates an annotated graph G representing a molecule. Nodes and edges of G are associated with annotations denoting atom type and bond type respectively. The discriminator takes both samples from the dataset and the generator and learns to distinguish them. Both xxx and xxxx are trained using improved WGAN such that the generator learns to match the empirical distribution and eventually outputs valid molecules.

The reward network is used to approximate the reward function of a sample and optimize molecule generation towards non-differentiable metrics using reinforcement learning. Dataset and generated samples are inputs of , differently from the discriminator, it assigns scores to them (e.g., how likely the generated molecule is to be soluble in water). The reward network learns to assign a reward to each molecule to match a score provided by an external software. The discriminator is then trained using the WGAN objective while the generator uses a linear combination of the WGAN loss and the RL loss (Fig. 12.6).

Result MolGAN was evaluated against some neural network-based drug generation models in a range of experiments on established benchmarks using the following metrics: validity, novelty, and uniqueness. Validity is defined as the ratio between the number of valid and all generated molecules. Novelty measures the ratio between the set of valid samples that are not in the dataset and the total number of valid samples. Finally, uniqueness is defined as the ratio between the number of unique samples and valid samples and it measures the degree of variety during sampling.

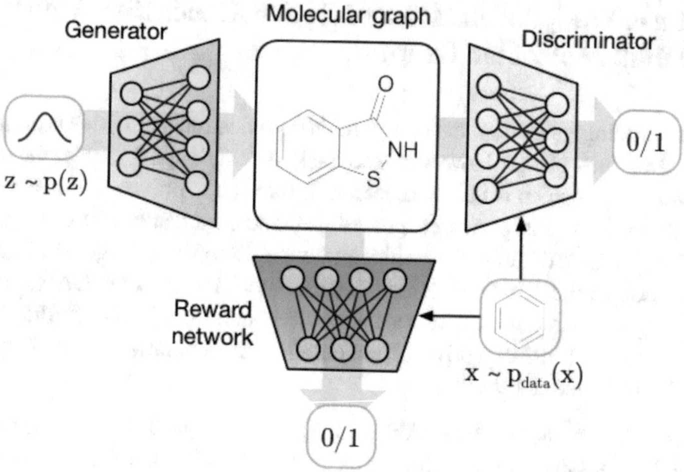

Fig. 12.6 Schema of MolGAN. A vector z is sampled from a prior and passed to the generator which outputs the graph representation of a molecule. The discriminator classifies whether the molecular graph comes from the generator or the dataset. The reward network tries to estimate the reward for the chemical properties of a particular molecule provided by an external software

Table 12.2 Comparison with different algorithms on QM9. Values are reported in percentages

Algorithm	Valid	Unique	Novel
CharacterVAE	10.3	67.5	90.0
GrammarVAE	60.2	9.3	80.9
GraphVAE	55.7	76.0	61.6
GraphVAE/imp	56.2	42.0	75.8
GraphVAE NoGM	81.0	24.1	61.0
MolGAN	98.1	10.4	94.2

Results on the full QM9 dataset are reported in Table 12.2. The MolGAN model has significantly higher validity and novelty scores compared with the VAE-based baselines. Notice that the VAEs optimize the evidence lower bound (ELBO) and there is no optimization of output validity. Moreover, since a part of the ELBO maximizes reconstruction of the observations, the novelty in the sampling process is not expected to be high since it is not optimized. However, in all reported methods novelty is $\geq 60\%$ and, in the case of CharacterVAE, 90%. Though CharacterVAE can achieve a high novelty score, it underperforms in terms of validity. For the uniqueness score, MolGAN is slightly higher compared to GrammarVAE, while the other baselines are superior in terms of this score.

12.6 Exercises

1. What is the main difference between GAN and VAE?
2. Which of the following is NOT true about GAN method?

   (a) GAN train two neural networks: Generator for generating synthetic examples, and Discriminator for differentiating synthetic and real examples.
   (b) The convergence of GAN model can be easily checked based on the loss function.
   (c) The input to the generator model is random noise.
   (d) The input to the discriminator model is synthetic examples and real examples.

3. Given the overall loss function as $\mathbb{E}_{x \sim p_{\text{data}}(x)}[\log D(x)] + \mathbb{E}_{z \sim p_z}(z)[\log(1 - D(G(z)))]$, which part of that is the generator's loss?

   (a) First term
   (b) Second term
   (c) Both term

4. which part of the loss function in previous question is the generator's loss?

   (a) First term
   (b) Second term
   (c) Both term

5. In MedGAN described in Chap. 12.3, what other neural network models are used besides GAN?

   (a) CNN
   (b) RNN
   (c) Feedforword neural network
   (d) Autoencoder

6. What exactly are the medical records generated by MedGAN?

   (a) Longitudinal electronic health records
   (b) Multi-hot disease category records
   (c) Clinical notes
   (d) Medical images

7. Which of the following is NOT true about VAE model?

   (a) VAE is a generative model for creating realistic data samples.
   (b) VAE has healthcare applications such as molecule generation.
   (c) The loss function in VAE is the exactly same as the loss function in standard autoencoder.
   (d) VAE has a strong probabilistic foundation.

8. Which of the following is NOT true about VAE model?

   (a) The encoder learns $q_\theta(z|x) \sim \mathcal{N}(\mu(x), \Sigma(x))$
   (b) The loss function of a data point x is $l_x = -\mathbb{E}_{x\sim D}[\log p(x|z) + \mathbb{D}_{KL}(q_\theta(z|x) \parallel p_\phi(z))]$
   (c) The decoder learns $p_\phi(x|z)$
   (d) A sampling step is required in order to produce the latent vector z.

9. In the probabilistic view of VAE, which expression corresponds to evidence lower bound (ELBO)? (Multiple correct choices)

   (a) $p_\phi(x) = \int p_\phi(x, z)dz$
   (b) $\mathbb{E}_{q_\theta(z|x)}\left[\log \frac{p_\phi(x,z)}{q_\theta(z|x)}\right]$
   (c) $\mathbb{E}_{q_\theta(z|x)}[\log p_\phi(x|z)] - \mathbb{D}_{KL}(q_\theta(z|x) \parallel p_\phi(z))$
   (d) $\mathbb{D}_{KL}(q_\theta(z|x) \parallel p\phi(z|x))$

10. What is the input to VAE model for drug molecule generation application described in Chap. 12.4? What baseline method do they compare against VAE model?

Bibliography

1. W.M. Abdelmoula, B. Balluff, S. Englert, J. Dijkstra, M.J.T. Reinders, A. Walch, L.A. McDonnell, B.P.F. Lelieveldt, Data-driven identification of prognostic tumor subpopulations using spatially mapped t-sne of mass spectrometry imaging data. Proc. Natil. Acad. Sci. **113**(43), 12244–12249 (2016)
2. D. Bahdanau, K. Cho, Y. Bengio, Neural machine translation by jointly learning to align and translate, in *3rd International Conference on Learning Representations, ICLR 2015, San Diego, May 7–9, 2015, Conference Track Proceedings*, ed. by Y. Bengio, Y. LeCun (2015)
3. T. Baumel, J. Nassour-Kassis, R. Cohen, M. Elhadad, N. Elhadad, Multi-Label classification of patient notes a case study on ICD code assignment, in *The Workshops of the Thirty-Second AAAI Conference on Artificial Intelligence* (2017)
4. I.M. Baytas, C. Xiao, X. Zhang, F. Wang, A.K. Jain, J. Zhou, Patient subtyping via time-aware LSTM networks, in *KDD'17: Proceedings of the 23rd ACM SIGKDD International Conference on Knowledge Discovery and Data Mining SIGKDD* (2017)
5. B.K. Beaulieu-Jones, C.S. Greene, Pooled Resource Open-Access ALS Clinical Trials Consortium, Semi-supervised learning of the electronic health record for phenotype stratification. J. Biomed. Inform. **64**, 168–178 (2016)
6. J. Bergstra, Y. Bengio, Random search for hyper-parameter optimization. J. Mach. Learn. Res. **13**, 281–305 (2012)
7. S. Biswal, H. Sun, B. Goparaju, M.B. Westover, J. Sun, M.T. Bianchi, Expert-level sleep scoring with deep neural networks. J. Am. Med. Inform. Assoc. **25**(12), 1643–1650 (2018)
8. S. Biswal, C. Xiao, L.M. Glass, E. Milkovits, J. Sun, Doctor2vec: dynamic doctor representation learning for clinical trial recruitment, in *AAAI Conference on Artificial Intelligence* (2020)
9. J. Bruna, W. Zaremba, A. Szlam, Y. LeCun, Spectral networks and locally connected networks on graphs, in *International Conference on Learning Representations* (2014)
10. N.D. Cao, T. Kipf, Molgan. An implicit generative model for small molecular graphs, In ICML 2018 workshop on Theoretical Foundations and Applications of Deep Generative Models (2018)
11. R.E. Carhart, D.H. Smith, R. Venkataraghavan, Atom pairs as molecular features in structure-activity studies: definition and applications. J. Chem. Inform. Comput. Sci. **25**, 64–73 (1985)
12. D.J. Cartwright, ICD-9-CM to ICD-10-CM codes: what? why? how? Adv. Wound Care **2**(10), 588–592 (2013)
13. Z. Che, D. Kale, W. Li, M.T. Bahadori, Y. Liu, Deep computational phenotyping, in *International Conference on Knowledge Discovery and Data Mining SIGKDD* (2015)

C. Xiao, J. Sun, *Introduction to Deep Learning for Healthcare*,
https://doi.org/10.1007/978-3-030-82184-5

14. Z. Che, S. Purushotham, K. Cho, D. Sontag, Y. Liu, Recurrent neural networks for multivariate time series with missing values (2016). arXiv:1606.01865
15. C. Che, C. Xiao, J. Liang, B. Jin, J. Zho, F. Wang, An RNN architecture with dynamic temporal matching for personalized predictions of parkinson's disease, in *SIAM on Data Mining* (2017)
16. Z. Che, Y. Cheng, S. Zhai, Z. Sun, Y. Liu, Boosting deep learning risk prediction with generative adversarial networks for electronic health records, in *2017 IEEE International Conference on Data Mining (ICDM)* (2017), pp. 787–792
17. J. Chen, T. Ma, C. Xiao, FastGCN: fast learning with graph convolutional networks via importance sampling, in *The International Conference on Learning Representations (ICLR)* (2018)
18. Y. Cheng, F. Wang, P. Zhang, J. Hu, Risk prediction with electronic health records: a deep learning approach, in *Proceedings of the 2016 SIAM International Conference on Data Mining* (2016)
19. K. Cho, B. van Merrienboer, C. Gulcehre, D. Bahdanau, F. Bougares, H. Schwenk, Y. Bengio, Learning phrase representations using rnn encoder-decoder for statistical machine translation, in *Conference on Empirical Methods in Natural Language Processing (EMNLP)* (2014)
20. K. Cho, B. van Merrienboer, D. Bahdanau, Y. Bengio, On the properties of neural machine translation: encoder-decoder approaches (2014). CoRR, abs/1409.1259
21. K. Cho, B. van Merrienboer, C. Gulcehre, D. Bahdanau, F. Bougares, H. Schwenk, Y. Bengio, Learning phrase representations using RNN Encoder–Decoder for statistical machine translation, in *Proceedings of the 2014 Conference on Empirical Methods in Natural Language Processing (EMNLP)* (Association for Computational Linguistics, Stroudsburg, 2014), pp. 1724–1734
22. K. Cho, B. van Merrienboer, C. Gulcehre, D. Bahdanau, F. Bougares, H. Schwenk, Y. Bengio, Learning phrase representations using RNN Encoder-Decoder for statistical machine translation, in *Proceedings of the 2014 Conference on Empirical Methods in Natural Language Processing (EMNLP)* (2014)
23. E. Choi, M. Bahadori, A. Schuetz, W.F. Stewart, J. Sun, Doctor AI: predicting clinical events via recurrent neural networks, in *Proceedings of Machine Learning for Healthcare* (2016)
24. E. Choi, M.T. Bahadori, E. Searles, C. Coffey, M. Thompson, J. Bost, J. Tejedor-Sojo, J. Sun, Multi-layer representation learning for medical concepts, in *International Conference on Knowledge Discovery and Data Mining (SIGKDD)* (2016)
25. E. Choi, M.T. Bahadori, J. Sun, J. Kulas, A. Schuetz, W. Stewart, Retain: an interpretable predictive model for healthcare using reverse time attention mechanism, in *30th Conference on Neural Information Processing Systems (NIPS)* (2016)
26. E. Choi, A. Schuetz, W.F. Stewart, J. Sun, Medical concept representation learning from electronic health records and its application on heart failure prediction (2016). https://arxiv.org/abs/1602.03686
27. Y. Choi, C.Y.-I. Chiu, D. Sontag, Learning low-dimensional representations of medical concepts, in *AMIA Summits on Translational Science Proceedings* (2016)
28. E. Choi, M.T. Bahadori, L. Song, W.F. Stewart, J. Sun, Gram: graph-based attention model for healthcare representation learning, in *International Conference on Knowledge Discovery and Data Mining SIGKDD* (2017)
29. E. Choi, S. Biswal, B. Malin, J. Duke, W.F. Stewart, J. Sun, Generating multi-label discrete electronic health records using generative adversarial networks (2017). arXiv:1703. 06490
30. E. Choi, A. Schuetz, W.F. Stewart, J. Sun, Using recurrent neural network models for early detection of heart failure onset. J. Am. Med. Inform. Assoc. **24**(2), 361–370 (2017)
31. E. Choi, C. Xiao, W. Stewart, J. Sun, MiME: multilevel medical embedding of electronic health records for predictive healthcare, in *Advances in Neural Information Processing Systems*, ed. by S. Bengio, H. Wallach, H. Larochelle, K. Grauman, N. Cesa-Bianchi, R. Garnett, vol. 31 (Curran Associates, Red Hook, 2018), pp. 4547–4557
32. G.D. Clifford, C. Liu, B. Moody, L.-W.H. Lehman, I. Silva, Q. Li, A. Johnson, R.G. Mark, AF classification from a short single lead ECG recording: the physionet/computing in cardiology challenge 2017. Comput. Cardiol. **44**, 1 (2017)

33. R. Collobert, J. Weston, L. Bottou, M. Karlen, K. Kavukcuoglu, P. Kuksa, Natural language processing (almost) from scratch. J. Mach. Learn. Res. **12**, 2493–2537 (2011)
34. M.E. Cowen, D.J. Dusseau, B.G. Toth, C. Guisinger, M.W. Zodet, Y. Shyr, Casemix adjustment of managed care claims data using the clinical classification for health policy research method. Med. Care **36**(7), 1108–1113 (1998)
35. J. Davis, M. Goadrich, The relationship between precision-recall and ROC curves, in *Proceedings of the 23rd International Conference on Machine Learning, ICML'06* (ACM, New York, 2006), pp. 233–240
36. F. Dernoncourt, J.Y. Lee, O. Uzuner, P. Szolovits, De-identification of patient notes with recurrent neural networks. J. Am. Med. Inform. Assoc. **24**(3), 596–606 (2017)
37. J. Devlin, M.-W. Chang, K. Lee, K. Toutanova, BERT: pre-training of deep bidirectional transformers for language understanding, in *Proceedings of NAACL-HLT 2019* (2019), pp. 4171–4186
38. I.D. Dinov, Volume and value of big healthcare data. J. Med. Stat. Inform. **4**, 3 (2016)
39. E. Dong, H. Du, L. Gardner, An interactive web-based dashboard to track COVID-19 in real time. Lancet Infect. Dis. **20**(5), 533–534 (2020)
40. D. Duvenaud, D. Maclaurin, J. Aguilera-Iparraguirre, R. Gómez-Bombarelli, T. Hirzel, A. Aspuru-Guzik, R.P. Adams, Convolutional networks on graphs for learning molecular fingerprints, in *Advances in Neural Information Processing Systems (NIPS 2015)*, vol. 28 (2015)
41. D. Duvenaud, D. Maclaurin, J. Aguilera-Iparraguirre, R. Gómez-Bombarelli, T. Hirzel, A. Aspuru-Guzik, R.P. Adams, Convolutional networks on graphs for learning molecular fingerprints, in *Proceedings of the 28th International Conference on Neural Information Processing Systems - Volume 2, NIPS'15* (MIT Press, Cambridge, 2015), pp. 2224–2232
42. B. Ehteshami Bejnordi, M. Veta, P. Johannes van Diest, B. van Ginneken, N. Karssemeijer, G. Litjens, J.A.W.M. van der Laak, The CAMELYON16 Consortium, Diagnostic assessment of deep learning algorithms for detection of lymph node metastases in women with breast cancer. JAMA **318**(22), 2199–2210 (2017)
43. C. Esteban, S.L. Hyland, G. Rätsch, Real-valued (medical) time series generation with recurrent conditional GANs (2017). https://arxiv.org/abs/1706.02633
44. A. Esteva, B. Kuprel, R.A. Novoa, J. Ko, S.M. Swetter, H.M. Blau, S. Thrun, Dermatologist-level classification of skin cancer with deep neural networks. Nature **542**, 115 (2017)
45. A. Esteva, B. Kuprel, R.A. Novoa, J. Ko, S.M. Swetter, H.M. Blau, S. Thrun, Dermatologist-level classification of skin cancer with deep neural networks. Nature **542**(7639), 115–118 (2017)
46. C. Farabet, C. Couprie, L. Najman, Y. Lecun, Learning hierarchical features for scene labeling. IEEE Trans. Pattern Anal. Mach. Intell. **35**(8), 1915–1929 (2013)
47. W. Fedus, I. Goodfellow, A.M. Dai, MaskGAN: better text generation via filling in the blank, in *International Conference on Learning Representations* (2018)
48. T. Fu, C. Xiao, J. Sun, CORE: automatic molecule optimization using copy & refine strategy. Proc. AAAI Conf. Artif. Intell. **34**(1), 638–645 (2020)
49. J. Futoma, J. Morris, J. Lucas, A comparison of models for predicting early hospital readmissions. J. Biomed. Inform. **56**(C), 229–238 (2015)
50. J. Gao, C. Xiao, L.M. Glass, J. Sun, COMPOSE: cross-modal pseudo-siamese network for patient trial matching, in *Proceedings of the 26th ACM SIGKDD International Conference on Knowledge Discovery & Data Mining, KDD'20* (Association for Computing Machinery, New York, 2020), pp. 803–812
51. J. Gao, R. Sharma, C. Qian, L.M. Glass, J. Spaeder, J. Romberg, J. Sun, C. Xiao, Stan: spatio-temporal attention network for pandemic prediction using real-world evidence. J. Am. Med. Inform. Assoc. **28**(4), 733–743 (2021)
52. P.V. Gehler, A.D. Holub, M. Welling, The rate adapting poisson model for information retrieval and object recognition, in *Proceedings of the 23rd International Conference on Machine Learning* (ACM, New York, 2006), pp. 337–344

53. J. Gehring, M. Auli, D. Grangier, D. Yarats, Y.N. Dauphin, Convolutional sequence to sequence learning (2017). CoRR, abs/1705.03122
54. J. Gilmer, S.S. Schoenholz, P.F. Riley, O. Vinyals, G.E. Dahl, Neural message passing for quantum chemistry, in *ICML'17: Proceedings of the 34th International Conference on Machine Learning*, vol. 70 (2017), 1263–1272
55. M. Glavatskikh, J. Leguy, G. Hunault, T. Cauchy, B. Da Mota, Dataset's chemical diversity limits the generalizability of machine learning predictions. J. Cheminform. **11**(1), 69 (2019)
56. J. Gligorijevic, D. Gligorijevic, M. Pavlovski, E. Milkovits, L. Glass, K. Grier, P. Vankireddy, Z. Obradovic, Optimizing clinical trials recruitment via deep learning. J. Am. Med. Inform. Assoc. **26**, 1195–1202 (2019)
57. R. Gómez-Bombarelli, J.N. Wei, D. Duvenaud, J.M. Hernández-Lobato, B. Sánchez-Lengeling, D. Sheberla, J. Aguilera-Iparraguirre, T.D. Hirzel, R.P. Adams, A. Aspuru-Guzik, Automatic chemical design using a Data-Driven continuous representation of molecules. ACS Cent. Sci. **4**(2), 268–276 (2018)
58. I. Goodfellow, J. Pouget-Abadie, M. Mirza, B. Xu, D. Warde-Farley, S. Ozair, A. Courville, Y. Bengio, Generative adversarial nets, in *Advances in Neural Information Processing Systems*, ed. by Z. Ghahramani, M. Welling, C. Cortes, N.D. Lawrence, K.Q. Weinberger, vol. 27 (Curran Associates, Red Hook, 2014), pp. 2672–2680
59. T.R. Goodwin, S.M. Harabagiu, Deep learning from EEG reports for inferring underspecified information. AMIA Jt. Summits. Transl. Sci. Proc. **2017**, 112–121 (2017)
60. A. Graves, G. Wayne, M. Reynolds, T. Harley, I. Danihelka, A. Grabska-Barwińska, S.G. Colmenarejo, E. Grefenstette, T. Ramalho, J. Agapiou, et al., Hybrid computing using a neural network with dynamic external memory. Nature **538**(7626), 471 (2016)
61. V. Gulshan, L. Peng, M. Coram, M. C. Stumpe, D. Wu, A. Narayanaswamy, S. Venugopalan, K. Widner, T. Madams, J. Cuadros, R. Kim, R. Raman, P.C. Nelson, J.L. Mega, D.R. Webster, Development and validation of a deep learning algorithm for detection of diabetic retinopathy in retinal fundus photographs. JAMA **316**(22), 2402–2410 (2016)
62. J. Hachmann, R. Olivares-Amaya, S. Atahan-Evrenk, C. Amador-Bedolla, R.S. Sánchez-Carrera, A. Gold-Parker, L. Vogt, A.M. Brockway, A. Aspuru-Guzik, The harvard clean energy project: large-scale computational screening and design of organic photovoltaics on the world community grid. J. Phys. Chem. Lett. **2**(17), 2241–2251 (2011)
63. W. Hamilton, Z. Ying, J. Leskovec, Inductive representation learning on large graphs, in *Advances in Neural Information Processing Systems*, ed. by I. Guyon, U.V. Luxburg, S. Bengio, H. Wallach, R. Fergus, S. Vishwanathan, R. Garnett, vol. 30 (Curran Associates, Red Hook, 2017), pp. 1024–1034
64. W.L. Hamilton, R. Ying, J. Leskovec, Inductive representation learning on large graphs (2017). CoRR, abs/1706.02216
65. A.Y. Hannun, P. Rajpurkar, M. Haghpanahi, G.H. Tison, C. Bourn, M.P. Turakhia, A.Y. Ng, Cardiologist-level arrhythmia detection and classification in ambulatory electrocardiograms using a deep neural network. Nat. Med. **25**(1), 65 (2019)
66. K. He, X. Zhang, S. Ren, J. Sun, Deep residual learning for image recognition (2015). CoRR, abs/1512.03385
67. K. He, X. Zhang, S. Ren, J. Sun, Deep residual learning for image recognition. In *IEEE Conference on Computer Vision and Pattern Recognition CVPR* (2016)
68. G. Hinton, R. Salakhutdinov, Reducing the dimensionality of data with neural networks. Science **313**(5786), 504–507 (2006)
69. G.E. Hinton, R.R. Salakhutdinov, Replicated softmax: an undirected topic model, in *Advances in Neural Information Processing Systems* (2009), pp. 1607–1614
70. G. Hinton, L. Deng, D. Yu, G. Dahl, A.-R. Mohamed, N. Jaitly, A. Senior, V. Vanhoucke, P. Nguyen, B. Kingsbury, et al., Deep neural networks for acoustic modeling in speech recognition. IEEE Signal Process. Mag. **29**, 82–97 (2012)
71. S. Hochreiter, J. Schmidhuber, Long short-term memory. Neural Comput. **9**(8), 1735–1780 (1997)

72. S. Hochreiter, J. Schmidhuber, Long short-term memory. Neural Comput. **9**(8), 1735–1780 (1997)
73. S. Hong, C. Xiao, T. Ma, H. Li, J. Sun, MINA: multilevel knowledge-guided attention for modeling electrocardiography signals, in *Proceedings of the Twenty-Eighth International Joint Conference on Artificial Intelligence, IJCAI-19* (International Joint Conferences on Artificial Intelligence Organization, 2019), pp. 5888–5894
74. Z. Hu, Z. Yang, X. Liang, R. Salakhutdinov, E.P. Xing, Toward controlled generation of text, in *Proceedings of the 34th International Conference on Machine Learning*, ed. by D. Precup, Y.W. Teh. Proceedings of Machine Learning Research, International Convention Centre, Sydney, 06–11 Aug 2017, PMLR, vol. 70 (2017), pp. 1587–1596
75. G. Huang, Z. Liu, L. van der Maaten, K.Q. Weinberger, Densely connected convolutional networks, in *2017 IEEE Conference on Computer Vision and Pattern Recognition (CVPR)* (2016)
76. A.N. Jagannatha, H. Yu, Bidirectional RNN for medical event detection in electronic health records, in *Proceedings of the 2016 Conference of the North American Chapter of the Association for Computational Linguistics: Human Language Technologies* (Association for Computational Linguistics, Stroudsburg, 2016), pp. 473–482
77. A.N. Jagannatha, H. Yu, Structured prediction models for RNN based sequence labeling in clinical text. Proc. Conf. Empir. Methods Nat. Lang. Process. **2016**, 856–865 (2016)
78. J.T. James, A new, evidence-based estimate of patient harms associated with hospital care. J. Patient Saf. **9**(3), 122–128 (2013)
79. S. Jean, K. Cho, R. Memisevic, Y. Bengio, On using very large target vocabulary for neural machine translation, in *Proceedings of the 53rd Annual Meeting of the Association for Computational Linguistics and the 7th International Joint Conference on Natural Language Processing (Volume 1: Long Papers)* (Association for Computational Linguistics, Stroudsburg, 2015), pp. 1–10
80. W. Jin, R. Barzilay, T.S. Jaakkola, Junction tree variational autoencoder for molecular graph generation (2018). CoRR, abs/1802.04364
81. A.E. Johnson, T.J. Pollard, L. Shen, H.L. Li-wei, M. Feng, M. Ghassemi, B. Moody, P. Szolovits, L.A. Celi, R.G. Mark, Mimic-iii, a freely accessible critical care database. Sci. Data **3**, 160035 (2016)
82. A.E.W. Johnson, T.J. Pollard, L. Shen, L.-W.H. Lehman, M. Feng, M. Ghassemi, B. Moody, P. Szolovits, L.A. Celi, R.G. Mark, MIMIC-III, a freely accessible critical care database. Sci. Data **3**, 160035 (2016)
83. H.J. Kam, H.Y. Kim, Learning representations for the early detection of sepsis with deep neural networks. Comput. Biol. Med. **89**, 248–255 (2017)
84. S. Kearnes, K. McCloskey, M. Berndl, V. Pande, P. Riley, Molecular graph convolutions: moving beyond fingerprints. J. Comput. Aided Mol. Des. **30**(8), 595–608 (2016)
85. S.K. Kearsley, S. Sallamack, E.M. Fluder, J.D. Andose, R.T. Mosley, R.P. Sheridan, Chemical similarity using physiochemical property descriptors. J. Chem. Inform. Comput. Sci. **36**, 118–127 (1996)
86. L. Khedher, J. Ramírez, J.M. Górriz, A. Brahim, F. Segovia, Early diagnosis of alzheimer's disease based on partial least squares, principal component analysis and support vector machine using segmented MRI images. Neurocomputing **151**, 139–150 (2015)
87. D. Kingma, M. Welling, Auto-encoding variational bayes (2013). arXiv:1312.6114
88. T. Kipf, M. Welling, Semi-supervised classification with graph convolutional networks, in *International Conference on Learning Representations* (2016)
89. T. Kipf, M. Welling, Variational graph auto-encoders (2016). https://arxiv.org/abs/1611.07308
90. A. Krizhevsky, I. Sutskever, G.E. Hinton, Imagenet classification with deep convolutional neural networks, in *Proceedings of the 25th International Conference on Neural Information Processing Systems - Volume 1, NIPS'12* (Curran Associates, Red Hook, 2012), pp. 1097–1105
91. M. Kuhn, I. Letunic, L.J. Jensen, P. Bork, The SIDER database of drugs and side effects. Nucleic Acids Res. **44**(D1), D1075–9 (2016)

92. A. Kumar, O. Irsoy, P. Ondruska, M. Iyyer, J. Bradbury, I. Gulrajani, V. Zhong, R. Paulus, R. Socher, Ask me anything: dynamic memory networks for natural language processing, in *International Conference on Machine Learning* (2016), pp. 1378–1387
93. M.J. Kusner, B. Paige, J.M. Hernández-Lobato, Grammar variational autoencoder, in *The International Conference on Machine Learning (ICML)* (2017)
94. T.A. Lasko, J.C. Denny, M.A. Levy, Computational phenotype discovery using unsupervised feature learning over noisy, sparse, and irregular clinical data. PLoS One **8**(6), 1–13 (2013)
95. H. Le, T. Tran, S. Venkatesh, Dual memory neural computer for asynchronous two-view sequential learning, in *Proceedings of the 24rd ACM SIGKDD International Conference on Knowledge Discovery and Data Mining* (ACM, New York, 2018), pp. 1637–1645
96. Y. Lecun, L. Bottou, Y. Bengio, P. Haffner, Gradient-based learning applied to document recognition, in *Proceedings of the IEEE* (1998), pp. 2278–2324
97. L. Li, W.-Y. Cheng, B.S. Glicksberg, O. Gottesman, R. Tamler, R. Chen, E.P. Bottinger, J.T. Dudley, Identification of type 2 diabetes subgroups through topological analysis of patient similarity. Sci. Transl. Med. **7**(311), 311ra174–311ra174 (2015)
98. Y. Li, D. Tarlow, M. Brockschmidt, R. Zemel, Gated graph sequence neural networks, in *The International Conference on Learning Representations (ICLR)* (2015)
99. J. Li, D. Zhou, Y. Shi, J. Yang, S. Chen, Q. Wang, P. Hui, Application of weighted gene co-expression network analysis for data from paired design. Sci. Rep. **8**, 622 (2018)
100. Q. Lin, S.-Q. Ye, X.-M. Huang, S.-Y. Li, M.-Z. Zhang, Y. Xue, W.-S. Chen, Classification of epileptic EEG signals with stacked sparse autoencoder based on deep learning, in *Intelligent Computing Methodologies*, ed. by D.-S. Huang, K. Han, A. Hussain. Lecture Notes in Computer Science, vol. 9773 (Springer, Cham, 2016), pp. 802–810
101. R. Lindsey, A. Daluiski, S. Chopra, A. Lachapelle, M. Mozer, S. Sicular, D. Hanel, M. Gardner, A. Gupta, R. Hotchkiss, H. Potter, Deep neural network improves fracture detection by clinicians. Proc. Natl. Acad. Sci. USA **115**(45), 11591–11596 (2018)
102. Z.C. Lipton, D.C. Kale, C. Elkan, R. Wetzel, Learning to diagnose with LSTM recurrent neural networks, in *The International Conference on Learning Representations (ICLR)* (2015)
103. Q. Liu, M. Allamanis, M. Brockschmidt, A.L. Gaunt, Constrained graph variational autoencoders for molecule design, in *Proceedings of the 32Nd International Conference on Neural Information Processing Systems, NIPS'18* (Curran Associates, Red Hook, 2018), pp. 7806–7815
104. X. Lv, Y. Guan, J. Yang, J. Wu, Clinical relation extraction with deep learning. Int. J. Hybrid Inform. Technol. **9**(7), 237–248 (2016)
105. J. Ma, R.P. Sheridan, A. Liaw, G.E. Dahl, V. Svetnik, Deep neural nets as a method for quantitative structure–activity relationships. J. Chem. Inform. Model. **55**(2), 263–274 (2015). PMID: 25635324
106. F. Ma, R. Chitta, J. Zhou, Q. You, T. Sun, J. Gao, Dipole: diagnosis prediction in healthcare via attention-based bidirectional recurrent neural networks, in *Proceedings of the 23rd ACM SIGKDD International Conference on Knowledge Discovery and Data Mining, KDD'17* (ACM, New York, 2017), pp. 1903–1911
107. T. Ma, J. Chen, C. Xiao, Constrained generation of semantically valid graphs via regularizing variational autoencoders, in *Proceedings of the 32Nd International Conference on Neural Information Processing Systems, NIPS'18* (Curran Associates, Red Hook, 2018), pp. 7113–7124
108. T. Ma, C. Xiao, J. Zhou, F. Wang, Drug similarity integration through attentive multi-view graph auto-encoders, in *Proceedings of the Twenty-Seventh International Joint Conference on Artificial Intelligence, IJCAI 2018, July 13–19, 2018, Stockholm* (2018), pp. 3477–3483
109. L.V.D. Maaten, G. Hinton, Visualizing data using t-SNE. J. Mach. Learn. Res. **9**, 2579–2605 (2008)
110. T. Mikolov, I. Sutskever, K. Chen, G.S. Corrado, J. Dean, Distributed representations of words and phrases and their compositionality, in *Neural Information Processing Systems (NIPS)* (2013)

111. T. Mikolov, I. Sutskever, K. Chen, G.S. Corrado, J. Dean, Distributed representations of words and phrases and their compositionality, in *Advances in Neural Information Processing Systems*, ed. by C.J.C. Burges, L. Bottou, M. Welling, Z. Ghahramani, K.Q. Weinberger, vol. 26 (Curran Associates, Red Hook, 2013), pp. 3111–3119
112. A. Miller, A. Fisch, J. Dodge, A.-H. Karimi, A. Bordes, J. Weston, Key-value memory networks for directly reading documents, in *Empirical Methods in Natural Language Processing* (2016), pp. 1400–1409
113. R. Miotto, L. Li, B. Kidd, J. Dudley, Deep patient: an unsupervised representation to predict the future of patients from the electronic health records. Sci. Rep. **6**, 26094 (2016)
114. J. Mullenbach, S. Wiegreffe, J. Duke, J. Sun, J. Eisenstein, Explainable prediction of medical codes from clinical text, in *Proceedings of the North American Chapter of the Association for Computational Linguistics (NAACL)* (2018)
115. A. Ng, Sparse autoencoders (2010). https://web.stanford.edu/class/cs294a/sparseAutoencoder.pdf
116. P. Nguyen, T. Tran, S. Venkatesh, Finding algebraic structure of care in time: a deep learning 316 approach, in NeurIPS ML4H workshop (2017)
117. J. Pennington, R. Socher, C. Manning, Glove: global vectors for word representation, in *Proceedings of the 2014 Empirical Methods in Natural Language Processing (EMNLP)* (2014), pp. 1532–1543
118. T. Pham, T. Tran, D. Phung, S. Venkatesh, DeepCare: a deep dynamic memory model for predictive medicine, in *Advances in Knowledge Discovery and Data Mining*. Lecture Notes in Computer Science (Springer, Cham, 2016), pp. 30–41
119. T. Pham, T. Tran, D. Phung, S. Venkatesh, Predicting healthcare trajectories from medical records: a deep learning approach. J. Biomed. Inform. **69**, 218–229 (2017)
120. Z. Qiao, A. Bae, L.M. Glass, C. Xiao, J. Sun, FLANNEL: Focal loss based neural network ensemble for COVID-19 detection. J. Am. Med. Inform. Assoc. **28**(3), 444–452 (2020)
121. R. Ramakrishnan, P.O. Dral, M. Rupp, O.A. von Lilienfeld, Quantum chemistry structures and properties of 134 kilo molecules. Sci. Data **1**, 140022 (2014)
122. J. Read, B. Pfahringer, G. Holmes, E. Frank, Classifier chains for multi-label classification, in *Joint European Conference on Machine Learning and Knowledge Discovery in Databases* (Springer, Berlin, 2009), pp. 254–269
123. S. Reed, Z. Akata, X. Yan, L. Logeswaran, B. Schiele, H. Lee, Generative adversarial text to image synthesis, in *Proceedings of the 33rd International Conference on Machine Learning, 20–22 Jun 2016*, ed. by M.F. Balcan, K.Q. Weinberger. Proceedings of Machine Learning Research (PMLR), vol. 48 (ACM, New York, 2016), pp. 1060–1069
124. D. Rogers, M. Hahn, Extended-connectivity fingerprints. J. Chem. Inf. Model. **50**(5), 742–754 (2010)
125. V.L. Roger, S.A. Weston, M.M. Redfield, J.P. Hellermann-Homan, J. Killian, B.P. Yawn, S.J. Jacobsen, Trends in heart failure incidence and survival in a community-based population. JAMA **292**(3), 344–350 (2004)
126. L. Ruddigkeit, R. Deursen, L. Blum, J. Reymond, Enumeration of 166 billion organic small molecules in the chemical universe database gdb-17. J. Chem. Inf. Model **52**, 2864–2875 (2012)
127. D.E. Rumelhart, G.E. Hinton, R.J. Williams, Learning internal representations by error propagation, in *Parallel Distributed Processing: Explorations in the Microstructure of Cognition*, vol. 1 (MIT Press, Cambridge, 1986), pp. 318–362
128. T.N. Sainath, A. Mohamed, B. Kingsbury, B. Ramabhadran, Deep convolutional neural networks for LVCSR, in *2013 IEEE International Conference on Acoustics, Speech and Signal Processing* (2013), pp. 8614–8618
129. T. Salimans, I. Goodfellow, W. Zaremba, V. Cheung, A. Radford, X. Chen, Improved techniques for training gans, in *Neural Information Processing Systems (NIPS)* (2016), pp. 2226–2234
130. Y. Sasaki, The truth of the F-measure. *Teach Tutor Mater* (2007)

131. K.T. Schütt, F. Arbabzadah, S. Chmiela, K.R. Müller, A. Tkatchenko, Quantum-chemical insights from deep tensor neural networks. Nat. Commun. **8**, 13890 (2017)
132. N.H. Shah, N. Bhatia, C. Jonquet, D. Rubin, A.P. Chiang, M.A. Musen, Comparison of concept recognizers for building the open biomedical annotator. BMC Bioinf. **10**(suppl 9), S14 (2009)
133. J. Shang, T. Ma, C. Xiao, J. Sun, Pre-training of graph augmented transformers for medication recommendation, in *Proceedings of the 28th International Joint Conference on Artificial Intelligence, IJCAI'19* (AAAI Press, Macao, 2019), pp. 5953–5959
134. J. Shang, C. Xiao, T. Ma, H. Li, J. Sun, Gamenet: graph augmented memory networks for recommending medication combination, in *AAAI Conference on Artificial Intelligence (AAAI)* (2019)
135. W.H. Shrank, T.L. Rogstad, N. Parekh, Waste in the US health care system: estimated costs and potential for savings. JAMA **322**(15), 1501–1509 (2019)
136. K. Simonyan, A. Zisserman, Very deep convolutional networks for large-scale image recognition (2014). arXiv:1409.1556
137. J. Snoek, H. Larochelle, R.P. Adams, Practical bayesian optimization of machine learning algorithms, in *Proceedings of the 25th International Conference on Neural Information Processing Systems - Volume 2, NIPS'12* (Curran Associates, Red Hook, 2012), pp. 2951–2959
138. T. Sterling, J.J. Irwin, ZINC 15–ligand discovery for everyone. J. Chem. Inf. Model. **55**(11), 2324–2337 (2015)
139. J.M. Stokes, K. Yang, K. Swanson, W. Jin, A. Cubillos-Ruiz, N.M. Donghia, C.R. MacNair, S. French, L.A. Carfrae, Z. Bloom-Ackermann, V.M. Tran, A. Chiappino-Pepe, A.H. Badran, I.W. Andrews, E.J. Chory, G.M. Church, E.D. Brown, T.S. Jaakkola, R. Barzilay, J.J. Collins, A deep learning approach to antibiotic discovery. Cell **180**(4), 688–702.e13 (2020)
140. A. Stubbs, C. Kotfila, Ö. Uzuner, Automated systems for the de-identification of longitudinal clinical narratives: overview of 2014 i2b2/UTHealth shared task track 1. J. Biomed. Inf. **58**, S11–S19 (2015)
141. S. Sukhbaatar, A. Szlam, J. Weston, R. Fergus, Weakly supervised memory networks (2015). CoRR, abs/1503.08895
142. S. Sukhbaatar, J. Weston, R. Fergus, et al., End-to-end memory networks. In *Neural Information Processing Systems (NIPS)* (2015)
143. Q. Suo, H. Xue, J. Gao, A. Zhang, Risk factor analysis based on deep learning models, in *Proceedings of the 7th ACM International Conference on Bioinformatics, Computational Biology, and Health Informatics* (ACM, New York, 2016), pp. 394–403
144. H. Suresh, P. Szolovits, M. Ghassemi, The use of autoencoders for discovering patient phenotypes (2017). arxiv-1703.07004
145. I. Sutskever, O. Vinyals, Q.V. Le, Sequence to sequence learning with neural networks, in *Proceedings of the 27th International Conference on Neural Information Processing Systems - Volume 2, NIPS'14* 2014 (MIT Press, Cambridge, 2014), pp. 3104–3112
146. C. Szegedy, W. Liu, Y. Jia, P. Sermanet, S. Reed, D. Anguelov, D. Erhan, V. Vanhoucke, A. Rabinovich, Going deeper with convolutions, in *IEEE Conference on Computer Vision and Pattern Recognition (CVPR)* (2015)
147. C. Szegedy, V. Vanhoucke, S. Ioffe, J. Shlens, Z. Wojna, Rethinking the inception architecture for computer vision, in *2016 IEEE Conference on Computer Vision and Pattern Recognition (CVPR)*, (2016), pp. 2818–2826
148. D. Szklarczyk, A. Santos, C. Mering, L. Jensen, P. Bork, M. Kuhn, Stitch 5: augmenting protein-chemical interaction networks with tissue and affinity data. Nucl. Acids Res. **44**(D1), D380–384 (2016)
149. D. Szklarczyk, J.H. Morris, H. Cook, M. Kuhn, S. Wyder, M. Simonovic, A. Santos, N.T. Doncheva, A. Roth, P. Bork, L.J. Jensen, C. von Mering, The STRING database in 2017: quality-controlled protein-protein association networks, made broadly accessible. Nucl. Acids Res. **45**(D1), D362–D368 (2017)

150. T. Tantimongcolwat, T. Naenna, C. Isarankura-Na-Ayudhya, M.J. Embrechts, V. Prachayasittikul, Identification of ischemic heart disease via machine learning analysis on magnetocardiograms. Comput. Biol. Med. **38**(7), 817–825 (2008)
151. E. Taskesen, M.J.T. Reinders, M. Robinson-Rechavi, 2d representation of transcriptomes by t-sne exposes relatedness between human tissues. PloS One **11**(2), e0149853 (2016)
152. N. Tatonetti, P. Patrick, R. Daneshjou, R. Altman, Data-driven prediction of drug effects and interactions. Sci. Transl. Med. **4**(125), 125ra31–125ra31 (2012)
153. N.P. Tatonetti, P.P. Ye, R. Daneshjou, R.B. Altman, Data-driven prediction of drug effects and interactions. Sci. Transl. Med. **4**(125), 125ra31 (2012)
154. J.H. Thean, A.J. Hall, R.J. Stawell, Uveitis in herpes zoster ophthalmicus. Clin. Experiment. Ophthalmol. **29**(6), 406–410 (2001)
155. P. Thodoroff, J. Pineau, A. Lim, Learning robust features using deep learning for automatic seizure detection, in *Machine Learning for Healthcare Conference* (2016), pp. 178–190
156. J.J. Titano, M. Badgeley, J. Schefflein, M. Pain, A. Su, M. Cai, N. Swinburne, J. Zech, J. Kim, J. Bederson, J. Mocco, B. Drayer, J. Lehar, S. Cho, A. Costa, E.K. Oermann, Automated deep-neural-network surveillance of cranial images for acute neurologic events. Nat. Med. **24**(9), 1337–1341 (2018)
157. T. Tran, D. Phung, S. Venkatesh, Mixed-variate restricted boltzmann machines, in *Asian Conference on Machine Learning* (2011), pp. 213–229
158. M. P. A. C. (U.S.), *Report to the Congress: promoting greater efficiency in Medicare* (Medicare Payment Advisory Commission, Washington, DC, 2007). https://iucat.iu.edu/iuk/8044570
159. L. van der Maaten, G. Hinton, Visualizing data using t-SNE. J. Mach. Learn. Res. **9**, 2579–2605 (2008)
160. A. Vaswani, N. Shazeer, N. Parmar, J. Uszkoreit, L. Jones, A.N. Gomez, L. Kaiser, I. Polosukhin, Attention is all you need, in *Conference on Neural Information Processing Systems* (2017)
161. P. Veličković, G. Cucurull, A. Casanova, A. Romero, P. Lio, Y. Bengio, Graph attention networks. arXiv:1710.10903 **1**(2), (2017)
162. P. Veličković, L. Karazija, N.D. Lane, S. Bhattacharya, E. Liberis, P. Liò, A. Chieh, O. Bellahsen, M. Vegreville, Cross-modal recurrent models for human weight objective prediction from multimodal time-series data (2017). arXiv:1709.08073
163. P. Vincent, H. Larochelle, I. Lajoie, Y. Bengio, P.-A. Manzagol, Stacked denoising autoencoders: learning useful representations in a deep network with a local denoising criterion. J. Mach. Learn. Res. **11**, 3371–3408 (2010)
164. A.M. Virshup, J. Contreras-García, P. Wipf, W. Yang, D.N. Beratan, Stochastic voyages into uncharted chemical space produce a representative library of all possible drug-like compounds. J. Am. Chem. Soc. **135**(19), 7296–7303 (2013)
165. W.-Q. Wei, R.M. Cronin, H. Xu, T.A. Lasko, L. Bastarache, J.C. Denny, Development and evaluation of an ensemble resource linking medications to their indications. J. Am. Med. Inform. Assoc. **20**(5), 954–961 (2013)
166. J. Weston, S. Chopra, A. Bordes, Memory networks, in *International Conference on Learning Representations* (2015)
167. C. Xiao, P. Zhang, W.A. Chaovalitwongse, J. Hu, F. Wang, Adverse drug reaction prediction with symbolic latent dirichlet allocation, in *Proceedings of the Thirty-First AAAI Conference on Artificial Intelligence (AAAI)* (2017)
168. S. Xie, R. Girshick, P. Dollár, Z. Tu, K. He, Aggregated residual transformations for deep neural networks, in *2017 IEEE Conference on Computer Vision and Pattern Recognition (CVPR)* (2017), pp. 5987–5995
169. A. Yahi, R. Vanguri, N. Elhadad, N.P. Tatonetti, Generative adversarial networks for electronic health records: a framework for exploring and evaluating methods for predicting Drug-Induced laboratory test trajectories. Front Public Health **8**, 164 (2017)
170. B. Yan, Y. Wang, Y. Li, Y. Gong, L. Guan, S. Yu, An EEG signal classification method based on sparse auto-encoders and support vector machine, in *2016 IEEE/CIC International Conference on Communications in China (ICCC)* (2016), pp. 1–6

171. H. Yang, J.M. Garibaldi, Automatic detection of protected health information from clinic narratives. J. Biomed. Inform. **58**, S30–S38 (2015)
172. K. Yang, K. Swanson, W. Jin, C. Coley, P. Eiden, H. Gao, A. Guzman-Perez, T. Hopper, B. Kelley, M. Mathea, A. Palmer, V. Settels, T. Jaakkola, K. Jensen, R. Barzilay, Analyzing learned molecular representations for property prediction. J. Chem. Inf. Model. **59**(8), 3370–3388 (2019)
173. Y. Yuan, G. Xun, K. Jia, A. Zhang, A multi-view deep learning method for epileptic seizure detection using short-time fourier transform, in *Proceedings of the 8th ACM International Conference on Bioinformatics, Computational Biology,and Health Informatics*, (ACM, New York, 2017), pp. 213–222
174. Y. Zhang, R. Chen, J. Tang, W. F. Stewart, J. Sun, LEAP: learning to prescribe effective and safe treatment combinations for multimorbidity, in *Proceedings of the 23rd ACM SIGKDD International Conference on Knowledge Discovery and Data Mining, KDD'17* (ACM, New York, 2017), pp. 1315–1324
175. Z. Zhang, P. Cui, W. Zhu, Deep Learning on Graphs: A Survey. IEEE Trans. Knowl. Data Eng. IEEE Computer Society, Los Alamitos, CA, USA, 1, 1–1, 1558–2191 (2018)
176. X. Zhang, C. Xiao, L. M. Glass, J. Sun, DeepEnroll: patient-trial matching with deep embedding and entailment prediction, in *Proceedings of The Web Conference 2020, WWW'20* (Association for Computing Machinery, New York, 2020), pp. 1029–1037
177. Z. Zhu, C. Yin, B. Qian, Y. Cheng, J. Wei, F. Wang, Measuring patient similarities via a deep architecture with medical concept embedding, in *IEEE 16th International Conference on Data Mining (ICDM)* (2016)
178. M. Zitnik, M. Agrawal, J. Leskovec, Modeling polypharmacy side effects with graph convolutional networks. Bioinformatics **34**(13), i457–i466 (2018)